Care of the Sick Neonate
A Quick Reference
for Health Care Providers

Paulette S. Haws, MSN, RNC, NNP
Neonatal Nurse Practitioner
Christiana Care Health Services, Inc.
Newark, Delaware

D1611695

LIPPINCOTT WILLIAMS & WILKINS
A **Wolters Kluwer** Company
Philadelphia • Baltimore • New York • London
Buenos Aires • Hong Kong • Sydney • Tokyo

Senior Acquisitions Editor: Patricia Casey
Managing Editor: Barclay Cunningham
Editorial Assistant: Megan Klim
Production Editor: Danielle Litka
Senior Production Manager: Helen Ewan
Art Director: Carolyn O'Brien
Design: Holly Reid-McLaughlin
Cover: Vasiliky Kiethas
Manufacturing Manager: William Alberti
Indexer: Gaye Tarallo
Compositor: Lippincott Williams & Wilkins
Printer: R.R. Donnelly-Crawfordsville

9 8 7 6 5 4 3 2 1

Library of Congress Cataloging-in-Publication Data
Care of the sick neonate : a quick reference for health care providers /
[edited by] Paulette S. Haws
        p. cm.
Includes bibliographical references and index.
   ISBN 0-7817-3496-7 (alk. paper)
   1.   Neonatal intensive care. 2.   Infants (Premature)--Care. 3.   Infants
(Newborn)--Care. 4.   Infants (Newborn)--Diseases. 5.
Pregnancy--Complications.   I. Haws, Paulette S.
   RJ250.C285 2003
   618.92'01--dc21   2002043444

Care has been taken to confirm the accuracy of the information presented and to describe generally accepted practices. However, the authors, editors, and publisher are not responsible for errors or omissions or for any consequences from application of the information in this book and make no warranty, express or implied, with respect to the content of the publication.

The authors, editors, and publisher have exerted every effort to ensure that drug selection and dosage set forth in this text are in accordance with the current recommendations and practice at the time of publication. However, in view of ongoing research, changes in government regulations, and the constant flow of information relating to drug therapy and drug reactions, the reader is urged to check the package insert for each drug for any change in indications and dosage and for added warnings and precautions. This is particularly important when the recommended agent is a new or infrequently employed drug.

Some drugs and medical devices presented in this publication have Food and Drug Administration (FDA) clearance for limited use in restricted research settings. It is the responsibility of the health care provider to ascertain the FDA status of each drug or device planned for use in his or her clinical practice.

LWW.com

For Janet and Robin

Thank you...and again, thank you

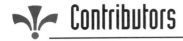# Contributors

Ann Marie Bodi, MSN, RNC, NNP
Neonatal Nurse Practitioner
Christiana Care Health Services, Inc.
Newark, Delaware
CHAPTER 21: Eyes and Ears

Susan E. Cheeseman, MSN, RNC, NNP
Neonatal Nurse Practitioner
Christiana Care Health Services, Inc.
Newark, Delaware
CHAPTER 11: Hematology

Cheryl A. Cloud, MSN, RNC, CRNP
Neonatal Nurse Practitioner
Christiana Care Health Services, Inc.
Newark, Delaware
CHAPTER 8: Nutrition

Patricia A. Coates, MSN, RNC, NNP
Neonatal Nurse Practitioner
Christiana Care Health Services, Inc.
Newark, Delaware
**CHAPTER 17: Genitourinary and
Renal Disorders**

Paulette S. Haws, MSN, RNC, NNP
Neonatal Nurse Practitioner
Christiana Care Health Services, Inc.
Newark, Delaware

Kathy Keen, MSN, RNC, NNP
Neonatal Nurse Practitioner
Christiana Care Health Services, Inc.
Newark, Delaware
**CHAPTER 17: Genitourinary and
Renal Disorders**

Cynthia J. Kelley, MSN, RNC, NNP
Neonatal Nurse Practitioner
Christiana Care Health Services, Inc.
Newark, Delaware
CHAPTER 10: Infectious Diseases

Robin R. Maguire, MSN, RNC, NNP
Neonatal Nurse Practitioner
Christiana Care Health Services, Inc.
Newark, Delaware
**CHAPTER 18: Metabolic and Endocrine
Disorders**

Donna DiSciascio Mann, MSN, RNC, NNP
Neonatal Nurse Practitioner
Christiana Care Health Services, Inc.
Newark, Delaware
CHAPTER 16: Gastrointestinal Disorders

Theresa M. McGreevy, MSN, RNC, NNP
Neonatal Nurse Practitioner
Christiana Care Health Services, Inc.
Newark, Delaware
CHAPTER 14: Cardiovascular Disorders

Karen M. O'Leary, MSN, RNC, NNP
Neonatal Nurse Practitioner
Christiana Care Health Services, Inc.
Newark, Delaware
**CHAPTER 20: Skin and Mucous Membrane
Lesions**

Karen L. Williams, MSN, RNC, NNP
Neonatal Nurse Practitioner
Christiana Care Health Services, Inc.
Newark, Delaware
**CHAPTER 12: Hepatic Diseases and
Hyperbilirubinemia**

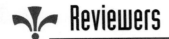 # Reviewers

Deborah Winders Davis, DNS, RNC
Associate Professor
Department of Pediatrics
School of Medicine
University of Louisville
Louisville, Kentucky

Michele T. Renaud, RN, MSN, PhD
Assistant Professor, Director, ASBN Program
Duke University School of Nursing
Durham, North Carolina

Frances R. Ward, RN, MSN
Doctoral Candidate in Nursing
University of Pennsylvania
Philadelphia, Pennsylvania

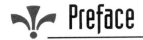 # Preface

Care of the Sick Neonate: A Quick Reference for Health Care Providers is not just another clinical handbook.

How many of us remember the calculations for the a-A gradient, body surface area (m^2), PGE_1 or insulin infusions, or mg/kg/minute of glucose? Do we remember the difference between alloimmune and autoimmune thrombocytopenia and which platelets (maternal versus random donor) are appropriate for transfusion? How does symmetrical versus asymmetrical intrauterine growth restriction affect our management of the infant? Few of us remember all that we hear or read. For that reason, this book was written with you and myself in mind.

The impetus behind *Care of the Sick Neonate* began while I was attending a neonatal nurse practitioner graduate program. Finding that there were so many bits of valuable information to help me manage the care of sick infants, I started jotting them all down on paper. As I garnered more worthy information in school and early on in my work, the jots on paper were gathered into a notebook that I fondly called my "book of all." Through the years, the "book of all" has been engaged by many a practitioner, nurse, resident, fellow, and attending physician. Because of its usefulness in providing instant and accessible answers to some very needed information, some of my colleagues suggested that it be published.

The goal of this book, as it always has been, is to assist all practitioners survive a NICU night call, a difficult transport, or a delivery room situation by providing easy-to-find answers to clinical questions. It provides a compilation of basic prenatal, perinatal, and neonatal information to those health care professionals (in particular, nurse practitioners, residents, and staff nurses) who plan and implement care for sick neonates. This book is not designed to supply complex maternal/neonatal pathophysiology, nor is it a comprehensive guide to every disease found in the neonatal period. Rather, it is a book of basic information covering most common neonatal diseases, health management strategies and interventions, and mathematical calculations.

It follows that the book's merits lay in its succinctness, in its userfriendly outline format, in its well-referenced, logically arranged sections (Pregnancy and Labor, Delivery Room Management, Neonatal Management, and Appendices), and in its compact size.

To those colleagues who urged me into this project and helped to transform it into its present form, I gratefully acknowledge their encouragement and support. I extend my deepest gratitude to my NNP colleagues at Christiana Care Hospital, especially Robin Maguire, who saw the value in this book, encouraged me to persevere through it, and enthusiastically stepped in to contribute their time and expertise, thus completing the project by authoring 10 chapters. It is time for us to pass it on to you.

Paulette S. Haws, MSN, RNC, NNP

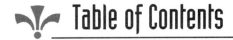 # Table of Contents

PART I

PREGNANCY AND LABOR

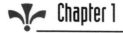 **Chapter 1**

Antenatal Testing

Paulette S. Haws, MSN, RNC, NNP

Part A: Several maternal serologic tests, as well as cervical, rectal, and urine cultures, are routinely performed during prenatal care. These diagnostic studies are designed to (1) identify maternal and fetal risk factors and (2) aid in managing the pregnancy to have an optimal maternal/fetal outcome.

I. Serology and urine

A. Blood type (ABO & Rh) and antibody screen: performed to identify pregnancies at risk for fetal hemolytic disease

1. ABO typing: ABO disease is more likely with the following combinations: m**O**ther is type **O** and b**AB**y is type **A**, **B**, or **AB**. ABO incompatibility in the fetus can occur with the first pregnancy; subsequent pregnancies have approximately the same risk for occurrence.

2. Rh determination (Christmas & Slotnick, 2000; Whitehurst, 1999): Rh sensitization occurs when an Rh-negative woman produces anti-Rh (D) IgG antibody as a result of exposure to Rh-positive blood through either a transfusion or previous pregnancy. First pregnancies have < 1% risk of fetal Rh disease unless the mother has been previously sensitized. Subsequent pregnancies are at a higher risk for Rh disease.

3. Antibody screen: women are screened for the presence of D (Rh) antigen on erythrocytes by direct antibody testing (DAT) and anti-Rh and other unusual antibodies in their serum by antibody screen (Indirect Coombs).

   a. Maternal titers measuring the amount of anti-Rh antibodies should be drawn to determine the degree of isoimmunization. If early maternal anti-D titer is ≥ 1:16, then an amniocentesis is recommended at 26 weeks' gestation to perform ΔOD 450 (Perry, 2000).

   b. Antibody titer is repeated at 26 to 28 weeks' gestation for all Rh-negative women. If the titer remains negative, then RhoGAM is administered. If the titer is positive, RhoGAM is not given because it will be ineffective. The pregnancy should then be managed to minimize the effects of fetal hemolytic disease and hydrops (Chan & Winkle, 1999; Scoggin & Morgan, 1998).

4. Neonatal complications of Rh/ABO group incompatibilities: hydrops fetalis; hemolysis and anemia; hypoxia; and hyperbilirubinemia and kernicterus

B. Complete blood count (CBC) with differential: determines the presence of maternal anemia and thrombocytopenia.
   1. Etiology of anemia includes (Terrone, 2000): relative dilutional anemia; increased blood loss (eg, placenta previa); decreased erythrocyte production (eg, folic acid, iron, or vitamin B_{12} deficiency); and increased erythrocyte destruction (eg, spherocytosis and porphyria and hemolytic anemia, elevated liver enzymes, and low platelet count [HELLP syndrome]).
   2. Etiology of thrombocytopenia includes (Heaman, 2000): decreased platelet production; increased peripheral platelet consumption; and increased platelet destruction (eg, idiopathic thrombocytopenia purpura [ITP]—antiplatelet antibody production with resultant destruction of the mother's platelets). In pregnancy, the most common causes are pregnancy-induced hypertension (PIH), systemic lupus erythematosus (SLE), and ITP.
C. Drug screening: perinatal drug use includes not only illegal drug use but also abusive use of prescription medications, tobacco, alcohol, and over-the-counter (OTC) drugs.
   1. Screening: careful documentation of legitimate prescription and OTC medications should be done so that positive toxicology results are not misinterpreted. Drugs or chemicals can be detected in blood, urine, saliva, amniotic fluid, hair, and meconium.
   2. Drug classifications:
      a. Amphetamines (Evans, 2000) stimulate the sympathetic nervous system and produce a euphoria similar to that of cocaine. Amphetamines are detectable in body fluids for 24 to 72 hours.
      b. Barbiturates are hypnosedatives (eg, phenobarbital) taken prenatally for sedation, treatment of hypertension, and seizure control (Kopecky & Koren, 1998). Neonatal abstinence syndrome symptoms begin at approximately 1 week of age.
      c. Cocaine blocks norepinephrine and dopamine uptake, with resultant exaggerated sympathetic stimulation; euphoria occurs as a result of excess dopamine in the central nervous system (CNS). Cocaine is present in body fluids for 24 to 60 hours (Evans, 2000), and screening is commonly performed on urine samples.
      d. Hallucinogenics: lysergic acid diethylamide (LSD), phencyclidine (PCP), and marijuana (cannabis) (Evans, 2000)
         (1) LSD: detectable in body fluids for 2 hours to 2 weeks after ingestion
         (2) PCP: detectable in body fluids for up to 7 days
         (3) Marijuana: present in body fluids for 2 to 8 weeks
      e. Opiates (heroin and methadone) induce euphoria and sedation and are highly addictive in both mother and fetus (Evans, 2000; Kopecky & Koren, 1998; Putman & Smith, 2000). Opiates remain in body fluids for 36 to 72 hours.
         (1) Onset of withdrawal symptoms: heroin (onset is 6 to 12 hours; average peak is 48 to 72 hours; subacute

symptoms persist postnatally for 4 to 6 months); methadone (onset is 36 to 72 hours; average peak is 6 days; subacute symptoms persist postnatally for 4 to 6 months)

D. Glucose screening: maintaining normal serum glucose levels throughout pregnancy through diet or insulin decreases the risk of intrauterine death and neonatal morbidity.

   1. Some practitioners universally screen all women early in pregnancy for diabetes mellitus, because 50% of all cases of gestational diabetes are missed when screening is based on risk factors alone.

   2. Selective screening is recommended at 24 to 28 weeks' gestation with the following risk factors: > 25 years old; family history of diabetes; glycosuria; maternal hypertension; and/or previous macrosomic, malformed, or stillborn infant.

E. Urinalysis: urinalysis will aid in screening for diabetes, PIH, and renal disease by detecting the presence of glucose, ketones, and protein. Additionally, the presence of red blood cells (RBCs), white blood cells (WBCs), and bacteria will help to detect a urinary tract infection (UTI).

II. Bacterial, protozoan, and viral screenings

A. *Chlamydia trachomatis* (Pickering, 2000) is an obligate intracellular bacterial organism.

   1. Transmission: transplacental transmission (eg, cesarean section with intact membranes) and vertically during a vaginal delivery

   2. Diagnosis: isolation of the organism from a cervical specimen

   a. Women should be screened early in pregnancy and again late in the third trimester.

   b. Women < 25 years of age and those with multiple partners are at higher risk for chlamydial infection and are also at a greater risk for concurrent gonorrhea infection.

   3. Neonatal complications: conjunctivitis presents within the first few days to several weeks of life; pneumonia presents between 2 and 19 weeks of age.

B. Gonorrhea (Moran, 2000; Pickering, 2000; Rivlin, 2000) is caused by a gram-negative, oxidase-positive diplococci (*Neisseria gonorrhoeae*).

   1. Transmission: among adults, transmission is commonly through sexual contact. Transmission to the fetus occurs during the birth process through an infected birth canal.

   2. Diagnosis: isolating the organism from an endocervical culture

   a. Screening should occur with the first prenatal visit and be repeated late in the third trimester.

   b. Maternal evaluation for concurrent chlamydial and syphilis infections is recommended.

   3. Maternal pregnancy complications include: premature rupture of membranes; preterm labor and delivery; and chorioamnionitis.

   4. Neonatal clinical manifestations include: purulent conjunctivitis that appears within 5 days of life and disseminated disease (bacteremia, arthritis, meningitis, and endocarditis).

C. Group B streptococcus (GBS) (Pickering, 2000): gram-positive diplococcus bacteria

1. Transmission: vertical transmission from mother to fetus occurs shortly before or during delivery.
2. Diagnosis (Gonik & McNamara, 1997): GBS bacteria can be isolated from vaginal, rectal, and urine cultures. Screening for GBS colonization with lower vaginal and anorectal cultures is recommended for all women at 35 to 37 weeks' gestation.
3. Treatment: it is recommended that women who have GBS bacteria be treated at the time of diagnosis and during labor with penicillin G or ampicillin (drugs of choice).
4. Neonatal clinical manifestations include:
   a. Infant may be asymptomatic.
   b. Early-onset GBS sepsis usually occurs within 24 hours after birth but has a range of 0 to 6 days. Symptoms include: respiratory distress syndrome (RDS), pneumonia, shock, poor perfusion, circulatory collapse, lethargy, temperature instability, meningitis, and feeding intolerance.
   c. Late-onset GBS sepsis usually occurs within 3 to 4 weeks after birth but ranges from 7 days to 3 months. Symptoms include: pneumonia, bacteremia, meningitis, osteomyelitis, septic arthritis, and cellulitis.
D. Hepatitis B virus (HBV) (Pickering, 2000): a DNA-containing, 42-nm hepadnavirus
   1. Transmission: occurs as a result of infected blood product transfusions, sharing nonsterilized needles, percutaneous and mucous membranes exposure to infected blood and body fluids, and sexual activity. Congenital infection occurs as a result of vertical transmission during pregnancy and childbirth.
   2. Screening: serologic screening should occur early in pregnancy and be repeated in third trimester for those hepatitis B surface antigen (HBsAg)-negative women who are at high risk for HBV exposure. Serologic antigen tests detect HBsAg and hepatitis B e antigen (HBeAg); assays detect antibody to HBsAg (anti-HBs), total antibody to hepatitis B core antigen (anti-HBc), IgM antibody to core antigen (IgM anti-HBc), and HBeAg antibody.
      a. HBsAg positive → indicates HBV is present; patient is infectious; earliest marker; antigen used in hepatitis B vaccine.
      b. HBeAg positive → infectious (high degree of infectivity); generally persists from 3 to 6 weeks; beyond 10 weeks is indicative of a carrier state.
      c. Anti-HBs positive → indicates HBV immunity; occurs from infection or vaccine; usually not present in carriers.
      d. Anti-HBc positive → indicates past or current HBV infection; does not develop in response to vaccine.
      e. IgM anti-HBc → indicates acute or recent HBV infection (including HBsAG-negative persons during "window" phase of infection).
      f. Antibody to HBe (anti-HBe) → identifies HBsAG carriers; low infectivity.
   3. Neonatal treatment and complications (Pickering, 2000) (refer to Chapter 10: Infectious Diseases)

E. Herpes simplex virus (HSV) (Landry, 1999; Pickering, 2000): an enveloped double-stranded DNA virus
   1. Transmission to the fetus occurs during vaginal delivery through contact with an infected genital tract or by an ascending infection through seemingly intact membranes. Fetal transmission is more likely (33%–50%) with primary maternal infection. The risk of fetal transmission is 0% to 5% with reactivated maternal infection.
   2. Maternal diagnosis:
      a. Suspicion: observation of cervical, vaginal, or external genital lesions
      b. Presumptive: fluorescent antibody or Papanicolaou smear of vesicular fluid
      c. Definitive: positive vesicle culture
   3. Maternal clinical manifestations: maternal infection may be asymptomatic. Cesarean section is recommended for women with active genital herpes lesions.
   4. Neonatal clinical manifestation include:
      a. Disseminated disease (25% of cases) with multiple organ involvement, especially the liver and lungs
      b. Localized CNS disease (35% of cases)
      c. Localized disease to skin, eyes, and mouth (40% of cases)
F. HIV: a human retrovirus (HIV-1 is common in the United States; HIV-2 is more common in Africa)
   1. Transmission (Pickering, 2000): in adults, transmission occurs through sexual contact and percutaneous and/or mucous membrane exposure to infected blood or body fluids. In fetuses, vertical transmission occurs before or at the time of delivery, and through breastfeeding.
   2. Diagnosis is positive when the presence of the HIV-1 organism is confirmed by the ELISA (enzyme-linked immunosorbent assay) and Western Blot assay serologic tests.
   3. Screening is recommended with initial prenatal blood tests. Neonatal HIV infection decreases by two thirds when there is prenatal administration of zidovudine (AZT, Retrovir) beginning at 14 to 34 weeks' gestation, intravenous AZT administration during the perinatal period, and oral AZT administration to the infant for 6 weeks after birth (Pickering, 2000).
   4. Clinical manifestations of HIV infection in the neonatal period are rare.
G. Rubella (Pickering, 2000) is an RNA virus (Rubivirus) in the *Togaviridae* family.
   1. Transmission occurs through exposure to infected nasopharyngeal secretions. In the fetus, transmission occurs transplacentally (Landry, 1999). Significant damage occurs with first-trimester transmission; rare disease occurs with second-trimester transmission.
   2. Screening: maternal immune status is determined through serologic (IgG specific) rubella antibody titers (Kenner & Lott, 1994).

Immunization is given after delivery to rubella-susceptible women.

3. Neonatal clinical manifestations include (Pickering, 2000): ophthalmologic defects (cataracts, glaucoma, and retinopathy); sensorineural deafness; cardiac (patent ductus arteriosus [PDA] and peripheral pulmonary artery stenosis); intrauterine growth restriction (IUGR), mental retardation, and microcephaly; and hepatosplenomegaly, anemia, and jaundice.

H. Syphilis (Pickering, 2000) is caused by a thin motile fragile spirochete (*Treponema pallidum*) that survives outside of the host for only a brief period of time.

   1. Transmission: transplacental transmission occurs any time during pregnancy or at birth.
   2. Definitive diagnosis: spirochete identification by microscopic darkfield examination or direct fluorescent antibody test of lesion exudate/tissue
   3. Presumptive diagnosis:
      a. Nontreponemal tests: Venereal Disease Research Laboratories (VDRL) slide test; rapid plasma reagin (RPR); and automated reagin test (ART). Positive nontreponemal tests should be confirmed by a specific treponemal test. False positive nontreponemal tests may occur with acute viral/bacterial infections, recent vaccination, collagen disease, malaria, and tuberculosis.
      b. Treponemal tests: fluorescent treponemal antibody absorption (FTA-ABS) and microhemagglutination test for *T. pallidum* (MHA-TP)
   4. Screening: maternal screening is recommended early in pregnancy. Screening should be repeated at 28 weeks for high-risk patients. After completion of antibiotic therapy, a repeat RPR should be drawn on the mother to ensure a decrease in titers.
   5. Maternal complications include: stillbirth and preterm labor and delivery.
   6. Neonatal clinical manifestations include: refer to Chapter 10: Infectious Diseases.

I. Toxoplasmosis (Carlson & Dattel, 2000; Pickering, 2000) is caused by a protozoan parasite (*Toxoplasma gondii*).

   1. Transmission to humans occurs through the ingestion of poorly cooked meat or handling infected cat feces. Congenital transplacental transmission most often occurs with a primary maternal infection.
   2. Diagnosis: identification of the protozoan in tissue sections, smears, or body fluid; demonstrating an eight-fold rise in antibody titers (IgM or IgG)
      a. IgG-specific antibodies peak 1 to 2 months after infection and are positive indefinitely.
      b. IgM-specific antibodies are detectable 2 weeks after infection, peak in 1 month and then decline, and are undetectable within 6 to 9 months.
      c. IgA antibody levels decline to undetectable concentrations sooner than IgM antibody levels.

3. Neonatal clinical manifestations (Kenner & Lott, 1994): refer to Chapter 10: Infectious Diseases.

Part B. Maternal serologic testing, chorionic villus sampling, amniotic fluid analysis, and percutaneous umbilical blood sampling are available to identify pregnancies at risk for genetic disorders. Additionally, maternal and fetal well-being are evaluated through external fetal monitoring and ultrasonography.

I. Genetic testing

A. Serology (Cunningham et al., 1997; Dickerman & Park, 1992; Shulman, 1992):

1. Carrier state for Tay-Sachs disease (eastern European [Ashkenazic] Jewish heritage; French-Canadian or Cajun descent): hexosaminidase A (serum or leukocytes)
2. α-Thalassemia (Chinese and Southeast Asian ancestry): mean corpuscular volume (MCV) $<$ 80 fL; normal hemoglobin electrophoresis; normal iron (Fe) studies
3. β-Thalassemia (Mediterranean ancestry, ie, Greek, Italian, and Sephardic Jews): MCV $<$ 80 fL; hemoglobin electrophoresis ↑ A_2; normal Fe studies
4. Sickle cell trait or disease (Black ancestry): hemoglobin S electrophoresis showing hemoglobin AS or SS
5. Cystic fibrosis (Caucasian): allele-specific oligonucleotide probes, polymerase chain reaction, and linkage analysis of affected families through the use of restriction fragment polymorphism and Southern blotting
6. Maternal serum α-fetoprotein (MSAFP) and triple screen: the
   a. MSAFP, unconjugated estriol (UE), and β-human chorionic gonadotropin (β-HCG) are performed on maternal serum. MSAFP and UE are fetal liver products found in the amniotic fluid that enter maternal circulation and can be detected and measured. These three markers are evaluated singly or in combination with one another to determine risk for chromosomal abnormalities, CNS malformations, and open neural tube and ventral wall defects. Additionally, maternal age is considered to determine risk for trisomy 21 (Chan & Winkle, 1999; Cunningham et al., 1997; Jasper, 2000; Wynn, 1992).
   b. Timing: MSAFP or triple screen is usually performed at 15 to 19 weeks' gestation; follow-up for abnormal MSAFP or triple screen results include amniocentesis, fetal ultrasonography, and genetic counseling (Table 1.1).

B. Chorionic villi sampling (CVS) is performed between 9 and 12 weeks (Jasper, 2000) to carry out genetic studies and gender determination.

1. Procedure: under ultrasound guidance a sample of chorionic villi from the placenta is aspirated either transvaginally with a catheter or transabdominally with a spinal needle.
2. Risks include: chromosomal mosaicism (due to mixture of retrieved fetal and maternal cells); limb anomalies (more common when performed at approximately 8 weeks); miscarriage;

TABLE 1.1. Triple Screen

α-Fetoprotein	Unconjugated Estriol	β-Human Chorionic Gonadotropin
Decreased levels indicate risk for Trisomy 18 Trisomy 13 Trisomy 21	Decreased levels indicate risk for Trisomy 18 Trisomy 21	Decreased levels indicate risk for Trisomy 18
Elevated levels Anencephaly Open neural tube defects Ventral wall defects Multifetal pregnancies Esophageal, intestinal, and urinary obstruction Liver and renal dysfunction Intrauterine fetal demise		Elevated levels indicate risk for Trisomy 21

chorioamnionitis; premature rupture of membranes; oligohydramnios; and fetomaternal hemorrhage.

  C. Amniocentesis is used to diagnose and/or treat maternal and fetal problems (Dickerman & Park, 1992; Jasper, 2000; Ladewig et al., 1998).

    1. Early in pregnancy (between 15 and 17 weeks' gestation) amniocentesis is used for the following: diagnosis of ventral wall and open neural tube defects through the detection of elevated levels of acetylcholinesterase and α-fetoprotein; and chromosomal/genetic and metabolic disease evaluation through chromosomal analysis, enzyme analysis, and metabolite levels.

    2. Later in pregnancy amniocentesis is used for the following:

      a. Confirmation of amnionitis

      b. Evaluating fetal lung maturity:

        (1) Lecithin/sphingomyelin (L/S) ratio > 2:1 indicates fetal lung maturity (false-positive L/S ratio possible in the IDM; a ratio of > 3:1 may be necessary to indicate lung maturity for the IDM).

        (2) Phosphatidlyglycerol (PG) usually appears at approximately 35 weeks' gestation. The presence of PG is a better marker of lung maturity than the L/S ratio.

        (3) Amniotic creatinine levels (increased levels are present later in gestation) of 2 mg/dL indicate lung maturity.

        (4) Lamellar body count (LBC) (also known as FLM [fetal lung maturity]): lamellar bodies carry surfactant and a count of 30,000 to 55,000/μl is suggestive of lung maturity (Jasper, 2000).

      c. Evaluating Rh-sensitized pregnancies through ΔOD 450 readings (refer to Chapter 3 for further details)

      d. Performing fluid reduction in pregnancies complicated by polyhydramnios

3. Procedure: amniocentesis is performed under ultrasound guidance by inserting a needle transabdominally through the uterine wall and into the amniotic sac. Amniotic fluid and fetal cells are retrieved, grown, and/or analyzed for the above-mentioned screening tests.

4. Risks include: maternal infection; PROM; spontaneous abortion; and needle injury to fetus.

D. Percutaneous umbilical blood sampling (PUBS) is used to make prenatal diagnoses (Hess, Hess, Floyd, & Fraser, 2000) (eg, hemophilia A and B; karyotyping; RBC isoimmunization; suspected congenital infection by obtaining IgM levels; and suspected fetal anemia) and fetal transfusions.

1. Timing: PUBS is usually performed after 19 weeks' gestation but is possible as early as 16 weeks' gestation, although it is technically difficult with earlier gestation.

2. Procedure is performed under ultrasound guidance. By way of a transabdominal approach, the umbilical cord is punctured and fetal blood is sampled.

3. Maternal and fetal risks include: maternal infection; maternal sensitization; fetal hemorrhage and death; PROM; and preterm labor and possible delivery.

II. Fetal well-being

A. Nonstress test (NST) is performed after 28 weeks' gestation to indirectly assess uteroplacental function (Chan & Winkle, 1999).

1. Procedure: external fetal monitoring assesses fetal heart rate (FHR) accelerations in relation to fetal activity. Baseline heart rate variability indicates a healthy fetal CNS and normal parasympathetic/sympathetic influences on cardiac output (Uebel & Lott, 1999).

2. Results:
   a. Reactive NST indicates a well-oxygenated fetus with an intact CNS; FHR increases by 15 bpm at least two times and lasting ≥ 15 seconds during a 20-minute testing period.
   b. Nonreactive NST indicates possible chronic hypoxia leading to acidosis and asphyxia; changes in FHR fail to meet criteria within 40 minutes.

B. Contraction Stress Test (CST) and Oxytocin Challenge Test (OCT) (Uebel & Lott, 1999) are performed after 28 weeks' gestation to evaluate fetal oxygen reserves and placental sufficiency as indicators for tolerance of labor.

1. Procedure: to perform the CST or OCT, contractions are induced by nipple stimulation or intravenous oxytocin administration. It is necessary to have three or more contractions in 10 minutes, with each contraction lasting 40 to 60 seconds. The FHR should increase with the contractions; there should be no decelerations.

2. Results:
   a. Negative CST: no late decelerations with adequate contractions; indicates good fetal outcome.

   b. Positive CST: presence of late decelerations (indicative of uteroplacental insufficiency) with two or more contractions in 10 minutes; indicates poor fetal outcome.
   c. Equivocal/suspicious CST: presence of variable decelerations (indicative of cord compression); repeat CST in 24 hours.
   3. Risks include (Murray, Canfield, & Harmon, 1986): uterine hyperstimulation, premature labor, and fetal bradycardia.
C. Obstetric ultrasound imaging (OUI) is used to evaluate the uterus, placenta, and fetus.
   1. Aids in the prenatal diagnosis of fetal malformations such as CNS anomalies (eg, neural tube defects, hydrocephalus); abdominal wall defects (after 13 weeks' gestation) and intestinal atresias; skeletal deformities and dysplasias; cardiac anomalies; pulmonary hypoplasia, diaphragmatic hernia; renal agenesis and dysplasias; and ascites.
   2. Timing and accuracy of ultrasounds (Chambers, 1995):
      a. First trimester ultrasound is accurate ± 5 days for estimated date of confinement (EDC).
      b. Second trimester ultrasound is accurate ± 7 days for EDC.
      c. Third trimester ultrasound is accurate ± 2 to 3 weeks for EDC.
   3. Types of scans include Level I scan (or basic scan) and Level II scan (or targeted scan):
      a. Level I scan is usually performed to evaluate fetal size, weight, gross anatomy, FHR and rhythm, placental placement, amniotic fluid volume (AFV), fetal number, and presentation.
      b. Level II scan is usually performed if more detailed information is needed for suspected fetal anomalies.
D. Biophysical profile (BPP) is performed to assess fetal well-being in relation to uteroplacental sufficiency.
   1. Timing: the BPP is performed after 28 weeks' gestation.
      a. Fetal development progresses from muscle tone (7th week) → general movement (8th week) → fetal breathing (10th week) → sucking (12th week) → heart rate reactivity (28th week).
      b. Chronic/acute hypoxia causes loss of these behaviors in reverse order of appearance (HR reactivity → sucking → fetal breathing → general movement → muscle tone).
   2. Procedure: to perform this test, external fetal monitoring is used to complete the NST portion of the BPP and ultrasonography is used to determine fetal breathing, movements, tone, and AFV (Table 1.2).
E. Doppler flow studies are performed to diagnose fetal IUGR through the evaluation of umbilical venous and arterial blood flow velocity and the calculation of the systolic:diastolic (S/D) ratio. Results include (Gregor, Paine, & Johnson, 1991):
   1. Normal S/D ratio is 3.0 after 30 weeks' gestation.
   2. Increasing S/D ratio is indicative of IUGR.
   3. Absent diastolic flow is abnormal due to uteroplacental insufficiency or compromised cord circulation.

TABLE 1.2. Biophysical Profile

Parameter	Outcome	Present	Absent
Nonstress test (NST)	**Reactive** NST: fetal heart rate increases by 15 beats/min at least 2 times and lasts ≥15 sec during a 20-min testing period. **Nonreactive** NST: does not meet criteria within 40 min.	2	0
Fetal breathing movements	≥ 1 episode of ≥ 30 sec in duration in 30 min	2	0
Fetal body movements	≥ 3 discrete body or limb movements in 30 sec	2	0
Fetal muscle tone	≥ 1 episode of extension with return to flexion (limb[s] or trunk)	2	0
Amniotic fluid volume	≥ 1 fluid pocket in 2 perpendicular planes of ≥ 2 cm	2	0

Interpretation	Score	Recommendations
	8-10: normal infant with low risk for chronic asphyxia	**8-10:** repeat weekly; twice weekly with diabetics or ≥ 42 wk Deliver infant if score = 8 **and** oligohydramnios
	4-6: suspected chronic asphyxia	**6:** repeat in 24 h Deliver infant if score = 6 **or** oligohydramnios
	0-2: strong suspicion of chronic asphyxia	**0-4:** deliver infant

Adapted from Jasper, M. L. (2000). Antepartum fetal assessment. In S. Mattson & J. E. Smith (Eds.), *Core curriculum for maternal-newborn nursing.* (2nd ed., pp. 127–160). Philadelphia: WB Saunders; and Ladewig, P. W., London, M. L., & Olds, S. B. (1998). *Maternal-newborn nursing care* (4th ed.). Menlo Park, CA: Addison Wesley Longman, Inc.

▼ References

Carlson, E. J., & Dattel, B. J. (2000). Infectious disease complications. In A. T. Evans & K. R. Niswander (Eds.), *Manual of obstetrics* (6th ed., pp. 163–198). Philadelphia: Lippincott Williams & Wilkins.

Chambers, S. E. (1995). An overview of ultrasound in obstetrics. In G. B. Reed, A. E Claireaux, & F. Cockburn (Eds.), *Diseases of the fetus and newborn* (2nd ed., pp. 877–882). London: Chapman & Hall Medical.

Chan, P. D., & Winkle, C. L. (1999). *Gynecology and obstetrics 1999-2000 edition.* Laguna Hills, CA: Current Clinical Strategies Publishing.

Christmas, J. T., & Slotnick, R. N. (2000). Isoimmunization. In A. T. Evans & K. R. Niswander (Eds.), *Manual of obstetrics* (6th ed., pp. 330–336). Philadelphia: Lippincott Williams & Wilkins.

Cunningham, F. G., MacDonald, P. C., Gant, N. F., Leveno, K. J., Gilstrap, L. C., Hankins, G. D. V., & Clark, S. L., (Eds.). (1997). *Williams obstetrics* (20th ed.). Norwalk, CT: Appleton & Lange.

Dickerman, L. H., & Park, V. M. (1992). Cytogenetic and molecular aspects of genetic disease and prenatal diagnosis. In A. A. Fanaroff & R. J. Martin (Eds.), *Neonatal-perinatal medicine: Diseases of the fetus and infant* (5th ed., pp 57–79). St. Louis: Mosby Year Book.

Evans, A. T. (2000). Perinatal drug use. In A. T. Evans & K. R. Niswander (Eds.), *Manual of obstetrics* (6th ed., pp. 27–39). Philadelphia: Lippincott Williams & Wilkins.

Gegor, C. L., Paine, L. L., & Johnson, T. R. B. (1991). Antepartum fetal assessment: a nurse-midwifery perspective. *Journal of Nurse-Midwifery, 36*(3), 164.

Gonik, B., & McNamara, M. F. (1997). Intrapartum-associated infectious complications. In R. K. Creasy (Ed.), *Management of labor and delivery* (pp. 527–543). Malden, MA: Blackwell Science.

Heaman, M. (2000). Other medical complications. In S. Mattson & J. E. Smith (Eds.), *Core curriculum for maternal-newborn nursing.* (2nd ed., pp. 564–606). Philadelphia: WB Saunders.

Hess, L. W., Hess, D. B., Floyd, R. C., & Fraser, R. F. (2000). Antepartum diagnosis of fetal anomalies. In M. E. Rivlin & R. W. Martin (Eds.), *Manual of clinical problems in obstetrics and gynecology* (5th ed., pp. 211–214). Philadelphia: Lippincott Williams & Wilkins.

Jasper, M. L. (2000). Antepartum fetal assessment. In S. Mattson & J. E. Smith (Eds.), *Core curriculum for maternal-newborn nursing* (2nd ed., 127–160). Philadelphia: WB Saunders.

Kenner, C., & Lott, J. W. (1994). Types of microorganisms. In J. W. Lott (Ed.), *Neonatal infection: Assessment, diagnosis, and management* (pp. 65–112). Petaluma, CA: NICU Ink.

Kopecky, E. A., & Koren, G. (1998). Maternal drug abuse: effects on fetus and neonate. In R. A. Polin & W. P. W. Fox (Eds.), *Fetal and neonatal physiology* (2nd ed., pp. 203–220). Philadelphia: W.B. Saunders.

Ladewig, P. W., London, M. L., & Olds, S. B. (1998). *Maternal-newborn nursing care* (4th ed.). Menlo Park, CA: Addison Wesley Longman, Inc.

Landry, N. (1999). Uncomplicated antepartum, intrapartum, and postpartum care. In J. Deacon & P. O'Neill (Eds.), *Core curriculum for neonatal intensive care nursing* (2nd ed., pp. 2–17). Philadelphia: WB Saunders.

Moran, B. A. (2000). Maternal infections. In S. Mattson & J. E. Smith (Eds.), *Core curriculum for maternal-newborn nursing* (2nd ed., pp. 419–448). Philadelphia: WB Saunders.

Murray, M. L., Canfield, S., & Harmon, J. (1986). Nipple stimulation-contraction stress test for the high-risk patient. In *Maternal and child nursing, 11,* 331.

Perry, K. G. (2000). Rh isoimmunization. In M. E. Rivlin & R. W. Martin (Eds.), *Manual of clinical problems in obstetrics and gynecology* (5th ed., pp. 101–104). Philadelphia: Lippincott Williams & Wilkins.

Pickering, L. K. (Ed.). (2000). *2000 Red book: Report of the committee on infectious diseases* (25th ed.). Elk Grove Village, IL: American Academy of Pediatrics.

Putman, M., & Smith, J. E. (2000). The drug-dependent neonate. In S. Mattson & J. E. Smith (Eds.), *Core curriculum for maternal-newborn nursing* (2nd ed., pp. 730–743). Philadelphia: WB Saunders.

Rivlin, M. E. (2000). Gonorrhea. In M. E. Rivlin & R. W. Martin (Eds.), *Manual of clinical problems in obstetrics and gynecology* (5th ed., pp. 277–281). Philadelphia: Lippincott Williams & Wilkins.

Scoggin, J., & Morgan, G. (1998). *Practice guidelines for obstetrics and gynecology.* Philadelphia: Lippincott.

Shulman, L. P. (1992). Perspectives on counseling in maternal serum alpha-fetoprotein screening. In S. Elias & J. L. Simpson (Eds.), *Maternal serum screening for fetal genetic disorders* (pp. 121–131). New York: Churchill Livingstone, Inc.

Terrone, D. A. (2000). Anemias and hemoglobinopathies in pregnancy. In M. E. Rivlin & R. W. Martin (Eds.), *Manual of clinical problems in obstetrics and gynecology* (5th ed., pp. 108–113). Philadelphia: Lippincott Williams & Wilkins.

Uebel, P., & Lott, J. W. (1999). A case study of antenatal distress and consequent neonatal respiratory distress. *Neonatal Network, 18*(5), 65.

Whitehurst, R. M. (1999). Blood abnormalities. In T. L. Gomella, M. D. Cunningham,
F. G. Eyal, & K. E. Zenk (Eds.), *Neonatology: Management, procedures, on-call
problems, diseases, drugs* (4th ed., pp. 314–334). Stamford, CT: Appleton & Lange.
Wynn, R. M. (Ed.) (1992). *Obstetrics and gynecology the clinical core* (5th ed.).
Philadelphia: Lea & Febiger.

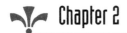

Chapter 2

Intrapartum

Paulette S. Haws, MSN, RNC, NNP

Part A: To accurately understand and communicate information regarding a patient's pregnancy history and progress during labor, correct terminology should be used.

I. Pregnancy
    A. Gravidity and parity (Cunningham, et al, 1997; Ladewig, London, & Olds, 1998; Turley, 2000):
        1. Gravidity is the total number of pregnancies.
            a. Primigravida is a woman pregnant for the first time.
            b. Multigravida is a woman who has had two or more pregnancies.
        2. Parity is the total number of pregnancies carried beyond 20 weeks' gestation, regardless of fetal outcome.
            a. Primapara is a woman who has had one pregnancy lasting more than 20 weeks' gestation.
            b. Multipara is a woman who has had two or more pregnancies lasting more than 20 weeks' gestation.
            c. Parity is further subdivided into four categories: term, preterm, abortion, and living children (eg, G9 P2345 = 9 pregnancies; 2 term, 3 premature, 4 abortions, 5 living).

II. Labor
    A. Dilation and effacement (Ladewig, London, & Olds, 1998; Turley, 2000; Wolcott & Conry, 2000):
        1. Dilation is the process whereby the external cervical os opens as a result of pressure applied by the presenting part and uterine muscle contractions. Dilation proceeds from 0 cm (external os is closed) to 10 cm (external os is totally dilated).
        2. Effacement occurs when the internal os is drawn up into the lower uterine segment and the cervical canal shortens from approximately 3 cm (0% effaced) to a thin orifice (100% effaced).
            a. Primaparas: effacement normally begins before labor; therefore, preceding dilation.
            b. Multiparas: effacement may only begin after the onset of labor, after dilation.
    B. Engagement: occurs when the widest diameter of the presenting part (eg, the biparietal diameter of the fetal head during a vertex presentation) passes to a level below the pelvic inlet (usually 0 station).
    C. Presentation: position of the fetus during labor and the anatomic part lying nearest the cervix. Fetal positions include (Cunningham et al., 1997; Turley, 2000; Wolcott & Conry, 2000):
        1. Cephalic presentation is classified according to the relationship of the head to the fetal body.

    a. Vertex (or occiput) (95%–96% of all deliveries at term): the head is sharply flexed with the chin in contact with the thorax.

    b. Face: neck is sharply extended and the face is the primary presenting part.

    c. Brow: usually a transient position that converts to either vertex or face presentation before delivery

  2. Breech (3%–4% of all deliveries at term)

    a. Types of breech presentation include: complete (flexed hips and knees); frank (flexed hips, knees extended over the anterior portion of the body); footling (extended hip or hips, extended knee or knees); and kneeling (extended hips, flexed knees).

    b. Increased fetal morbidity and mortality

  3. Transverse presentation: occurs when the buttocks or head is prevented from entering the lower pelvis. The shoulder is usually the presenting part (0.3%–0.4% of all deliveries at term). Expect maternal and/or fetal injury with vaginal delivery.

D. Station: the relationship of the presenting part of the infant to the level of the mother's ischial spines (landmark for the midpelvis) (Wolcott & Conry, 2000)

  1. 0 station: presenting part is at the level of the ischial spines; in vertex presentation the widest part of the fetal head, ie, the biparietal diameter, has passed through the pelvic inlet.

  2. "Minus" station: presenting part is above the ischial spines; at − 3 the presenting part is 3 cm above the spine and is described as "floating."

  3. "Plus" station: presenting part is below the ischial spines; at + 3 the presenting part is on the perineum and may be visible during a contraction.

Part B: Parturition, the process of giving birth to a child, progresses through stages. Fetal well-being is followed by way of electronic fetal monitoring, and, during the birthing process, the mother may require analgesia and anesthesia depending upon the mode of delivery.

I. Stages of labor

There are three classic stages of labor and a fourth stage of labor (Cunningham et al., 1997; Pritchard, 1985; Smith, 2000; Wolcott & Conry, 2000).

A. First stage of labor (dilation)

  1. The first stage of labor begins when the uterine contractions have enough frequency, intensity, and duration to cause cervical effacement and dilation. The stage ends with full cervical dilation.

  2. The first stage of labor is further divided into three phases: latent, active, and transition (Table 2.1).

B. Second stage of labor (infant expulsion): begins with full dilation of the cervix and ends with expulsion of the infant.

  1. Contractions occur every 2 to 3 minutes and last for 60 to 90 seconds.

  2. There is full dilation (10 cm) and effacement (100%).

  3. Station ranges from 0 to + 3.

  4. Intensity of contractions is 80 to 100 mmHg.

TABLE 2.1. First Stage of Labor

	Latent	Active	Transition
Contractions	Irregular; every 5–10 min	Every 2–5 min	Every 2–3 min
Duration of contractions	30–45 sec	45–60 sec	60–90 sec
Intensity of contractions	25–40 mmHg by intrauterine pressure catheter (IUPC)	50–70 mmHg by IUPC	70–90 mmHg by IUPC
Dilation	0–3 cm	4–7 cm	8–10 cm
Rate of dilation	Variable length of time, but may extend up to 20 h	~1.2 cm/h for primapara ~1.5 cm/h for multipara	
Effacement	0%–40%	40%–80%	80%–100%
Station		−2 to 0	−1 to +1

    C. Third stage of labor (placental expulsion): begins with infant expulsion and ends with expulsion of delivery of placenta and fetal membranes.

    D Fourth stage of labor (immediately postpartum): the first few hours immediately after delivery when myometrial contractions and retraction, as well as vessel thrombosis, occur to effectively control bleeding from the placental implantation site

II. Essentials of fetal monitoring (Berkowitz & Nageotte, 2000; Chan & Winkle, 1999):

    A. Fetal heart rate (FHR)

        1. Normal FHR ranges from 120 to 160 beats per minute (bpm).

        2. Bradycardia, as evidenced by deceleration on a fetal monitor tracing, is the initial response to hypoxia.

        3. Tachycardia may occur with prolonged severe hypoxia. It is also a response to maternal fever, chorioamnionitis, and congenital heart disease.

        4. Cardiac arrhythmia

            a. Irregular pattern appearance repeats itself.

            b. Usually benign if baseline variability and reactivity are present. Often resolves after birth.

            c. May signify underlying cardiac anomaly.

    B. Deceleration

        1. Early deceleration

            a. Occurs as a result of a *fetal head compression* that decreases cerebral blood flow. At the end of a contraction, cerebral blood flow returns and the deceleration ends. Early deceleration is usually benign.

    b. Occurs more frequently with primigravidas and cephalopelvic disproportion.

    c. Appearance of early deceleration on fetal monitor tracing

        (1) Uniformly shaped deceleration with minimal amplitude

        (2) FHR rarely drops fewer than 30 bpm below the baseline.

        (3) Deceleration is usually in phase with the uterine contraction: slow onset beginning early in the contraction cycle; reaches nadir with the peak of the contraction; returns slowly to baseline, usually before the end of the contraction; and long-term variability (LTV) and short-term variability (STV) are usually present.

2. Late deceleration

    a. Occurs as a result of hypoxia caused by *uteroplacental insufficiency*. Etiology of uteroplacental insufficiency includes: chronic maternal disease (eg, diabetes mellitus [DM], systemic lupus erythematosus [SLE], hypertension [HTN], or pregnancy-induced hypertension [PIH]); hypotension associated with blood loss (eg, placental abruption or uterine rupture), anesthesia, medications, or drug use; maternal drug use; maternal smoking; placenta that is small, aged, calcified, or deteriorated; and uterine hyperstimulation.

    b. Appearance of a late deceleration on a fetal monitor tracing

        (1) U-shaped with low amplitude; pattern is smooth and persistent.

        (2) The fall in FHR is usually 10 to 30 bpm below baseline; the depth of the deceleration does not always indicate the severity of fetal hypoxia; decelerations may deepen as fetal hypoxia becomes more severe.

        (3) Onset of a late deceleration is gradual, occurring after the onset of the contraction (up to 30 seconds after the initiation of the contraction); reaches its nadir long after the peak of the contraction; returns to baseline after the end of the contraction.

        (4) LTV and STV are usually decreased or absent.

        (5) Persistent late decelerations are nonreassuring.

3. Variable deceleration

    a. Occurs as a result *of umbilical cord compression*, decreased umbilical cord perfusion, baroreceptor stimulation with a vagal response, and *hypoxia and hypercarbic* conditions.

    b. Appearance of a variable deceleration on a fetal monitor tracing

        (1) Variable shapes (W, U, V)

        (2) FHR often drops significantly below the baseline. Variable decelerations are either mild (duration < 30 seconds or FHR not < 80 bpm regardless of the duration of the variable), moderate (FHR 70 to 80 bpm, regardless of the duration of the variable), or severe (FHR < 70 bpm for > 60 seconds).

        (3) Onset of the deceleration is abrupt and variable, ie, before, after, or coinciding with the onset of the contraction; return to baseline is abrupt.

(4) Commonly associated with preaccelerations and postaccelerations (or shoulders)

c. Reassuring variable: duration < 45 seconds; rapid return to baseline; normal LTV and STV

d. Nonreassuring variable

(1) Duration > 60 seconds; FHR < 70 bpm; slow return to baseline; loss of STV

(2) Treatment for nonreassuring fetal monitor tracings (Chan & Winkle, 1999): determine the cause for the fetal pattern; institute measures to correct the primary problem and improve fetal oxygenation and placental perfusion.

C. Acceleration (Chan & Winkle, 1999; Cunningham et al., 1997; Schmidt, 2000):

1. Accelerations are common changes in heart rate, often seen in early labor and in association with variable decelerations. They occur as a result of fetal movement, tactile stimulation secondary to uterine contraction or examination, and umbilical cord occlusion. Usually accelerations are reassuring, indicating the fetus is not acidotic.

2. Appearance of an acceleration on fetal monitor tracing

a. FHR increases 10 to 15 bpm above the baseline. (Reactivity, ie, increased FHR of 10 to 15 bpm lasting for > 15 seconds in response to fetal activity or tactile stimulation, is present after 28 to 30 weeks' gestation.)

b. Abrupt onset

c. Variability is usually present.

d. May occur with the uterine contraction.

e. May occur in association with variable decelerations as preaccelerations and/or postaccelerations (or overshoots or shoulders).

f. Decreased or absent variability

D. Variability

1. STV

a. Refers to the "instantaneous change in fetal heart rate from one beat to the next. This variability is a measure of the time interval between cardiac systoles" (Cunningham et al., 1997). Time interval for STV is measured in milliseconds (Schmidt, 2000).

b. Etiology of absent STV includes: hypoxia; neurogenic causes (eg, maternal medications, fetal anomalies).

c. Appearance of STV on fetal monitor is assessed by the roughness or smoothness of the FHR line tracing.

(1) Present STV: rough line tracing secondary to beat-to-beat changes

(2) Absent STV: smooth line tracing secondary to fewer beat-to-beat changes

2. LTV

a. Refers to the "oscillatory changes that occur during the course of 1 minute and result in the waviness of the baseline. The normal frequency of such waves is 3 to 5 cycles per minute" (Cunningham et al., 1997).

    b. Etiology of LTV changes (Schmidt, 2000):
      (1) Normal LTV: fetus is awake, active, or experiencing rapid eye movement (REM) sleep.
      (2) Marked LTV: early sign of mild hypoxia
      (3) Decreased LTV: hypoxia, fetal neurogenic abnormalities, and altered sleep states
    c. Appearance of LTV on fetal monitor tracing (Berkowitz & Mageotte, 2000; Schmidt, 2000):
      (1) Normal/average: amplitude change 6 to 25 bpm
      (2) Marked/saltatory: amplitude change > 25 bpm
      (3) Decreased/minimal: amplitude change 0 to 5 bpm
      (4) Absent: amplitude change < 2 bpm
  3. Sinusoidal pattern
    a. "Sine wave oscillates at 5 to 30 beats of amplitude and 3 to 6 cycles per minute" (Schmidt, 2000).
    b. Associated fetal problems include: fetal anemia and/or hypoxia; Rh sensitization; and acute fetomaternal hemorrhage.
    c. Appearance of sinusoidal pattern on fetal monitor tracing: undulating pattern; spontaneous onset; absent STV; and no accelerations

III. Obstetric analgesia and anesthesia

  A. Indications: maternal obstetric analgesia and anesthesia is administered to relieve pain from uterine contractions and vaginal or abdominal delivery. Ideally, obstetric analgesia and anesthesia do not deleteriously affect effective uterine contractions, maternal expulsive efforts, or maternal and fetal well-being.

  B. Analgesia (Wolcott & Conry, 2000): pain management during labor and delivery is an important part of the birthing process. Pain control methods, such as psychoprophylaxis (eg, antenatal instruction regarding methods to maintain concentration and self-control) and alternate pain management tactics (eg, use of professional support persons such as a nurse, nurse midwife, or doula; massage therapy, acupressure, and therapeutic touch; music and aromatherapy; and positioning techniques) are invaluable. Regarding chemoprophylaxis, it is essential to use the appropriate narcotic or analgesic agent at the appropriate time during labor.

    1. First stage of labor (latent phase): mild sedation with short-acting barbiturate or ataractic (eg, hydroxyzine, secobarbital, or sodium pentobarbital); they will not slow the labor process.

    2. Second stage of labor (active phase): narcotics are administered parenterally; oral analgesics should be avoided. Narcotics cross the placenta and may depress the fetus.

  C. Regional anesthesia

    1. Epidural anesthesia: epidural anesthesia allows ambulation during the first stage of labor and effective pushing during the second stage of labor.

      a. Procedure (Wolcott & Conry, 2000): hydrate mother with 500 to 1000 mL nondextrose intravenous solution before placement of epidural catheter. A plastic catheter is threaded into the epidural space between L_2 and S_1. A test dose is adminis-

tered to ensure proper catheter placement; a full dose is subsequently given for regional block or surgical anesthesia.
   b. Contraindications include (Wolcott & Conry, 2000): maternal infection in lumbar area; septicemia; coagulopathy, especially thrombocytopenia; neurologic disorders; and hypovolemia.
   c. Maternal complications include (Cunningham et al., 1997): hypotension and decreased cardiac output; cardiorespiratory arrest; neurologic complications; urinary retention; and adverse drug reactions.
   d. Fetal complications: no fetal effects unless there is maternal hypotension resulting in decreased placental blood flow
2. Spinal (subarachnoid) anesthesia
   a. Low spinal anesthesia (or saddle block) (Cunningham, 1997; Wolcott & Conry, 2000) is an excellent form of pain control during a vaginal delivery.
      (1) Procedure: to prevent maternal hypotension, a fluid bolus of 300 to 500 mL should be administered before injecting the spinal anesthesia. A local anesthetic is injected into the subarachnoid space at L_4-L_5 or L_5-S_1, resulting in motor and sensory nerve blockage.
   b. High spinal anesthesia (Cunningham, 1997, Wolcott & Conry, 2000) is used for pain control during abdominal delivery.
      (1) Procedure: to prevent maternal hypotension, a fluid bolus of 300 to 500 mL should be administered before injecting the spinal anesthesia into the subarachnoid space at L_4-L_5 or L_5-S_1.
   c. Contraindications include: maternal infection in lumbar area; septicemia; coagulopathy; neurologic disorders; hypovolemia; placenta previa and placental abruption; and fetal distress.
   d. Maternal complications include: hypotension and decreased cardiac output; cardiorespiratory arrest; neurologic sequelae; urinary retention; and adverse drug reactions.
   e. Fetal effects: decreased placental blood flow secondary to maternal hypotension
3. Paracervical block (Cunningham et al., 1997; Wolcott & Conry, 2000) provides excellent pain control from uterine contractions, especially during the first stage of labor.
   a. Procedure: an anesthetic agent is injected into each side of the cervix to block Frankenhäuser's ganglion.
   b. Fetal complications include bradycardia secondary to possible "toxicity from the local anesthetic uterine artery vasoconstriction, or hypercontractility of the uterus" (Wolcott & Conry, 2000).
4. Pudendal block (Cunningham et al., 1997; Smith, 2000; Wolcott & Conry, 2000) provides pain control during spontaneous vaginal delivery, outlet forceps delivery, episiotomy, and episiotomy repair.
   a. Procedure: an anesthetic agent is injected through the right and left sacrospinous ligaments, thereby blocking the pudendal nerve near the ischial spines.
   b. Maternal complications include: inadvertent intravascular injection of anesthetic agent leading to possible systemic toxi-

city and seizures; hematoma secondary to blood vessel perforation; and infection at injection site.

c. Fetal complications: rare or none

5. Local infiltration (Smith, 2000) is used for pain control for actual vaginal delivery and episiotomy and subsequent repair.

a. Procedure: the perineum is injected with a local anesthetic agent.

D. General anesthesia

1. Indication: balanced general anesthesia, which is a combination of nitrous oxide (N_2O), oxygen, a halogenated agent (eg, isoflurane), a short-acting barbiturate (eg, thiopental), and a muscle relaxant (eg, succinylcholine) used for analgesia and altering consciousness, is used to perform tracheal intubation, cesarean section, and some forceps delivery.

2. Maternal complications include (Cunningham et al., 1997): aspiration pneumonia; failed intubation; hepatitis and hepatic necrosis associated with the use of halogenated hydrocarbons; and increased blood loss when halogenated hydrocarbons are used.

3. Fetal complications: respiratory depression

IV. Operative deliveries

A. Assisted vaginal deliveries (forceps and vacuum)

1. Indications include (Rosemond & Fedrizzi, 2000; Smith, 2000):

a. Maternal reasons: failure to progress secondary to inadequate force of contractions or inadequate pushing techniques; maternal physical condition (eg, cardiomyopathy, pulmonary disease, intrapartum infection, neurologic disorder); and maternal fatigue

b. Fetal reasons: fetal distress; fetal malposition; macrosomia; preterm infant (eg, possible cranial damage with prolonged pushing); and prolapsed cord, placental abruption, or nonreassuring fetal monitor tracing

2. Prerequisites for assisted delivery (forceps and vacuum) include: empty bladder; fetal head is engaged; fully dilated cervix; no cephalopelvic disproportion; and ruptured membranes.

3. Maternal complications include (Cunningham et al., 1997; Vaughan & Gillogley, 2000): lacerations of vagina, perineum, rectum, or bladder; hemorrhage secondary to lacerations; pelvic hematomas; urinary retention; and urinary tract infection.

4. Fetal complications include:

a. Forceps: asphyxia and death; brachial plexus injuries; cephalohematomas; facial palsies and lacerations; and skull fractures and intracranial hemorrhage

b. Vacuum: asphyxia; brachial plexus injury; cephalohematoma; hyperbilirubinemia; intracranial and retinal hemorrhage; and subgaleal hemorrhage

B. Cesarean section

1. Cesarean section is classically defined as the birth of a fetus through an abdominal wall incision (laparotomy) and uterine wall incision (hysterotomy) (Cunningham et al., 1997).

2. Indications include (Cunningham et al., 1997; Smith, 2000): abnormal fetal presentation (eg, breech or transverse lie) or size

(macrosomia); dystocia or failure of labor to progress; fetal distress, disease, or anomaly; maternal conditions that compromise fetal well-being (eg, placenta previa, abruption, or active herpes lesions); and repeat cesarean section.

3. Procedure: analgesia and anesthesia is provided with either a regional block (epidural or high spinal anesthesia) or balanced general anesthesia. Types of abdominal incision include (Culbert, 2000): low transverse incisions (90% of cesarean sections) that are made through the lower, less muscular portion of the uterus, which is less likely to rupture with subsequent pregnancies; classic incisions that are made through the upper uterine segment and allow rapid uterine entry and extraction of the fetus (these incisions are at higher risk for increased blood loss during surgery and uterine rupture with subsequent pregnancies and labor).

4. Maternal complications include: complications associated with regional or general anesthesia; hemorrhage; infection; and uterine rupture with subsequent pregnancies attempting a vaginal birth after cesarean section.

5. Fetal complications include: respiratory depression with the use of general anesthesia; incisional trauma made when entering the uterus; blood loss if the uterine incision is made through anterior placenta; fetal injury due to the extraction process; transient tachypnea of the newborn; and respiratory distress syndrome.

▼ References

Berkowitz, K., & Nageotte, M. P. (2000). Intrapartum fetal monitoring. In A. T. Evans & K. R. Niswander (Eds.), *Manual of obstetrics* (6th ed., pp. 313–329). Philadelphia: Lippincott Williams & Wilkins.

Chan, P. D., & Winkle, C. R. (1999). *Gynecology and obstetrics 1999-2000 edition*. Laguna Hills, CA: Current Clinical Strategies Publishing.

Culbert, S. A. (2000). Cesarean birth. In J. E. Rivlin & R. W. Martin (Eds.), *Manual of clinical problems in obstetrics and gynecology* (5th ed., pp. 163–168). Philadelphia: Lippincott Williams & Wilkins.

Cunningham, F. G., MacDonald, P. C., Fant, N. F., Leveno, K. J., Gilstrap, L. C., Hankins, G. D. V., & Clark, S. L. (Eds.). (1997). *Williams obstetrics* (20th ed.). Norwalk, CT: Appleton & Lange.

Ladewig, P. W., London, M. L., & Olds, S. B. (1998). *Maternal-newborn nursing care: The nurse, the family, and the community* (4th ed.). Menlo Park, CA: Addison-Wesley.

Pritchard, J. A., MacDonald, P. C, & Gant, N. F. (1985). *Williams obstetrics* (17th ed.). Norwalk, CT: Appleton-Century-Crofts.

Rosemond, R. L., & Fedrizzi, R. P. (2000). Forceps and vacuum extraction. In A. T. Evans & K. R. Niswander (Eds.), *Manual of obstetrics* (6th ed., pp. 160–168). Philadelphia: Lippincott Williams & Wilkins.

Schmidt, J. (2000). Intrapartum fetal assessment. In S. Mattson & J. E. Smith (Eds.), *Core curriculum for maternal-newborn nursing* (2nd ed., pp. 271–299). Philadelphia: WB Saunders.

Smith, K. V. (2000). Normal childbirth. In S. Mattson & J. E. Smith (Eds.), *Core curriculum for maternal-newborn nursing* (2nd ed., pp. 241–270). Philadelphia: WB Saunders.

Turley, G. M. (2000). Essential forces and factors in labor. In S. Mattson & J. Smith (Eds.), *Core curriculum for maternal-newborn nursing* (2nd ed., pp. 204–240). Philadelphia: WB Saunders.

Vaughan, M. C., & Gillogley, K. M. (2000). Abnormal labor and delivery. In A. T. Evans & K. R. Niswander (Eds.), *Manual of obstetrics* (6th ed., pp. 425–439). Philadelphia: Lippincott Williams & Wilkins.

Wolcott, H. D., & Conry J. A. (2000). Normal labor. In A. T. Evans & K. R. Niswander (Eds.), *Manual of obstetrics* (6th ed., pp. 392–424). Philadelphia: Lippincott Williams & Wilkins.

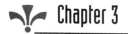 **Chapter 3**

High-Risk Pregnancies and Deliveries

Paulette S. Haws, MSN, RNC, NNP

The topics discussed in this chapter are those conditions—maternal, fetal, or both—that place the well-being of the mother and/or infant at risk, not only during the pregnancy but also during delivery.

A. ABO incompatibility:
1. ABO disease is more likely with the following combinations: m**O**ther is type **O** with anti-A or anti-B in her serum; the b**AB**y is A, **B**, or **AB** blood type. ABO disease occurs with first pregnancies and frequently with subsequent pregnancies.
2. Diagnosis: prenatal maternal blood typing and infant blood typing and direct antibody testing (DAT)
3. Fetal outcomes include (Whitehurst, 1999):
   a. Hemolytic anemia (mild) and reticulocytosis. Onset of jaundice within 24 hours of life.
   b. Infant's direct antiglobulin (Coombs) may be weakly positive and then become negative at day of life (DOL) 2-3. Infant's indirect Coombs' test will identify presence of maternal isoantibody.

B. Rh (D) sensitization occurs when a woman who is Rh negative produces anti-Rh (D) IgG antibody after exposure to Rh-positive blood through either a transfusion or a previous pregnancy. Women are screened for the presence of D (Rh) antigen on erythrocytes by DAT and other unusual antibodies in their serum by antibody screen (Indirect Coombs) (Cunningham et al., 1997; Glass, 2000; Jasper, 2000).
1. Diagnosis:
   a. Antibody screen: maternal antibody levels determine the amount of isoimmunization. Rh antibody titer (albumin agglutination technique) of $\geq 1:16$ places the fetus at risk for hemolytic anemia. If early maternal anti-D titer is $\geq 1:16$, then an amniocentesis is recommended at 26 weeks to perform ΔOD 450 (Perry, 2000).
   b. ΔOD 450: maternal antibodies (anti-Rh) cross the placenta and destroy fetal red blood cells (RBCs). Bilirubin, a breakdown product of destroyed RBCs, is measured in the amniotic fluid (optical density [OD] Δ450 mμ) and the ΔOD 450 result, combined with gestational age, predicts the amount of fetal hemolysis.
2. Maternal treatment: antibody titer is repeated at 26 to 28 weeks' gestation for all women who are Rh negative.
   a. Negative titer: maternal administration of anti-D immune globulin (RhoGAM) at 28 weeks' gestation, and within 72 hours after delivery, amniocentesis, chorionic villus sampling

(CVS), percutaneous umbilical blood sampling (PUBS), and/or fetomaternal hemorrhage

   b. Positive titer: RhoGAM is not given because it is ineffective. The pregnancy is then managed to minimize the effects of fetal hemolytic disease and hydrops (Chan & Winkle, 1999; Scoggin & Morgan, 1998).

  3. Fetal outcome includes: hydrops fetalis (hemolytic anemia, congestive heart failure [CHF], pleural effusions and respiratory distress, ascites, and hypoalbuminemia); hyperbilirubinemia.

  C. Advanced maternal age (AMA): defined as older than 35 years. Women of AMA have a higher incidence of chronic illness (eg, arthritis, diabetes, hypertension [HTN], uterine fibroids) that can affect pregnancy course and outcome (Deitch, 2000); there are also potential psychosocial concerns. Additionally, there is an increased risk of delivering an infant with a chromosomal abnormality, as demonstrated in Table 3.1 (Carcio, 1999).

  D. Antenatal bleeding: classified as either chronic or acute blood loss and is the result of multiple fetal, maternal, placental, uterine, and/or cord conditions.

   1. Uteroplacental conditions:

    a. Placental abruption: partial or complete placental separation from the uterine wall before delivery

     (1) Maternal factors associated with placental abruption include: AMA; alcohol, tobacco, and illegal drug use (eg, cocaine); chronic HTN and pregnancy-induced HTN (PIH); multiple gestation; and previous history of an abruption.

     (2) A small abruption with minimal blood loss may be tolerated by the fetus; however, a large abruption leads to a decreased uteroplacental surface area, fetal asphyxia, and decreased fetal/maternal well-being. Intervention with a large abruption is immediate delivery to prevent perinatal asphyxia and/or death.

    b. Placenta previa: abnormally low placental implantation with partial or complete covering of internal cervical os

     (1) Fetal/neonatal outcomes: the extent of bleeding dictates the severity of the outcome. Infants may be anemic or, in the case of severe bleeding, experience fetal distress and/or demise (Ladewig, London, & Olds, 1998).

 TABLE 3.1. Chromosomal Abnormalities in Relation to Maternal Age

Age (yr)	Risk for Trisomy 21	Total Risk for Chromosomal Abnormality
20	1:667	1:526
30	1:952	1:385
40	1:106	1:83

(2) Intervention for complete previa includes fetal lung assessment at 35 to 36 weeks, with delivery via cesarean section; possible vaginal delivery with partial placenta previa.

c. Placenta accreta: placenta attaches abnormally to the uterine wall with complete or partial absence of the decidua basalis. Therefore, the placental villi invade the myometrium, posing a considerable maternal risk for hemorrhage, uterine rupture, and infection (Cunningham et al., 1997).

d. Fetomaternal transfusion: chronic blood loss from the fetal intravascular compartment across the placenta into the maternal intervillous space

  (1) Diagnosis: confirmed with the use of Kleihauer-Betke stain on maternal blood. Acid-resistant fetal cells, containing hemoglobin F, appear to be normally colored while maternal "ghost" cells, containing hemoglobin A, appear colorless (Mentzer & Glader, 1998).

  (2) Maternal clinical manifestations include isoimmunization and, with massive hemorrhage, transfusion reaction.

  (3) Neonatal clinical manifestations include pallor, anemia, and iron deficiency.

e. Fetofetal (twin-to-twin) transfusion:

  (1) Arterial-venous anastomosis: fetofetal transfusion occurs with monochorionic twins whose placenta contains an arterial-venous anastomosis between the twins, a condition that carries a high morbidity/mortality rate. A difference in hemoglobin > 4 to 5 g/dL between the twins is indicative of an arterial-venous anastomosis (Gilbert, 1998).

  (2) Venous-venous and arterial-arterial vascular connections between the fetuses have a lower incidence of morbidity.

  (3) Donor twin clinical manifestations and therapy include: anemia; pallor; lower birth weight than recipient twin; hypoglycemia; and oligohydramnios. Therapy involves volume replacement and/or transfusion to alleviate the anemia.

  (4) Recipient twin clinical manifestations and therapy include: polycythemia; plethora; higher birth weight than donor twin; hydrops fetalis; hyperbilirubinemia; and presence of hydramnios. Therapy includes partial exchange transfusion with fresh frozen plasma or normal saline to decrease the polycythemia.

f. Uterine rupture: *Uterine rupture is an obstetric emergency* associated with the following conditions (Austin & Sheridan, 2000; Carty, 1989): previous cesarean section (commonly with classic incision); oxytocin administration; parity > 4; epidural anesthesia; version; placental abruption; mid forceps delivery; abdominal trauma.

       (1) Maternal clinical manifestations include: abdominal pain and/or rigidity; vaginal bleeding; and hypovolemic shock.

       (2) Fetal clinical manifestations include: fetal distress secondary to impeded uteroplacental blood flow and possible fetal demise.

  2. Umbilical cord conditions:

    a. Cord length: Normal cord length at term is approximately 55 cm. An abnormally short cord (< 32 cm) may indicate a congenital anomaly/problem (eg, renal agenesis, pulmonary hypoplasia, and decreased fetal movement secondary to limb dysfunction) and increase the risk for placental abruption or cord rupture. An abnormally long cord increases the risk for cord prolapse and fetal entrapment (Kellogg, 1998).

    b. Velamentous cord insertion (Cunningham et al, 1997; Kellogg, 1998; Reed, Claireaux, & Cockburn, 1995) occurs when the cord implants at the edge of the placenta. The cord vessels separate in the membranes before reaching the placental margin and are surrounded solely by a fold of amnion, thereby exposing the vessels to an increased risk of compression by the presenting part or tearing when the membranes are ruptured. Fetal outcomes include: asymmetric head shape; fetal distress and/or fetal demise; and intrauterine growth restriction (IUGR).

    c. Cord accidents (eg, cord rupture, hematoma, tight nuchal or body cord, knotted cord, prolapse) interfere with placental blood flow to and from the fetus, with resultant fetal hypoperfusion, hypoxia, distress, and/or demise.

E. Diabetes mellitus (DM) (pregestational and gestational) (Chang & Winkle, 1999; de Veciana & Mason, 2000; Kalb, 2000; Martin, 2000):

  1. Definition: DM is an autoimmune disease characterized by hyperglycemia secondary to decreased pancreatic insulin production, decreased insulin release in response to a carbohydrate load, or impaired cellular response to insulin. Diabetes in pregnancy can be classified according to White's Classification or the American Diabetes Association Classification (Table 3.2).

  2. Pregestational (overt) DM: presents before conception and is traditionally classified as type 1 (insulin-dependent) or type 2 (non–insulin-dependent).

    a. Treatment: insulin is used to control overt DM during pregnancy because oral antihyperglycemic agents may be teratogenic to the fetus, especially during organogenesis.

    b. Insulin-dependent patients should be euglycemic at conception and throughout their first trimesters to decrease infant morbidity and mortality. Women with known or suspected overt DM should be screened during the first prenatal visit and then at 24 to 28 weeks' gestation if the first screening is negative.

  3. Gestational DM (GDM) is restricted to pregnant women whose onset of diabetes/impaired glucose tolerance occurs during pregnancy, usually in the third trimester. Treatment includes diet control or insulin.

TABLE 3.2. Diabetes Mellitus (DM) Classification Systems

White's Classification	American Diabetes Association Classification
A$_1$—GDM without insulin A$_2$—GDM requiring insulin B—onset ≥ 20 yr old; duration < 10 yr C—onset 10–19 yr old; duration 10–19 yr (no vascular disease) D—onset < 10 yr old; duration ≥ 20 yr or any onset/duration with retinopathy or hypertensive retinopathy F—nephropathy H—arteriosclerotic heart disease R—proliferative retinopathy or vitreous hemorrhage T—history of renal transplant	Type 1—characterized by β-cell destruction and insulin deficiency (IDDM or juvenile onset DM) Type 2—broad range resulting from insulin resistance and insulin deficiency to insulin secretory defect and insulin resistance (non-insulin dependent DM or adult onset DM) Other types—genetic defects of β-cells, pancreatic diseases, defects in insulin function GDM—alteration in glucose tolerance with onset during pregnancy

GDM = gestational diabetes mellitus; IDDM = insulin-dependent diabetes mellitus.

4. Glucose screening:
   a. Some practitioners universally screen all women early in pregnancy for DM because 50% of all cases of GDM are missed when screening is based on risk factors alone.
   b. Selective screening is recommended at 24 to 28 weeks' gestation with the following risk factors: > 25 years old; family history of diabetes; previous macrosomic, malformed, or stillborn infant; maternal HTN; and glycosuria.
   c. Maintaining normal serum glucose levels through diet or insulin decreases the risk of intrauterine death and neonatal morbidity. Adequate glucose control during pregnancy is generally accepted as the following: fasting serum glucose (60 to 90 mg/dL); two-hour postprandial glucose (< 120 mg/dL).
   d. Glucose screening procedure: give a 500-g glucose load and draw serum glucose after 1 hour. If the serum glucose is > 140 mg/dL, then a 3-hour glucose tolerance test is recommended.
   e. Three-hour glucose tolerance test procedure: obtain fasting serum glucose. If fasting serum glucose is ≥ 95 mg/dL then administer a 100-g glucose load and draw serum glucose levels after 1, 2, and 3 hours. Normal values: 1 hour (≤ 180 mg/dL); 2 hours (≤ 155 mg/dL); 3 hours (≤ 140 mg/dL).
5. Evaluation tools to determine fetal status and potential fetal outcomes:
   a. Fetal ultrasounds: early ultrasound for dates; ultrasound at 18 to 20 weeks to evaluate growth and fetal anatomy (especially

head and spine); echocardiogram at 20 to 23 weeks to evaluate congenital cardiac disease; repeat ultrasound at 28 to 32 weeks to reassess fetal growth and amniotic fluid index (AFI).

   b. Triple screen or maternal serum α-fetoprotein (MSAFP) at 15 to 20 weeks to evaluate fetus for chromosomal, neural tube, and abdominal wall defects. Amniocentesis is recommended if the triple screen or MSAFP are abnormal.

   c. Nonstress tests initiated between 28 and 34 weeks' gestation, depending upon the severity of maternal diabetes

   d. Biophysical profile during the third trimester to assess fetal well-being

   6. Fetal outcomes include: cardiac (septal hypertrophy); central nervous system (CNS) defects (neural tube, vertebral and skeletal anomalies, caudal regression); hypoglycemia and hypocalcemia; IUGR; macrosomia; meconium plug syndrome; polycythemia and hyperbilirubinemia; renal vein thrombosis; and respiratory distress.

F. Dystocia is defined as difficult labor secondary to maternal, fetal, and/or uterine/cervical causes. These problems include cephalopelvic disproportion; abnormal fetal size, anomaly, or presentation; vaginal scarring/atresia; cervical carcinoma; and uterine malformation, position, or masses.

G. Fetal anomalies: fetal anomalies diagnosed prenatally will affect the course of the pregnancy. Depending upon the certainty of diagnosis and fetal prognosis, the health care provider is obligated to offer alternatives regarding management of the pregnancy. These alternatives include aggressive management (eg, cesarean section for fetal distress or maternal complications and neonatal resuscitation); nonaggressive management (eg, no fetal monitoring or cesarean section for fetal distress); and termination of the pregnancy.

H. Hemoglobinopathies (Beers & Berkow, 1999; Cunningham et al., 1997): a group of diseases affecting erythrocytes due to the presence of one or more abnormally formed hemoglobin molecules

   1. Sickle cell disease (predominant in southeast Asian and African American populations) occurs as a result of a single amino acid substitution (valine for glutamate) in position 6 of the β chain.

   a. Maternal complications become more intense during pregnancy, with worsening anemia, vasoocclusive episodes with severe pain, increase in infections, pulmonary compromise, and PIH.

   b. Neonatal outcomes include spontaneous abortion, stillbirth, and IUGR. Neonates who inherit the trait are asymptomatic until later in infancy when HbF is replaced with HbA and HbS (Wong et al., 1999).

   2. Thalassemias are inherited RBC disorders characterized by impaired production of one or more of the peptide chains that are normal components of globin.

   a. α-Thalassemia (patients of Asian origin) is the result of reduced synthesis of the α chains of hemoglobin. α-Thalassemia is not associated with maternal morbidity. Infants with heterozygous α-thalassemia are usually healthy but develop hemolytic anemia in early infancy; infants with homozygous α-thalassemia usually die in utero or in the neonatal period.

b. β-Thalassemia (patients of Mediterranean, Italian, and Greek origin) is the result of reduced synthesis of the β chains of hemoglobin. Adults with β-thalassemia minor experience mild to moderate anemia, whereas those with β-thalassemia major are severely anemic and may not live beyond puberty. Infants with heterozygous β-thalassemia are asymptomatic, whereas those with homozygous β-thalassemia become severely anemic in the newborn period and fail to thrive.

3. Tay-Sachs (eastern European Jewish origin; French-Canadian and Cajun descent) is an inherited autosomal recessive lysosomal storage disorder. Most infants die by 2 to 5 years of age.

I. HTN (chronic and PIH):

1. Chronic (preexisting) renal disease occurs before 20 weeks' gestation. Maternal renal disease may be secondary to urinary tract infections (UTIs), glomerular disease, or systemic diseases (eg, diabetes, systemic lupus erythematosus [SLE]) (Bartram, Joffe, & Perry, 1998).

    a. Pregnancy outcomes depend upon presence of prepregnancy maternal HTN and renal insufficiency. Chronic HTN (sustained blood pressure [BP] > 140 mmHg systolic or > 90 mmHg diastolic) may lead to superimposed PIH.

    b. Neonatal outcomes include: IUGR secondary to uteroplacental insufficiency; prematurity; and fetal demise.

2. PIH: onset of symptoms occurs after 20 weeks' gestation. PIH is most often seen in the young and elderly primigravida.

    a. Maternal risk factors for PIH include (Chan & Winkle, 1999): antiphospholipid antibodies; chronic HTN and renal disease; DM; first pregnancy; multiple gestation; and SLE.

    b. Maternal outcomes include (Cloherty, 1998): CNS complications (eg, stroke, seizures, and blindness); hepatic failure; disseminated intravascular coagulopathy (DIC); pulmonary edema; and placental abruption.

3. Three subsets of PIH include (Bartram et al., 1998):

    a. Preeclampsia is PIH with renal involvement caused by maternal vasoconstriction, increased vascular resistance, and increased blood pressure. It is characterized by the classic triad of **HTN, proteinuria, and edema.** Resolution of preeclampsia is usually swift and complete after delivery.

    b. Eclampsia is PIH with CNS involvement leading to seizures. Maternal clinical manifestations result from hypoperfusion of the following: kidneys (HTN and proteinuria); liver (hepatic disorders and coagulopathies); brain (seizures); and uterus (uteroplacental insufficiency, placental vascular abnormalities, and placental abruption).

    c. HELLP syndrome is a severe form of PIH. The classic HELLP triad is maternal **h**emolytic anemia, **e**levated **l**iver enzymes, and **l**ow **p**latelet count. HELLP symptoms (maternal jaundice;

elevated blood urea nitrogen [BUN] and creatinine levels; right upper quadrant abdominal pain; and subcapsular liver hematoma) may appear before the HTN and proteinuria observed with preeclampsia.

   d. Neonatal outcomes are consistent for preeclampsia, eclampsia, and HELLP: hypotonia and respiratory depression secondary to maternal magnesium administration; hypoxemia and acidosis; IUGR; perinatal asphyxia and death; prematurity; and thrombocytopenia and neutropenia.

J. IUGR (symmetric and asymmetric) (Burlbow, 1996; Desai, 1999; Wheeler, 1997):

   1. Symmetric IUGR affects all organ systems equally, and growth restriction begins during the first trimester. The head circumference/abdominal circumference (HC/AC) ratio is normal. Etiology of symmetric IUGR includes: congenital abnormalities; congenital infection (eg, TORCH); genetic factors, such as parental physical constitution; and maternal conditions (see "Maternal risk factors" that follows).

   2. Asymmetric IUGR (or "head sparing" IUGR) reportedly occurs in late second and early third trimester. Blood is selectively shunted to the brain and other vital organs, with a resultant increased HC/AC ratio. Etiology of asymmetric IUGR includes: abnormal placental or uterine formation; discordant twins; maternal vascular disorders (HTN, DM, and PIH); and multiple gestation.

   3. Diagnosis: fetal growth restriction is diagnosed by plotting fetal measurements obtained from serial ultrasounds that are performed at 2- to 3-week intervals. IUGR is present when measurements fall *below the 10th percentile*.

   4. Maternal risk factors (Scoggin & Morgan, 1998; Sohl & Moore, 1998): alcohol, drug, and tobacco use/abuse; genetic (syndromes) and constitutional (small parental stature); infection (eg, rubella, cytomegalovirus [CMV], toxoplasmosis, syphilis, and malaria); malnutrition; high altitude environment; maternal conditions (eg, pulmonary, renal, or cardiac disease, and anemia); placental dysfunction; and uterine malformation

   5. Fetal outcomes (Gomella, Cunningham, Eyal, & Zenk, 1999): asphyxia, meconium aspiration, and persistent pulmonary hypertension; congenital malformation; hypoglycemia and hypocalcemia; increased risk of stillbirth; polycythemia; and temperature instability and decreased brown fat deposition

K. Multiple gestation pregnancy (Cunningham et al., 1993; Gilbert, 1998; Gomella et al., 1999; Scoggin & Morgan, 1998):

   1. Twins are the most common multiple gestation (4:1,000 pregnancies for monozygotic twins and 7:1,000 to 11:1,000 pregnancies for dizygotic twins). The frequency of naturally occurring higher multiple births is less than twinning, although multiple gestations secondary to ovulation induction and in vitro fertilization have increased during the past 2 decades.

   2. Types of twinning:

    a. Monozygotic twins derive from one ovum (identical). They are always the same gender: diamnionic, dichorionic (division within 72 hours of fertilization produces two embryos, two amnions, two chorions, and two placentas or one fused placenta); diamnionic, monochorionic (division between the fourth and eighth day produces two embryos, two amnions, one chorion, and one placenta); monoamnionic, monochorionic (division at 8 days after fertilization produces two embryos, one amnion, one chorion, and one placenta; these infants are at great risk for cord entanglement and accidents); and division later than 8 days after fertilization, when the embryonic disc has already formed, will result in incomplete cleavage and the formation of conjoined twins.

    b. Dizygotic twins are derived from two ova (fraternal). They may be the same or different genders. There are two amnions and two chorions and there is a thick dividing membrane between the chorions. They have two placentas or a single fused placenta.

  3. Potential maternal problems with multiple gestation pregnancies include: iron-deficiency anemia; polyhydramnios; placenta previa, abruption, postpartum hemorrhage; PIH; preterm labor, premature rupture of membranes (PROM); cord accidents; fetofetal transfusions; increased chance for congenital malformation; and fetal malpresentation.

L. Oligohydramnios and polyhydramnios (Kellogg, 1998; Wheeler, 1997):

  1. Oligohydramnios is defined as an AFI < 8 cm at term.

    a. Etiology of oligohydramnios includes: prolonged or chronic leaking of amniotic fluid and congenital anomalies (eg, renal agenesis, urinary outlet obstruction).

    b. Fetal outcomes include: pulmonary hypoplasia, contractures, and Potter's sequence.

  2. Polyhydramnios (or hydramnios) is defined as an AFI ≥ 25 cm.

    a. The etiology of polyhydramnios includes: the specific cause is largely unknown but is associated with fetal anomalies (eg, CNS defects and gastrointestinal [GI] obstructions); insulin-dependent pregestational and gestational diabetes; multiple gestation; and Rh isoimmunization.

    b. Complications include preterm labor, fetal malpresentation, and cord prolapse.

M. Rupture of membranes (ROM) and chorioamnionitis (Chan & Winkle, 1999; Moran, 1993; Scoggin & Morgan, 1998):

  1. PROM is the rupture of membranes before the onset of labor.

    a. Risk factors associated with PROM include: maternal infection (chorioamnionitis and UTIs); fetal malpresentation; previous cervical damage; previous history of PROM; maternal weight (pregravid obesity or low weight gain during pregnancy); smoking; AMA.

    b. Fetal/neonatal outcomes associated with PROM include: fetal compression syndrome, malpresentation, and neonatal sepsis.

2. Preterm PROM (pPROM) is the leaking of amniotic fluid before the 37th week of gestation. Prolonged rupture of membranes is often defined as rupture > 18 to 24 hours before delivery.
3. Chorioamnionitis is the inflammation of the chorion and amnion often associated with premature and/or prolonged rupture of membranes before labor, prenatal infection, and/or poor prenatal care.
    a. Common pathogens for chorioamnionitis include: chlamydia; *Escherichia coli*; group A and B streptococcus; *Haemophilus influenza*; and *Neisseria gonorrhoeae*.
    b. Clinical maternal manifestations of chorioamnionitis include: maternal fever/chills; uterine tenderness and pain; foul-smelling vaginal discharge; and uterine contractions.
    c. Fetal manifestations include: fetal tachycardia, fetal monitoring consistent with hypoxia, and neonatal sepsis.
    d. Interventions for chorioamnionitis include: appropriate maternal parenteral antimicrobial therapy and delivery of infant.
N. Preterm labor (PTL): the presence of regular uterine contractions with cervical dilation and effacement before 37 weeks' gestation (Chan & Winkle, 1999)
    1. Maternal factors contributing to PTL include: cervical incompetence and uterine deformities; fetal anomaly and fetal malpresentation; maternal infection (eg, chorioamnionitis and UTI); multiple gestation; polyhydramnios; PROM; and smoking, cocaine use, and poor prenatal care.
    2. Management for PTL includes: bed rest and hydration; pharmacologic intervention with tocolytic agents (eg, magnesium sulfate, terbutaline, and indomethacin) to suppress uterine contractions, implemented when PTL occurs before 34 weeks' gestation; and other adjunctive therapy (eg, corticosteroids and antibiotic prophylaxis for group B streptococcus).
    3. Neonatal outcome depends upon the gestational age and reason for the premature labor.
O. Postdates: a pregnancy whose duration is longer than 42 weeks (Scoggin & Morgan, 1998). Fetal outcomes include: anoxia secondary to uteroplacental insufficiency; dystocia as a result of macrosomia; fetal dysmaturity (eg, decreased subcutaneous fat, decreased weight:length ratio, little or no vernix, and peeling skin, long fingernails, and abundant hair growth) resulting from placental insufficiency; hypoglycemia; and meconium aspiration.
P. Substance use and abuse: perinatal drug use includes not only illegal drug use but also abusive use of prescription medications, tobacco, alcohol, and over-the-counter (OTC) drugs. Illegal, addicting, and recreational drug use and abuse is widespread but the exact extent is unknown. It crosses all socioeconomic, racial, and ethnic barriers, and most drug abuse includes more than one drug (Ladewig et al., 1998; Wheeler, 1997).
    1. Screening: drugs or chemicals can be detected in blood, urine, saliva, amniotic fluid, hair, and meconium. Careful documenta-

tion of legitimate prescription (eg, Demerol) and OTC medications (eg, cold medications containing ephedrine) taken by the mother should be done so that positive toxicology results are not misinterpreted.

2. Maternal and fetal outcomes depend upon the drug classifications.

   a. Alcohol increases the risk of fetal neurologic damage, lower birth weight, fetal alcohol syndrome, and spontaneous abortions. The amount of intrauterine alcohol exposure required to produce fetal neurological deficits has not been established. However, increased exposure is associated with more serious deficits.

   b. Tobacco use decreases uteroplacental perfusion, with resultant decreased fetal oxygenation. Smoking more than one-half pack a day increases the risk of experiencing preterm labor. Neonatal outcomes include lower birth weights and an increased risk of sudden infant death syndrome (SIDS).

   c. Cocaine causes maternal euphoria, energy, heightened sexual desire followed by anxiety, exhaustion, and depression. Fetal complications include spontaneous abortion, preterm labor and delivery, IUGR, abruption, and long-term behavioral problems.

   d. Heroin is addictive and associated with increased risk for preterm labor and delivery, IUGR, and neonatal abstinence syndrome.

   e. Fetal effects of marijuana, lysergic acid diethylamide (LSD), and amphetamines are undetermined.

Q. SLE: an autoimmune vascular collagen disease with mild to severe manifestations affecting connective tissue in multiple organ systems (Bartram et al., 1998; Gillerman, 1993)

   1. Maternal complications include:

      a. Multisystem symptoms: anemia, thrombocytopenia, and leukopenia; anorexia, vomiting, and weight loss; butterfly rash; carditis; CNS disturbances, fatigue, and fever; hepatitis and elevated liver enzymes; HTN and renal dysfunction; joint pain; positive ANA (antinuclear antibody) and decreased complement levels, positive anticardiolipin antibody, positive rheumatoid factor, and positive direct Coombs; and pulmonary effusions and associated pleural pain

      b. Increased risk for spontaneous abortions, stillbirth, and preterm labor

   2. Neonatal outcomes include: congenital heart block; IUGR and prematurity; transient lupus-like rash; and transient thrombocytopenia, leukopenia, and hemolytic anemia.

R. Thrombocytopenia (Cunningham et al., 1997; Heaman, 2000; Johnson & VanDorsten, 2000): platelet count < 150,000/μL

   1. Etiology: occurs as a result of either increased platelet destruction (eg, idiopathic thrombocytopenia purpura [ITP]), peripheral consumption of platelets (eg, DIC), or decreased platelet production.

2. Factors contributing to thrombocytopenia include: PIH; SLE; ITP (an autoimmune process whereby the mother produces antiplatelet antibodies that destroy her own platelets); obstetric bleeding requiring blood transfusions; consumptive coagulopathies; viral infections and septicemia; and anemias (eg, acquired hemolytic, megaloblastic, and aplastic).

3. Clinical manifestations include: petechiae; oozing from puncture sites; hematuria; hemoptysis; GI hemorrhage; and cerebral hemorrhage.

4. Interventions include: corticosteroids (1 mg/kg/d), which may improve platelet counts; IV immunoglobulin; and splenectomy for patients unresponsive to steroid therapy.

5. Neonatal effects include: transplacental acquisition of maternal platelet associated IgG antibodies with resultant thrombocytopenia (monitor infant's platelet count); and intracranial hemorrhage.

S. Thyroid disease (Kalb, 2000):

1. Hyperthyroidism: maternal hyperthyroidism (Grave's disease) occurs in approximately 1:500 to 1:1,000 pregnancies.

   a. Clinical manifestations of hyperthyroidism closely resemble characteristics of pregnancy (eg, increased metabolic rate, increased protein-bound iodine values, and increased iodine uptake), thereby making diagnosis difficult.

   b. Maternal treatment includes: surgery and antithyroid medications (eg, propylthiouracil [PTU] or methimazole).

   c. Maternal and fetal effects include: increased risk of spontaneous abortion and intrauterine fetal demise (IUFD) in untreated maternal hyperthyroidism; preterm labor and delivery; IUGR; and neonatal hypothyroidism secondary to maternal antithyroid medication administration. (Refer to Chapter 17 for more in-depth information regarding neonatal thyroid disease.)

2. Hypothyroidism: maternal hypothyroidism classifies as either primary or secondary hypothyroidism.

   a. Etiology of primary hypothyroidism includes: Hashimoto's thyroiditis; iodine deficiency; thyroid gland destruction secondary to radiation or surgery; and complications of antithyroid medications.

   b. Secondary hypothyroidism arises from pituitary-hypothalamic disease.

   c. Maternal clinical manifestations include: irregular menses and ovulation that often result in fertility problems; fatigue and lethargy; cold intolerance; headache; constipation; and paresthesias.

   d. Outcomes include: good maternal and fetal outcomes are expected with appropriate hormonal replacement (Levothyroxin); and increased risk of fetal morbidity/mortality with inadequate thyroid hormone replacement therapy during pregnancy.

▼ References

Austin, D. A., & Sheridan, M. E. (2000). Labor and delivery at risk. In S. Mattson & J. E. Smith (Eds.), *Core curriculum for maternal-newborn nursing* (2nd ed., pp. 607–635). Philadelphia: WB Saunders.

Bartram, J., Joffe, G. M., & Perry, L. (1998). Prenatal environment: effect on neonatal outcome. In G. B. Merenstein & S. L. Gardner (Eds.), *Handbook of neonatal intensive care* (4th ed., pp. 9–29). St. Louis: Mosby.

Beers, M. H., & Berkow, R. (Eds.). (1999). *The Merck manual of diagnosis and therapy* (17th ed.). Whitehouse Station, NJ: Merck Research Laboratories.

Burlbow, J. (1996). Intrauterine growth restriction. *OB-GYN Ultrasound Today*, 3(1), 30–32.

Carcio, H. A. (1999). *Advanced health assessment of women: Clinical skills & procedures*. Philadelphia: Lippincott.

Carty, E. M. (1989). Ruptured uterus. In E. R. Knor (Ed.), *Decision making in obstetrical nursing* (pp. 136–137). Toronto: BC Decker, Inc.

Chan, P. D., & Winkle, C. R. (1999). *Gynecology and obstetrics 1999-2000 edition*. Laguna Hills, CA: Current Clinical Strategies Publishing.

Cloherty, J. P. (1998). Maternal conditions that affect the fetus. In J. P. Cloherty & A. R. Stark (Eds.), *Manual of neonatal care* (4th ed., pp. 11–29). Philadelphia: Lippincott-Raven.

Cunningham, F. G., MacDonald, P. C., Gant, N. F., Leveno, K. J., Gilstrap, L. C., Hankins, G. D. V., & Clark, S. L. (Eds.). (1997). *Williams obstetrics* (20th ed.). Norwalk, CT: Appleton & Lange.

Deitch, K.V. (2000). Age-related concerns. In S. Mattson & J. E. Smith (Eds.), *Core curriculum for maternal-newborn nursing* (2nd ed., pp. 116–125). Philadelphia: WB Saunders.

Desai, M. S. (1999). Intrauterine growth retardation. In T. L. Gomella, M D. Cunningham, F. G. Eyal, & K. E. Zenk (Eds.), *Neonatology: Management, procedures, on-call problems, diseases, and drugs* (4th ed., pp. 441–446). Stamford, CT: Appleton & Lange.

de Veciana, M., & Mason, M. E. (2000). Endocrine disorders. In A. T. Evans & K. R. Niswander (Eds.), *Manual of obstetrics* (6th ed., pp. 127–147). Philadelphia: Lippincott Williams & Wilkins.

Gilbert, W. M. (1998). Placental function and diseases: the placenta, fetal membranes, and umbilical cord. In H. W. Taeusch & R. A. Ballard (Eds.), *Avery's diseases of the newborn* (7th ed., pp. 57–64). Philadelphia: WB Saunders.

Gillerman, H. (1993). Other medical complications. In S. Mattson, & J. E. Smith (Eds.), *Core curriculum for maternal-newborn nursing* (pp. 565–612). Philadelphia: WB Saunders.

Glass, S. M. (2000). Hematologic disorders. In J. Deacon & P. O'Neill (Eds.), *Core curriculum for neonatal intensive care nursing* (2nd ed., pp. 383–412). Philadelphia: WB Saunders.

Gomella, T. L, Cunningham, M. D., Eyal, F. G., & Zenk, K. E. (Eds.). (1999). *Neonatology: Management, procedures, on-call problems, diseases, drugs* (4th ed.). Stamford, CT: Appleton & Lange.

Heaman, M. (2000). Other medical complications. In S. Mattson & J. E. Smith (Eds.), *Core curriculum for maternal-newborn nursing* (pp. 564–606). Philadelphia: WB Saunders.

Jasper, M. L. (2000). Antepartum fetal assessment. In S. Mattson & J. E. Smith (Eds.), *Core curriculum for maternal-newborn nursing* (2nd ed., pp. 127–160). Philadelphia: WB Saunders.

Johnson, D. D., & VanDorsten, P. (2000). Immunologic disorders complicating pregnancy. In A. T. Evans & K. R. Niswander (Eds.), *Manual of obstetrics* (6th ed., pp. 229–234). Philadelphia: Lippincott Williams & Wilkins.

Kalb, K. A. (2000). Endocrine and metabolic disorders. In S. Mattson & J. E. Smith (Eds.), *Core curriculum for maternal-newborn nursing* (2nd ed., pp. 473–508). Philadelphia: WB Saunders.

Kellogg, B. (1998). Placental development and functioning. In S. Mattson & J. E. Smith (Eds.), *Core curriculum for maternal-newborn nursing* (2nd ed., pp. 55–67). Philadelphia: WB Saunders.

Ladewig, P. W., London, M. L., & Olds, S. B. (1998). *Maternal-newborn nursing care: The nurse, the family, and the community* (4th ed.). Menlo Park, CA: Addison-Wesley.

Martin, R. W. (2000). Diabetes associated with pregnancy. In M. E. Rivlin & R. W. Martin (Eds.), *Manual of clinical problems in obstetrics and gynecology* (5th ed., pp. 74–76). Philadelphia: Lippincott Williams & Wilkins.

Mentzer, W. C., & Glader, B. E. (1998). Erythrocyte disorders in infancy. In H. W. Taeusch & R. A. Ballard (Eds.), *Avery's diseases of the newborn* (7th ed., pp. 1080–1111). Philadelphia: WB Saunders.

Moran, B. (1993). Maternal infections. In S. Mattson & J. E. Smith (Eds.), *Core curriculum for maternal-newborn nursing* (pp. 435–464). Philadelphia: WB Saunders.

Perry, K. G. (2000). Rh Isoimmunization. In M. E. Rivlin & R. W. Martin (Eds.), *Manual of clinical problems in obstetrics and gynecology* (5th ed., pp. 101–104). Philadelphia: Lippincott Williams & Wilkins.

Reed, G. B., Claireaux, A. E., & Cockburn, F. (Eds.). (1995). *Diseases of the fetus and newborn* (2nd ed.). London: Chapman & Hall Medical.

Scoggin, J., & Morgan, G. (1998). *Practice guidelines for obstetrics & gynecology.* Philadelphia: Lippincott.

Sohl, B., & Moore, T. R. (1998). Abnormalities of fetal growth. In H. W. Taeusch & R. A. Ballard (Eds.), *Avery's diseases of the newborn* (7th ed., pp. 90–101). Philadelphia: WB Saunders.

Wheeler, L. (1997). *Nurse-midwifery: A practical guide to prenatal & postpartum care.* Philadelphia: Lippincott.

Whitehurst, R. R. (1999). Blood abnormalities. In T. L. Gomella, M D. Cunningham, F. G. Eyal, & K. E. Zenk (Eds.), *Neonatology: Management, procedures, on-call problems, diseases, and drugs* (4th ed., pp. 314–334). Stamford, CT: Appleton & Lange.

Wong, D. L., Hockenberry-Eaton, M., Winkelstein, M. L., Wilson, D., Ahmann, E., & DiVito-Thomas, P. A. (Eds.). (1999). *Whaley & Wong's nursing care of infants and children* (6th ed.). St. Louis: Mosby.

PART II

DELIVERY ROOM MANAGEMENT

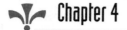 Chapter 4

Delivery Room Environment
Paulette S. Haws, MSN, RNC, NNP

I. Personnel
If at all possible, *before delivery*, introduce yourself to the mother, father, family, and significant others and explain to them who will be in attendance, why your presence at the delivery has been requested, and which interventions might be needed.

At each delivery there should be at least one person solely dedicated to the care of the infant and who is capable of initiating resuscitation. For a low-risk delivery, additional personnel skilled at performing cardiopulmonary resuscitation (CPR), intubation, peripheral or umbilical line insertion, and medication administration should be immediately available. For a high-risk delivery, a minimum of two people should be in attendance, solely dedicated to the care of the infant and capable of performing the techniques required for an infant resuscitation.

II. Equipment (*SOAPTIM*—a useful acronym borrowed from anesthesia):
A. **S** (suction): bulb syringe; wall suction set at 100 mmHg; meconium aspirator; suction catheters (5 FR or 6 FR, 8 FR, 10 FR, or 12 FR); and 8-FR feeding tube and 10 or 20 mL syringes

B. **O** (oxygen): ambu bag (flow-inflating bag or self-inflating bag with reservoir) attached to a 100% oxygen source; face masks (newborn and premature sizes); and oxygen tubing attached to a 100% oxygen source

C. **A** (airway): laryngoscope handle and blades (sizes 00, 0, and 1); extra bulbs and batteries; endotracheal tubes (2.0, 2.5, 3.0, 3.5, and 4.0 mm ID); stylets; oral airways (newborn and premature sizes); and tape

D. **P** (pharmacy [emergency medications]): epinephrine (1:10,000 solution); sodium bicarbonate 4.2% (0.5 mEq/mL); intravenous (IV) fluids (normal saline, Ringer's lactate, and Dextrose 10%); O-negative whole blood cross-matched with the mother's blood; and Narcan (0.4 mg/mL or 1 mg/mL solution)

E. **T** (table): warmer bed (prewarmed before delivery); and towels and blankets

F. **I** (IV catheters): catheters for peripheral IVs (24 gauge); umbilical catheters (3.5 FR and 5 FR) and insertion trays (sterile gloves, scalpel, umbilical tape, povidone-iodine solution, stopcocks, and suture material); butterfly catheters (23 and 25 gauge), three-way stopcocks, and various size syringes for emergency use during a thoracentesis and/or paracentesis

G. **M** (monitor and miscellaneous items): stethoscope; clock or watch with a second hand; cardiorespiratory monitor; pulse oximeter; gloves; cord clamp; and scissors

III. **Thermoregulation**
  A. Hypothermia:
    1. **Keep the baby warm.** Ideally, the newborn care area temperature should be kept between **75°F and 79°F** (23.8°C to 26.1°C) and humidity between 30% and 60% (Hauth & Merenstein, 1997). **Use warm blankets to dry the baby.**
    2. Neonates should be kept in a **neutral thermal environment** (ie, an environmental temperature at which a newborn infant's metabolic rate and oxygen consumption are kept at a minimum while maintaining a normal body temperature).
    3. Premature infants lose heat more easily than term infants secondary to:
       a. *Decreased brown fat storage* with decreased glycogen stores
       b. *Decreased tone*; therefore, unable to curl up and decrease the amount of skin exposed to a cooler environment
       c. *Increased head:body ratio*; therefore, allowing greater heat loss than term infants
    4. Hypothermia leads to a vicious cycle of . . . Acidosis → Hypoxia → Pulmonary hypertension → Acidosis . . .
    5. Complications of hypothermia (Eyal, 1999):
       a. Metabolic acidosis due to anaerobic metabolism for heat production (when glycogen stores are depleted and O_2 consumption increases), with resultant lactic acid production
       b. Pulmonary hypertension (HTN) secondary to pulmonary vasoconstriction, hypoxia, and acidosis
       c. Hypoglycemia secondary to depleted glycogen stores
       d. Clotting disorders (eg, disseminated intravascular coagulopathy [DIC], pulmonary hemorrhage); intraventricular hemorrhage
       e. Shock secondary to decreased systemic blood pressure and cardiac output; apnea and bradycardia
    6. Methods of heat loss:
       a. Evaporation (wet infants lose body heat to surrounding dry air)
       b. Conduction (warm infants lose body heat to cold surfaces in which they are in contact, such as cold mattresses and cool blankets)
       c. Convection (infants lose body heat when cool air flows over wet skin)
       d. Radiation (infants lose body heat to colder objects in the room)
    7. Rewarming methods (rapid versus slow) are controversial. Some authorities recommend rewarming at a rate no greater than 1°C/hr for term infants or 0.6°C/hr for infants < 1,200 g, < 28 weeks' gestation, or temperature < 32°C (89.6°F).
  B. Hyperthermia (core temperature > 99.5°F *or* > 37.5°C) (Eyal, 1999):
    1. Etiology: environmental (excessive infant bundling, loose skin temperature probe, high environmental temperature, or inappro-

priate servo-control settings); maternal fever during labor; infection (eg, herpes); dehydration; and opiate withdrawal

2. Clinical manifestations:
   a. Increased metabolic rate and oxygen consumption; tachycardia; tachypnea or periodic breathing and apnea
   b. Expect a "true fever" when there is a cool ambient or incubator temperature and cool extremities secondary to peripheral vasoconstriction.

3. Interventions:
   a. Determine the cause for the elevated temperature.
   b. Adjust the environmental temperature, adjust servocontrol settings, or remove excessive blankets.

▼References

Eyal, F. G. (1999). Temperature regulation. In T. L. Gomella, M. D. Cunningham, F. G. Eyal, & K. E. Zenk (Eds.), *Neonatology: Management, procedures, on-call problems, diseases, drugs* (4th ed., pp. 38–42). Stamford, CT: Appleton & Lange.

Hauth, J. C., & Merenstein, G. B. (Eds.). (1997). *Guidelines for perinatal care* (4th ed.). Elk Grove, IL: American Academy of Pediatrics; and Washington, DC: The American College of Obstetricians and Gynecologists.

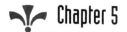 **Chapter 5**

Delivery Room Resuscitation

Paulette S. Haws, MSN, RNC, NNP

In the delivery room, time is of the essence. Evaluating the infant's condition and response to resuscitation and making decisions regarding further interventions is an ongoing process. Therefore, a *low-risk delivery* should be attended by a health care provider who is capable of initiating resuscitation. Additionally, personnel who are capable of performing all aspects of resuscitation should be immediately available. A *high-risk delivery* should be attended by at least two people who, together, are capable of providing complete resuscitation. The Neonatal Resuscitation Program (NRP) provides the algorithms for such resuscitations.

This chapter, whose purpose is to provide a synopsis of the salient points of the current guidelines for NRP (2000 edition), **does not replace** *the NRP textbook or the need to attend an NRP provider course.*

I. Steps in the neonatal resuscitation process

A. *Dry, suction, stimulate* (these procedures are performed simultaneously).
   1. *Dry* the infant and remove the wet towels.
      a. If meconium is present and with any of the following conditions, immediately intubate the trachea and remove secretions by applying suction (100 mmHg) directly to the endotracheal tube (ETT):
         (1) Apnea or poor respiratory effort
         (2) Heart rate (HR) is < 100 beats per minute (bpm).
         (3) Poor muscle tone
      b. Remove wet towels *after* the suction procedure.
   2. *Suction* the mouth first; suction the nose second.
      a. Bulb syringe should be sufficient to remove secretions.
      b. Vigorous suctioning of the oropharynx during the first few minutes of life can cause vagal stimulation with resultant profound bradycardia or apnea.
   3. *Stimulate* infant **only** by flicking feet, drying, or rubbing back; if the infant does not breathe, then begin positive pressure ventilation (PPV).
B. *Respirations, HR, color:*
   1. Evaluate *respirations*:
      a. Establish an airway. Clear the airway of secretions and place infant in "sniffing position."
      b. If apnea and/or gasping respiration **or** (HR) < 100 bpm, begin PPV with 100% O_2
         (1) First few breaths → > 30 cm H_2O pressure.
         (2) Subsequent breaths → 15 to 20 cm H_2O pressure

(3) Premature infants may require higher pressures due to decreased lung compliance and increased chest wall compliance.

c. Respiratory rate during PPV: 40 to 60 bpm
  (1) Breathe . . . two . . . three . . . Breathe . . . two . . . three . . . Breathe . . . two . . . three
  (2) Insert orogastric or nasogastric tube after several minutes of PPV to decompress the stomach.
  (3) If the infant fails to establish a spontaneous and/or effective breathing pattern after several minutes of bag/mask PPV, then endotracheal intubation should be considered.
  (4) Endotracheal tube sizes: see Table 5.1.

2. Evaluate HR:
  a. HR < 100 bpm → PPV with 100% O_2
    (1) Discontinue PPV when HR > 100, breathing, and pink.
    (2) Continue PPV with persistent apnea or ineffective respirations or HR < 100.
  b. HR < 60 after 30 seconds of PPV with 100% O_2 → begin chest compressions.
    (1) Three compressions: one manual breath (90 compressions and 30 breaths per minute).
    (2) One . . . and . . . two . . . and . . . three . . . and . . . breathe . . . and . . . one . . . and . . . two . . .and . . .
    (3) Place the tips of the two middle fingers or the flat part of the thumb on the lower third of the infant's sternum, above the xiphoid process, and compress to a depth of one-third the anteroposterior diameter of the chest. *Improper finger placement may result in fractured rib(s), lacerated liver, and pneumothorax.*
    (4) Discontinue chest compressions when HR > 60 bpm.
    (5) Continue PPV until HR > 100.

3. Observe *color*:
  a. Central cyanosis:
    (1) Regular respirations but cyanotic → provide free-flow 100% O_2 with flow-inflating bag (*self-inflating bags do not provide free-flow O_2*), O_2 tubing, or O_2 mask.
    (2) Persistent central cyanosis with 100% free-flow O_2 → consider a trial of PPV and/or diagnosis of cyanotic congenital heart disease.

4. Resuscitation algorithm: Figure 5.1

 TABLE 5.1. **Endotracheal Tube Sizes**

ETT Size (mm)	Weight (kg)	Gestational Age (wk)	Depth of Insertion (cm)
2.5	< 1	< 28	6–7
3.0	1–2	28–34	7
3.5	2–3	34–38	8
3.5–4.0	> 3	> 38	9

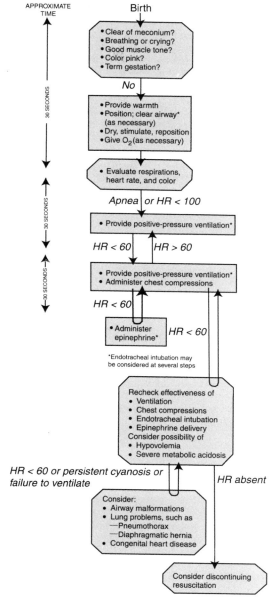

Figure 5-1. Neonatal resuscitation algorithm. Reprinted with permission from Kattwinkel, J. (Ed.). (2000). *Textbook of Neonatal Resuscitation*. (4th ed.). Elk Grove Villiage, IL: American Academy of Pediatrics and American Heart Association.

TABLE 5.2. Resuscitation Medications

Medication	Dosage	Route	Frequency/Comments
Epinephrine 1:10,000	0.1–0.3 mL/kg (0.01–0.03 mg/kg)	Endotracheal (ET) or IV; give rapidly	May repeat every 3 to 5 min
Volume expander: normal saline; Ringer's lactate; Whole blood (O neg cross-matched with mother's blood)	10 mL/kg	IV; give over 5 to 10 min	Repeat if signs of hypovolemia persist: pallor persisting after oxygenation, weak pulses, high or low heart rate, or poor response to resuscitation.
Sodium bicarbonate 4.2% solution (**8.4% solution: always dilute 1:1 with sterile H$_2$O**)	2 mEq/kg	IV; give slowly (1 mEq/kg/min)	Give NaHCO$_3$ if blood gases are available **or** suspected metabolic acidosis with prolonged resuscitation. **Infant must be well ventilated.**
Narcan (0.4 mg/mL) or (1 mg/mL)	0.1 mg/kg	IV, ET, IM, SQ; give rapidly	**Giving Narcan (naloxone) to a mother with an unknown drug history (opiates) may precipitate neonatal seizures.**

Adapted from Kattwinkel, J. (Ed). (2000). *Textbook of neonatal resuscitation* (4th ed.). Elk Grove Village, IL: American Academy of Pediatrics and American Heart Association.

TABLE 5.3. **APGAR Scores***

	0	1	2
Appearance (color)	Pale or cyanotic	Pink body with blue extremities	Completely pink
Pulse	Heart rate (HR) is absent	HR < 100	HR > 100
Grimace (reflex irritability)	No response	Facial grimace	Cough or gag
Activity (tone)	Limp	Slight flexion	Flexed position or active
Respirations	Absent	Slow, irregular	Crying, good air entry

*Scoring system developed by Dr. Virginia Apgar in 1953.

II. Resuscitation medications and response to resuscitation

A. Delivery room resuscitation medications (Kattwinkel, 2000): Table 5.2

B. NRP textbook (4th ed.) guidelines have offered the following recommendations for noninitiation and discontinuation of resuscitation:

    1. Noninitiation of resuscitation:

        a. Known lethal congenital defects (eg, anencephaly, trisomies 13 and 18)

        b. Birth weight < 400 g

        c. < 23 weeks' gestation

    2. Discontinuation of resuscitation efforts: no HR after 15 minutes in spite of the administration of proper resuscitation efforts

C. APGAR scores (Gomella, Cunningham, Eyal, & Zenk, 1999): APGAR scores are used solely for the purpose of describing how well an infant responded to resuscitation efforts, not to determine the need for resuscitation (Table 5.3).

▼ References

Gomella, T. L., Cunningham, M. D., Eyal, F. G., & Zenk, K. E. (Eds.). (1999). *Neonatology: Management, procedures, on-call problems, diseases, drugs* (4th ed.). Stamford, CT: Appleton & Lange.

Kattwinkel, J. (Ed). (2000). *Textbook of neonatal resuscitation* (4th ed.). Elk Grove Village, IL: American Academy of Pediatrics and American Heart Association.

PART III

NEONATAL MANAGEMENT

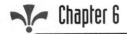

Chapter 6

Admission and Discharge

Paulette S. Haws, MSN, RNC, NNP

I. Admission: initial steps (listed alphabetically and not necessarily in order of performance) undertaken during admission to a special care nursery
  A. Admission note
  B. Admission orders include:
  1. Date and time
  2. Gestational age and birth weight
  3. Diagnoses
  4. Monitoring (eg, cardiorespiratory monitor, pulse oximetry)
  5. Intravenous (IV) fluids: peripheral or central access; solution; and rate
  6. Nutrition: nothing by mouth (NPO) or enteral feedings (formula, amount, frequency, and method)
  7. Respiratory support: oxyhood (O_2 concentration); nasal cannula (O_2 concentration and liter flow); nasal CPAP; or mechanical ventilation (eg, O_2 concentration, respiratory rate, inspiratory and peek expiratory pressures, and inspiratory time)
  8. Medications (eg, antimicrobials, hepatitis B prophylaxis, surfactant, vasopressors, sedation, and analgesia)
  9. Laboratory tests (eg, blood for hematologic and chemistry studies; blood, urine, cerebrospinal fluid [CSF], and body fluids for bacterial and viral cultures)
  10. Imaging studies (eg, x-rays, ultrasounds, computed tomography [CT] scan, magnetic resonance imaging [MRI], echocardiogram, and electroencephalograph [EEG])
  11. Consultations (eg, genetics, cardiology, ophthalmology, neurology, and social services)
  12. Other (eg, blood glucose testing such as Accu-chek®, daily weights, and strict intake and output recording)
  C. Appropriate stabilizing interventions (**STABLE®**—http://www. Stableprogram.com): S (sugar), T (temperature), A (assisted breathing), B (blood pressure), L (laboratory work), and E (emotional support)
  D. Consents must be obtained from the appropriate family member for the following: admission; blood product transfusion; invasive procedures; research protocols; surgery; or transfer to another facility.
  E. Implement a growth chart (provides important data for premature infants during their hospitalization).
  F. Physical examination:
  1. **Before touching the baby:**
     a. Observe overall physical appearance; obvious anomalies; color; work of breathing; and tone, posture, and movement.

      b. Listen (without and with a stethoscope).
  2. Proceed with a systematic head-to-toe assessment:
      a. Head: shape, fontanels, sutures, caput, cephalohematoma, lesions, bruising, hair whorl pattern, and skull deformities
      b. Face: symmetry, shape, frontal bossing, midface hypoplasia/flattening, and abnormal philtrum
      c. Eyes: size, spacing, conjunctiva, drainage, red reflex, and sclera
      d. Ears: shape, position, alignment, tags, and pits
      e. Nose: size, shape, nasal bridge, midline position, and patency of nares
      f. Mouth: clefts, thickness of the lips, color of oral secretion, and lesions
      g. Throat: position of trachea and masses
      h. Chest/respiratory: symmetry, clavicles, nipple spacing, size of breast buds, work of breathing, air entry, and breath sounds
      i. Cardiovascular: rate, rhythm, point of maximum impulse (PMI), murmurs (intensity and location), pulses (brachial and femoral), capillary refill, and color of skin and mucous membranes
      j. Abdomen: shape, cord (number of vessels), size of liver/kidneys/spleen, masses, bowel sounds, musculature, and abdominal wall defects
      k. Genitourinary: genitalia, penile abnormalities, testes, size of labia/clitoris, position and patency of anus, voiding and stooling, lesions
      l. Spine/neurologic: tufts, dimples, lesions, masses, and reflexes (suck, gag, Moro, and grasp)
      m. Musculoskeletal: range of motion, digits, tone, position at rest/crying, masses, and Ortolani & Barlow hip maneuvers
      n. Skin: color, texture, lesions, transparency, and birthmarks
  3. Procedure note (include the following essential elements in the note): name of procedure; purpose; method; specimens collected; complications; and patient tolerance
G. Update family/significant others (offer written materials).

II. Discharge: because discharge planning often begins on the day of admission, the following is a list of those items that may appear on the discharge orders or a discharge summary
A. Age in days; gestational age, or postconceptional age
B. Discharge diagnoses
C. Discharge measurements: weight, length, head circumference (HC), and growth percentiles
D Name of the primary caretaker
E. Feeding (formula, amount, frequency, and method)
F. Medications:
  1. Name, dosage, route, and frequency
  2. Provide prescriptions if necessary. Essential information in a prescription include:
      a. Drug name and concentration
      b. Dispense (amount)
      c. Sig: dose, route, frequency

    d. Signature

    e. Example: vitamin E suspension (50 IU/1 mL)
       Dispense: 1 bottle (100 mL)
       Sig: 1 mL PO BID

G. Monitoring devices (eg, home cardiorespiratory monitor, pulse oximetry)

H. Medical equipment (eg, feeding apparatus, oxygen tanks, ostomy supplies, and tracheostomy supplies)

I. Follow-up appointments:

    1. Pediatrician

    2. Home health nurse

    3. Medical specialists (eg, cardiologist, ophthalmologist, neurologist)

    4. Contact telephone numbers for the caregivers in case there are questions after discharge

    5. Provide a copy of the last chest x-ray for the primary caregiver to give to the pediatrician (eg, may be helpful to have a baseline x-ray for an infant with bronchopulmonary dysplasia).

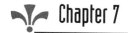 **Chapter 7**

Fluid and Electrolytes

Paulette S. Haws, MSN, RNC, NNP

Maintaining proper fluid and electrolyte balance, especially with the extremely premature infant, is of vital importance to his or her outcome. It is also a mathematical challenge. This chapter succinctly reviews the following: the function of the major electrolytes, deviations from normal serum values, etiologies and clinical manifestations of electrolyte imbalances, treatment modalities, useful mathematical calculations, and the concepts of anion gap, insensible water loss, and daily fluid requirements.

I. Anion gap (AG) (Choukair, 2000; Simmons, 1998)
  A. AG is the number of unaccounted extracellular anions, other than bicarbonate and chloride, needed to balance the positive charge of Na^+. Sodium, bicarbonate, and chloride are the major extracellular ions. A metabolic acidosis is the result of either excess acid or deficient buffering agents:
   1. Acidosis secondary to excess organic acid production increases the AG.
   2. Acidosis secondary to a loss of buffer does not result in an AG.
  B. Calculation: $AG = Na^+ - (Cl^- + CO_2^-)$; Normal value: 12 mEq/L $\pm$ 2 mEq/L
  C. Etiology of AG:
   1. Metabolic acidosis with an increased AG:
    a. Increased acid production: diabetic ketoacidosis; lactic acid; malnutrition; systemic diseases (diabetes mellitus [DM], cirrhosis, pancreatitis); and tissue hypoxia
    b. Inborn errors of metabolism (carbohydrates [CHOs], urea cycles, amino acids, organic acids)
    c. Other: acute and chronic renal failure; decreased acid excretion; nonsteroidal anti-inflammatory drug (NSAID) intoxication; and salicylate intoxication
   2. Metabolic acidosis with normal AG (hyperchloremic acidosis): diarrhea; hyperalimentation; loss of bicarbonate from the kidneys; loss of bicarbonate via gastrointestinal (GI) tract; small bowel or pancreatic drainage; and surgery for necrotizing enterocolitis (NEC)
II. Calcium (Ca^{++})
  A. Function: calcium is essential for the formation of bone and teeth, maintaining cell membrane permeability, enzyme reaction activation for muscle contraction (especially myocardial muscle) and nerve conduction, and coagulation (factor IV); calcium and phosphorus activity are interdependent.
  B. **Hypocalcemia**: total serum calcium (tCa) < 7 mg/dL *or* serum ionized calcium (iCa) < 4.4 mg/dL (1.1 mmol/L)
   1. Etiology (Rubin, 1998; Choukair, 2000):

  a. Early onset (within the first 2 days of life): asphyxia; infant of a diabetic mother; intrauterine growth restriction (IUGR); and prematurity

  b. Late onset (after first week of life): hyperphosphatemia and vitamin D deficiency

  c. Hypoparathyroidism: DiGeorge Syndrome (congenital absence or hypoplasia of the thymus and parathyroid glands); maternal hyperparathyroidism; and parathyroid agenesis

  d. Hypomagnesemia

  e. Renal tubular acidosis

  f. Other: bicarbonate infusion; diuretic drug therapy (furosemide); pancreatitis; and rapid transfusion with citrated blood

 2. Clinical manifestations:

  a. Early onset: apnea; irritability, jitteriness, and profound tetany; prolonged QT interval on electrocardiogram (ECG), arrhythmias; and seizures

  b. Late onset: rickets, bone demineralization, and bone fractures; and elevated alkaline phosphatase

 3. Treatment:

  a. Early onset:

   (1) Administer a parenteral infusion of 10% calcium gluconate for infants of diabetic mothers (IDM) and infants who are perinatally stressed/asphyxiated. Untoward effects include nephrolithiasis, cardiac arrhythmias, skin sloughs, and subcutaneous calcifications secondary to intravenous (IV) infiltrates.

   (2) Acute treatment for tetany/seizures is an **IV bolus of 10% calcium gluconate (1–2 mL/kg during 5–10 minutes)**—observe for bradycardia (Rubin, 1998).

   (3) Alkalotic infants being treated for pulmonary hypertension should have calcium supplementation via parenteral infusion when pH > 7.50.

   (4) Administer 10% calcium gluconate (100 mg/100 mL citrated blood exchanged) during exchange transfusion (Young & Mangum, 2000).

   (5) Serum calcium levels will not improve without normal serum magnesium levels.

  b. Late onset:

   (1) Provide adequate enteral nutrition.

   (2) When administering hyperalimentation use **calcium:phosphate ratios of 1.3:1 to 2:1** to promote adequate calcium and phosphate absorption.

   (3) Substitute thiazide diuretic for furosemide.

   (4) Vitamin D supplementation

C. **Hypercalcemia:** tCa > 11 mg/dL *or* iCa > 5.4 mg/dL (1.36 mmol/L)

 1. Etiology (Rubin, 1998; Silva-Neto, 1999): acute adrenal insufficiency; Fanconi's syndrome (inherited or acquired disorder characterized by proximal renal tubular dysfunction); hypervitaminosis A and D; iatrogenic reasons (eg, excessive calcium or vitamin D supplementation); malignancies; neonatal hyperparathyroid disorders; phosphate depletion; subcutaneous fat necrosis; thiazide diuretic therapy; and thyrotoxicosis

2. Clinical manifestations: abdominal cramping, nausea, vomiting; hypotonia, lethargy, seizures; polyuria, renal calculi; poor feeding and poor weight gain; and shortened QT interval, bradycardia

3. Treatment:
   a. Administer steroids for treatment of malignancies and hypervitaminosis D.
   b. Discontinue thiazide diuretic therapy; furosemide may be given to promote hypercalciuria.
   c. Hydrate infant to increase urine output and calcium excretion.
   d. Reduce calcium intake and discontinue vitamin D supplementation.
   e. Limit sunlight exposure.
   f. **Do not mix calcium gluconate with bicarbonate in the same IV fluids (it will form a precipitate).**

III. Magnesium (Mg^{++})

A. Function: magnesium catalyzes intracellular enzyme reactions (eg, muscle contraction and CHO metabolism) and is essential for parathyroid function and bone:serum calcium balance (Stokowski, 1999).

B. **Hypomagnesemia**: serum magnesium level < 1.52 mEq/L (0.75 mmol/L) (Silva-Neto, 1999)
   1. Etiology (Choukair, 2000; Koo & Tsang, 1999):
      a. Urinary losses secondary to: diuretics; hypercalcemia; and renal tubular acidosis
      b. GI losses secondary to: vomiting and diarrhea; short bowel syndrome; and malabsorption syndromes
      c. Endocrine disorders: DM; parathyroid hormone disorders (eg, maternal hyperparathyroidism); and hyperaldosterone disorders
      d. Other: decreased maternal magnesium levels; drugs (eg, aminoglycosides, loop diuretics); exchange transfusion with citrated blood; and increased phosphate intake
   2. Clinical manifestations (Stokowski, 1999): hypocalcemia that does not respond to calcium replacement therapy; tremors, irritability, and hyperreflexia; and seizures (usually unresponsive to anticonvulsants)
   3. Treatment for hypomagnesemia is the administration of parenteral magnesium sulfate

C. **Hypermagnesemia**: serum magnesium level > 2.3 mEq/L (1.15 mmol/L) (Silva-Neto, 1999)
   1. Etiology (Huttner, 1998): administration of magnesium-containing antacids; prenatal administration of magnesium sulfate for maternal pregnancy-induced hypertension (PIH) or preterm labor (PTL)
   2. Clinical manifestations: poor feeding, delayed GI motility and stooling, abdominal distention; lethargy and hypotonia; and respiratory depression

   3. Treatment:
      a. Delay enteral feedings until tone is improved and infant demonstrates better sucking ability.
      b. Remove exogenous magnesium.
      c. Respiratory support

IV. Phosphorus (P⁻)(Bakewell-Sachs, 1999; Gomella, Cunningham, Eyal, & Zenk, 1999; Tsang, Demarini, & Rath, 1998)

   A. Function: the function of phosphorus, an intracellular anion, includes the production of energy-transfer enzymes (eg, ATP and ADP), cell metabolism, erythrocyte function, and bone mineralization. The activity of phosphorus and calcium are interdependent.
   B. **Hypophosphatemia**: serum phosphorus < 4 mg/dL (1.29 mmol/L)
      1. Etiology: rickets/osteopenia of prematurity; inadequate intake of phosphorus; and familial hypophosphatemias (Fanconi's syndrome, x-linked hypophosphatemia, and vitamin D-resistant rickets)
      2. Clinical manifestation of hypophosphatemia is bone demineralization.
      3. Treatment:
         a. Increase calcium and phosphorus intake.
         b. Oral supplemental phosphate
         c. Provide fortified human milk or preterm milk formulas to premature infants.
   C. **Hyperphosphatemia**: serum phosphorus > 7 mg/dL (2.26 mmol/L)
      1. Etiology: ingestion of high phosphorus formulas; increased parenteral intake; decreased phosphorus excretion secondary to renal failure; and hormonal regulation defect (eg, hypoparathyroidism)
      2. Clinical manifestations: metastatic calcifications and hypocalcemia
      3. Treatment:
         a. Decrease parenteral phosphorus intake.
         b. Change to a low-phosphorus formula (eg, Similac PM 60/40).
         c. Administer calcium supplementation.

V. Potassium (K⁺)

   A. Function (Stokowski, 1999): potassium is the major intracellular cation and assists in the regulation of intracellular osmotic activity. Potassium is also essential in acid-base and water balance and muscle tissue function (especially myocardial tissue). Together with sodium, potassium regulates cell membrane potential. Ninety percent of potassium is intracellular, and the intracellular/extracellular distribution of K⁺ is determined by the sodium-potassium pump. Insulin, glucagon, and blood pH affect this distribution.
   B. **Hypokalemia**: serum potassium < 3.5 mEq/L
      1. Etiology (Gomella et al., 1999):
         a. Hyperaldosteronism (congenital Cushing's and congenital aldosteronism)
         b. Bartter's syndrome (potassium-wasting disorder with hypokalemia, normal blood pressure [BP], and elevated levels of aldosterone and renin)
         c. Increased potassium losses: drug-induced losses (eg, amphotericin B, thiazide diuretics, gentamicin, and carbenicillin)

and GI tract losses (eg, diarrhea, nasogastric (NG) tube drainage, vomiting, and pyloric stenosis)

d. Decreased serum potassium secondary to increased intracellular uptake: insulin infusion and alkalosis

e. Inadequate intake (either IV or oral)

f. Hypercalcemia and hypomagnesemia

g. Renal tubular defects

h. Medications (eg, terbutaline, albuterol, isoproterenol, and catecholamines)

2. Clinical manifestations (Gomella et al., 1999): arrhythmias may occur if hypokalemia is present during the use of digitalis; ileus; and muscle weakness and decreased deep tendon reflexes

3. Treatment:

a. Monitor ECG for ST segment depression, low-voltage T wave, and presence of U wave.

b. Increase potassium intake **(daily maintenance requirement ≈ 2–3 mEq/kg/day)**.

c. Potassium replacement for symptomatic hypokalemia: 0.5 to 1 mEq/Kg IV infuse over 1 hour (maximum concentration 40 mEq/L in PIV; 80 mEq/L for CVL) and then reassess (Young & Mangnum, 2000).

d. Correct pyloric stenosis.

e. Treat the cause of diarrhea or vomiting (replace NG losses mL/mL with .45% normal saline solution + KCl additive).

f. Treat the underlying disorder causing metabolic or respiratory acidosis.

C. Hyperkalemia: serum potassium > 5.5 mEq/dL

1. Etiology (Gomella et al., 1999): adrenal insufficiency; hemolysis; potassium-sparing diuretics; prematurity with renal immaturity; renal failure; respiratory or metabolic acidosis (Choukair, 2000); and tissue necrosis (eg, NEC)

2. Clinical manifestations:

a. ECG disturbances: as the serum K^+ increases (> 7.0 mEq/L) there will be ECG changes starting with a peaked T wave, loss of P wave, widening of the QRS, and ST depression. Bradycardia will ensue, advance to first degree atrioventricular (AV) block, ventricular arrhythmias, and cardiac arrest.

b. Lethargy, hypotonia, paresthesias, and tetany

3. Treatment:

a. Dialysis

b. Drug therapy (Choukair, 2000; Gomella et al., 1999; Young & Mangum, 2000):

(1) Calcium gluconate 10% (0.5–1 mEq/kg via IV over 5–10 minutes): decreases myocardial excitability.

(2) Sodium bicarbonate (1–2 mEq/kg via IV over 10 to 30 minutes): increases blood pH and forces potassium into the cells.

(3) Glucose and insulin IV infusions (0.01–0.1U regular insulin/kg/hour): drives potassium into the cells.

(4) Sodium polystyrene resin (Kayexalate) (1 g/kg PO q6h or PR q 2–6 h): 1 g of resin removes approximately 1 mEq of potassium.

    c. Exchange transfusion

    d. Remove potassium from IV fluids and discontinue potassium-containing medications.

VI. Sodium (Na⁺)

  A. Function: Sodium is the major extracellular cation. Along with other electrolytes, sodium is responsible for maintaining osmotic equilibrium between fluid compartments; functions in the active transport of sodium and potassium ions into and out of the cells via the sodium-potassium pump; assists in establishing a negative electrical potential within the cell membrane (Guyton & Hall, 1998; Stokowski, 1999).

  B. **Hyponatremia**: serum sodium < 130 mEq/L (Seri & Evans, 1998)

    1. Etiology:

      a. Volume overload (dilutional hyponatremia):

        (1) Excessive IV fluids (↑ urine output, ↓ urine osmolality, ↓ urine-specific gravity)

        (2) Fluid retention secondary to congestive heart failure (CHF) or paralysis (↓ urine output, ↓ urine sodium, ↑ urine osmolality, ↑ urine-specific gravity)

        (3) Renal and liver failure

      b. Increased sodium loss:

        (1) Diuretics, renal tubular sodium losses, hyperglycemia, adrenal insufficiency (↑ urine output, ↑ urine sodium, ↓ urine osmolality, ↓ urine-specific gravity)

        (2) GI losses and third spacing (↓ urine output, ↓ urine sodium, ↑ urine osmolality, ↑ urine-specific gravity)

      c. Decreased sodium intake **(daily maintenance requirement ≈ 2–4 mEq/kg/day)**

      d. **Syndrome of inappropriate antidiuretic hormone secretion** (SIADH) (Gomella et al., 1999): SIADH is associated with central nervous system (CNS) disorders, perinatal asphyxia, intraventricular hemorrhage (IVH), hydrocephalus, and meningitis.

        (1) Clinical manifestations of SIADH: ↓ urine output, urine osmolality > serum osmolality, ↓ serum sodium and ↓ serum osmolality, ↑ urinary sodium and ↑ specific gravity

        (2) Treatment for SIADH is fluid restriction.

      e. Drug-induced hyponatremia:

        (1) Diuretics leading to Na⁺ losses

        (2) Indomethacin leading to H_2O retention, thereby causing a dilutional hyponatremia

        (3) Opiates, carbamazepine, and barbiturates may lead to SIADH.

        (4) Hyperosmolar IV fluids leading to osmotic diuresis and salt-wasting

    2. Clinical manifestations: edema (in fluid overload); seizures (usually evident with serum Na⁺ < 120 mEq/L); and signs of dehydration (eg, poor skin turgor, dry mucous membranes, decreased urine output, increased urine-specific gravity, and depressed fontanel)

3. Treatment:
   a. Correct sodium deficit parenterally.
   b. Fluid restriction for volume overload and SIADH
   c. Increase sodium intake.
C. Hypernatremia: serum sodium > 150 mEq/L (Seri & Evans, 1998)
   1. Etiology:
      a. Dehydration: too little free water and increased insensible water loss through skin and lungs
      b. Increased sodium intake
      c. Diabetes insipidus (DI) (or vasopressin deficiency): a metabolic disorder due to decreased activity of the posterior lobe of the pituitary gland. The reabsorption of water from renal tubules due to activity of vasopressin (or antidiuretic hormone [ADH]) is either blocked or is the result of an ADH deficiency.
         (1) Etiology of DI includes: CNS insults, trauma, or tumor.
         (2) Clinical manifestations of DI (Keefer, 2000): ↓ specific gravity, ↑ serum sodium, ↑ urine output (renal tubules excrete water but hold onto sodium)
         (3) Treatment for DI: nasal or oral administration of DDAVP (desmopressin acetate) (Keefer, 2000)
   2. Clinical manifestations (Choukair, 2000): depressed deep tendon reflexes; lethargy, poor tone, poor feeding, irritability, and seizures; respiratory failure; and signs of dehydration (poor skin turgor, dry mucous membranes, decreased urine output, increased specific gravity, and depressed fontanel)
   3. The treatment for hypernatremia is replacement of free water.
D. Sodium calculations:
   1. Sodium (Na⁺) replacement (Gomella et al., 1999; Seri & Evans, 1998):
      a. (Na⁺ *desired* − Na⁺ *measured*) × (weight [kg] × 0.6) = amount (mEq) needed to correct deficit.
         (1) Give ≈ 1/2 this amount in 12 to 24 hours (some clinicians will infuse at a faster rate). Changes in serum sodium concentration should be limited to no more than 10 mEq/L in 24 hours.
      b. Example:
         (Na⁺ 132 mEq *desired* − Na⁺ 122 mEq *measured*) × (1.5 kg × 0.6) = 9 mEq
         Total amount needed to correct deficit: give ≈ 4.5 mEq in 12 to 24 hours.
   2. Free H₂O deficit or excess (Seri & Evans, 1998):
      a. (Na⁺ *desired* ÷ [Na⁺ *measured* − 1]) × (weight [kg] × 0.6) = amount (L) H₂O deficit or excess
      b. Example:
         (Na⁺ 132 mEq/L *desired* ÷ [Na⁺ 152 mEq/L *measured* − 1]) × (1.5 kg × 0.6) = 0.78 L deficit
   3. IV saline solutions:
      0.9% = sodium 0.154 mEq/mL (154 mEq/L)
      0.45% = sodium 0.077 mEq/mL (77 mEq/L)

0.25% = sodium 0.036 mEq/mL (36 mEq/L)

3% = sodium 0.5 mEq/mL (**use with caution!**)

4. Serum osmolality: osmolality (the concentration of osmotically active particles in solution expressed in terms of osmoles of solute per kilogram of solvent) is largely determined by the serum sodium concentration and is expressed as the number of particles/L. Normal serum values: 285–295 mOsm/L.

   a. Calculation:

   2 (serum Na$^+$ *mEq/L*) + [(serum glucose *mg/dL* ÷ 18) + (blood urea nitrogen [BUN] *mg/dL* ÷ 2.8)]

   b. Example:

   2 (140 mEq/L) + [(100 mg/dL ÷ 18) + (20 mg/dL ÷ 28)] = 286 mOsm/L

5. **Fractional excretion of Na$^+$** (FENa) (Simmons, 1998): FENa expresses the difference between glomerular filtration and tubular reabsorption of sodium.

   a. Newborns with FENa < 1% are oliguric secondary to prerenal factors (eg, hypotension or decreased cardiac output).

   b. Newborns with FENa > 2.5% usually present with acute renal failure or are receiving diuretic therapy.

   c. Infants < 32 weeks' gestation often have FENa > 2.5%, regardless of fluid and electrolyte balance.

   d. FENa = 100 × ([urine Na$^+$ × plasma creatinine] ÷ [plasma Na$^+$ × urine creatinine])

   e. Example:

   100 × ([6 × 1.1]) ÷ (130 × 24.]) = 1.43

VII. Chloride (Cl$^-$) (Tsang et al., 1998):

A. Function: Cl is a major extracellular anion and, in conjunction with sodium, maintains plasma volume; serum chloride and bicarbonate (HCO_3^-) concentrations are inversely related (when chloride is lost, bicarbonate increases, causing a metabolic alkalosis; when Cl levels increase, bicarbonate decreases, causing a metabolic acidosis).

B. **Hypochloremia**: serum chloride < 90 mEq/L (90 mmol/L)

   1. Etiology: decreased intake (occurs with soy formulas) and increased losses from GI or renal sources (prolonged vomiting or NG aspiration; renal losses secondary to diuretic therapy)

   2. Clinical manifestations: metabolic alkalosis; hypokalemia; and failure to thrive

   3. Treatment:

      a. Replace NG losses.

      b. Correct alkalosis, and consider changing diuretic therapy.

C. **Hyperchloremia**: serum chloride > 115 mEq/L (115 mmol/L)

   1. Etiology: bicarbonate depletion as a result of diarrhea or renal losses secondary to renal tubular acidosis; increased chloride intake (eg, excessive NaCl administration)

   2. Clinical manifestations: diarrhea leading to hyperchloremic metabolic acidosis

   3. Treatment:

      a. Discontinue NaCl administration.

      b. Replace free-water losses.

VIII. Insensible water loss (IWL)

A. IWL (nonmeasurable) occurs as a result of evaporation through the infant's mucous membranes and skin. Approximately 30% of water is lost from the respiratory tract and 70% from the skin. Premature infants have a larger IWL than term infants, secondary to an immature epithelial skin layer with poor keratinization, large water content, decreased subcutaneous fat, and a larger surface area:body weight ratio (Stokowski, 1999).

B. Factors that increase IWL (Bell & Oh, 1999; Ochikubo, 1999): prematurity (the amount of IWL is inversely proportional to the gestational age and weight of the infant); low environmental humidity; radiant warmer; high environmental temperature; hyperthermia; phototherapy; increased motor activity and crying; skin breakdown; abdominal wall and neural tube defects (before corrective surgery); tachypnea; and respiratory support without humidified gases

C. Factors that decrease IWL: applying patches to infant's skin to prevent breakdown; increasing ambient humidity to 40 to 50%; double-walled incubators; plastic blankets and heat shields; and respiratory support with humidified gases

D. IWL at varying birth weights (Alexander & Robin, 2000; Bell & Oh, 1999; Ochikubo, 1999):
   1. 750–1000 g → up to 85 mL/kg/day.
   2. 1000–1500 g → 30–65 mL/kg/day.
   3. 1500–2000 g → 15–30 mL/kg/day.

IX. Initial daily fluid requirements (general guidelines)

A. Term infant:
   1. Fluid intake (mL/kg/day):
      a. Day of life (DOL) 1 → 60–80 mL/kg/day
      b. DOL 2-3 → 80–120 mL/kg/day
      c. After DOL 3 → increase by 10 to 20 mL/kg/day up to ~160 mL/kg/day
   2. Weight loss: term infants can lose up to 10% to 15% of their birth weight during the first 3 to 5 days of life (Ochikubo, 1999).
   3. Electrolytes:
      a. Follow electrolytes and adjust fluids to keep serum sodium < 150 mEq/L.
      b. Usually not necessary to add supplemental sodium until DOL 2 to 3 when diuresis commences and serum sodium decreases
      c. Add supplemental potassium (1–2 mEq/kg/day) after **adequate urine output (1–2 mL/kg/hr)** is established.
      d. Follow tCa or iCa and add supplemental calcium as needed.
   4. Glucose:
      a. Follow serum glucose levels and adjust IV dextrose concentrations accordingly.
      b. Term infants usually require a **glucose infusion rate of 4–7 mg/kg/min** to remain euglycemic.
      c. Example:
         80 mL/kg/day of a 10% dextrose IV solution = 5.56 mg/kg/day glucose
   5. Renal: satisfactory urine output is approximately 1–2 mL/kg/hr.

B. Preterm infant:
1. Fluid intake (mL/kg/day):
   a. DOL 1:
      (1) < 1000 g (100–150 mL/kg/day).
      (2) 1000–1500 grams (80–100 mL/kg/day).
      (3) Preterm infants have a higher IWL than term infants, secondary to poor skin keratinization, thereby necessitating a larger fluid intake.
      (4) When calculating total fluids, be cognizant of medications, flushes, and fluids used in volume resuscitation for hypovolemia, acidosis, sepsis, or hypoglycemia.
      (5) Excessive fluid administration can exacerbate respiratory distress syndrome (RDS) and is associated with bronchopulmonary dysplasia (BPD), patent ductus arteriosus (PDA), and NEC (Stokowski, 1999).
   b. DOL 2 to 3:
      (1) < 1000 g (120–150 mL/kg/day)
      (2) 1000–1500 g (100–120 mL/kg/day)
   c. After DOL 3:
      (1) < 1000 g (140–190 mL/kg/day)
      (2) 1000–1500 g (140–160 mL/kg/day)
2. Weight loss: preterm infants may lose 10% to 20% of birth weight in the first week of life (Stokowski, 1999).
3. Electrolytes:
   a. Follow electrolytes closely and adjust fluids to maintain serum sodium < 150 mEq/L.
   b. Gradually add parenteral sodium on DOL 2 to 3 when diuresis commences and serum sodium decreases.
   c. Before adding potassium to parenteral fluid, establish **adequate urine output (1–2 mL/kg/hr)**.
   d. Body stores of calcium are low in preterm infants; therefore, add supplemental parenteral calcium (10% calcium gluconate, 200–800 mg/kg/day) (Young & Mangum, 2000).
4. Glucose (Stokowski, 1999):
   a. Follow serum glucose levels and adjust IV glucose concentrations accordingly.
   b. **Typical glucose infusion rate is 6–8 mg/kg/min.**
   c. Because premature infants usually have higher fluid requirements, they need lower IV glucose concentrations (D5W, D7½W) to maintain the same glucose infusion rate.
   d. Hyperglycemia (> 150 mg/dL) may lead to an osmotic diuresis and dehydration; hyperosmolar extracellular fluid in the brain may contribute to neurological damage and IVH.
5. Renal: satisfactory urine output is approximately 1–2 mL/kg/hr.

▼
References

Alexander, D. C., & Robin, B. (2000). Neonatology. In G. B. Avery, M. A. Fletcher, & M. G. MacDonald (Eds.), *Neonatology: Pathophysiology & management of the newborn* (5th ed., pp. 417–438). Philadelphia: Lippincott Williams & Wilkins.

Bakewell-Sachs, S. (1999). Neonatal nutrition. In J. Deacon & P. O'Neill (Eds.), *Core curriculum for neonatal intensive care nursing* (2nd ed., pp. 294–325). Philadelphia: WB Saunders.

Bell, E. F., & Oh, W. (1999). Fluid and electrolyte management. In G. B. Avery, M. A. Fletcher, & M. G. MacDonald (Eds.), *Neonatology: Pathophysiology & management of the newborn* (5th ed., pp. 345–361). Philadelphia: Lippincott Williams & Wilkins.

Choukair, M. K. (2000). Fluids and electrolytes. In G. K. Siberry & R. Iannone (Eds.), *The Harriet Lane handbook* (15th ed., pp. 229–250). St. Louis: Mosby.

Gomella, T. L., Cunningham, M. D., Eyal, F. G., & Zenk, K. E. (Eds.). (1999). *Neonatology: Management, procedures, on-call problems, diseases, and drugs* (4th ed.). Norwalk, CT: Appleton & Lange.

Guyton, A. C., & Hall, J. E. (Eds.). (1997). *Human physiology and mechanisms of disease* (6th ed.). Philadelphia: WB Saunders.

Huttner, K. M. (1998). Metabolic problems: Hypocalcemia, hypercalcemia, and hypermagnesemia. In J. P. Cloherty & A. R. Stark (Eds.), *Manual of neonatal care* (4th ed., pp. 553–562). Philadelphia: Lippincott-Raven.

Keefer, J. R. (2000). Common management issues. In G. K. Siberry & R. Iannone (Eds.), *The Harriet Lane handbook* (15th ed., pp. 207–228). St. Louis: Mosby.

Koo, W. W. K., & Tsang, R. C. (1999). Calcium and magnesium homeostasis. In G. B. Avery, M. A. Fletcher, & M. G. MacDonald (Eds.), *Neonatology: Pathophysiology & management of the newborn* (5th ed., pp. 715–738). Philadelphia: Lippincott Williams & Wilkins.

Ochikubo, C. (1999). Fluids and electrolytes. In T. L. Gomella, M. D. Cunningham, F. G. Eyal, & K. E. Zenk (Eds.), *Neonatology: Management, procedures, on-call problems, diseases, drugs* (4th ed., pp. 68–74). Stamford, CT: Appleton & Lange.

Rubin, L. P. (1998). Disorders of calcium and phosphorus metabolism. In H. W. Taeusch & R. A. Ballard (Eds.), *Avery's diseases of the newborn* (7th ed., pp. 1189–1206). Philadelphia: WB Saunders.

Seri, I., & Evans, J. (1998). Acid-base, fluid, and electrolyte management. In H. W. Taeusch & R. A. Ballard (Eds.), *Avery's diseases of the newborn* (7th ed., pp. 372–393). Philadelphia: WB Saunders.

Silva-Neto, G. (1999). Rickets and disorders of calcium and magnesium metabolism. In T. L. Gomella, M. D. Cunningham, F. G. Eyal, & K. E. Zenk (Eds.), *Neonatology: Management, procedures, on-call problems, diseases, drugs* (4th ed., pp. 524–532). Stamford, CT: Appleton & Lange.

Simmons, C. F. (1998). Fluid and electrolyte management. In J. P. Cloherty & A. R. Stark (Eds.), *Manual of neonatal care* (4th ed., pp. 87–100). Philadelphia: Lippincott-Raven.

Stokowski, L. C. (1999). Metabolic disorders. In J. Deacon & P. O'Neill (Eds.), *Core curriculum for neonatal care nursing* (2nd ed., pp. 326–356). Philadelphia: WB Saunders.

Tsang, R. C., Demarini, S., & Rath, L. L. (1998). Fluids, electrolytes, vitamins, and trace minerals. In C. Kenner, J. W. Lott, & A. A. Flandermeyer (Eds.), *Comprehensive neonatal nursing, a physiologic perspective* (2nd ed., pp. 336–353). Philadelphia: WB Saunders.

Young, T. E., & Mangum, B. (2000). *Neofax 2000* (13th ed.). Raleigh, NC: Acorn Publishing, Inc.

Chapter 8

Nutrition

Cheryl A. Cloud, MSN, RNC, CRNP, and Paulette Haws, MSN, RNC, NNP

Providing nutrition to preterm and ill term infants continues to be a challenge to newborn caregivers. These infants are abruptly removed from an intrauterine environment, where they receive a steady provision of maternal glucose, to an extrauterine environment consisting of intermittent enteral feedings (Ogata, 1999). The current standard for postnatal nutrition in preterm infants, according to the American Academy of Pediatrics (AAP), is to duplicate or match the normal fetal growth rate. There are three general categories of nutritional requirements: energy, provided by calories in the form of carbohydrates, proteins, and fats; minerals; and vitamins. This chapter reviews current recommendations for calculating and delivering these nutritional requirements.

I. Carbohydrates (CHO)

A. Calories:
   1. Forty percent to 50% of total daily calories should consist of CHO.
   2. Normal intravenous (IV) dextrose administration is **4–7 mg/kg/min**. (Too much glucose can lead to osmotic diuresis secondary to glucosuria.)
   3. IV dextrose (anhydrous) = 3.4 kcal/g.
   4. Oral glucose intake = 4 kcal/g.
   5. A % solution refers to the number of grams of dextrose per 100 mL.

B. Calculations:
   1. Formulas to determine the amount of glucose (mg/kg/min) being delivered via an IV solution (2 formulas) (Box 8.1).
   2. Formula used to increase dextrose concentration in IV fluids:
      a. 2 mL D50% + 98 mL IV fluid = ↑ dextrose concentration by 1%
      b. Example: 2 mL D50% + 98 mL D10% = 100 mL D11%
   3. Formula used to change % dextrose to maintain specific mg/kg/min:
      a. $\% \text{ dextrose} = \dfrac{\text{desired mg/kg/min} \times 1{,}440 \times \text{wt (kg)}}{\text{total mL/day}} = \dfrac{x}{1{,}000}$
      b. Example:
      $$\frac{5.6 \text{ mg/kg/min} \times 1{,}440 \times 3 \text{ kg}}{240 \text{ mL/day}} = \frac{100.8}{1{,}000} = 0.10 \ (10\%)$$
   4. Formula used to calculate the total calories/day obtained from CHO:
      a. Total mL/day × % dextrose (expressed as decimal) × 3.4 (calories/g) (Table 8.1).
      b. 240 mL/day × 0.06 × 3.4 = 48.96 calories/day from **CHO**

▼ **BOX 8.1** | **Formulas to Determine the Amount of Glucose Delivered (mg/kg/min)**

$$\text{mg/kg/min} = \frac{\text{IV rate} \times \% \text{ glucose (expressed as a whole number)} \times 0.167}{\text{weight (kg)}}$$

$$\text{eg,} \frac{10 \text{ mL/h} \times 10 \text{ (eg, 10\% glucose)} \times 0.167}{3 \text{ kg}} = 5.56 \text{ mg/kg/min}$$

$$\text{mg/kg/min} = \frac{\begin{array}{c} \text{volume} \\ \times \% \text{ dextrose (expressed as a decimal)} \\ \times 1{,}000 \text{ mL} \end{array}}{\text{weight (kg)}} = \frac{x}{1{,}440 \text{ (min/d)}}$$

$$\text{eg,} \frac{240 \text{ mL/d} \times 0.10 \times 1{,}000 \text{ mL}}{3 \text{ kg}} = \frac{8{,}000}{1{,}440} = 5.55 \text{ mg/kg/min}$$

  C. Hypoglycemia (Cloharty & Stark, 1998; Gomella, Cunningham, Eyal, & Zenk, 1999):
  1. Definition: blood glucose level < 40 mg/dL.
  2. Etiology (two basic etiologies): (Table 8.2)
  3. Clinical manifestations of hypoglycemia: apnea; cyanosis or pallor; feeble suck and poor feeding; lethargy, hypotonia, and weak cry; seizures; coma; temperature instability; and tremors, jitteriness, and irritability.
  4. Treatment for hypoglycemia:
    a. Infants at risk for hypoglycemia should have their blood glucose levels followed carefully. Verify and treat infants whose blood glucose is < 40 mg/dL.
    b. Treatment of asymptomatic infants varies with each institution: begin early feedings for term infants without risk factors; parenteral glucose for serum glucose levels < 25 mg/dL.

 TABLE 8.1 Caloric Content of Parenteral Dextrose

Dextrose Solution	Kcal/cc
D5W	0.17
D7.5W	0.255
D10W	0.34
D12.5W	0.425
D15W	0.51
D20W	0.68
D25W	0.85

From Gomella, T. L., Cunningham, M. D., Eyal, F. G., & Zenk, K. E., (Eds.). (1999). *Neonatology: Management, procedures, on-call problems, diseases, and drugs* (4th ed.). Norwalk, CT: Appleton & Lange.

TABLE 8.2 Etiologies for Hypoglycemia

Increased use of glucose stores/ excessive tissue use	Decreased glucose stores/ inadequate production
• Infant of a diabetic mother (associated problems include: caudal regression syndrome; macrosomia; hypoglycemia; IUFD; hypocalcemia; hyperviscosity or polycythemia; hyperbilirubinemia; RDS; cardiac outflow tract obstruction, septal hypertrophy, and cardiomyopathy) • IUGR • Erythroblastosis fetalis • Beckwith-Wiedemann syndrome • Islet cell hyperplasia • Insulin-producing tumors (nesidioblastosis) • Maternal drugs • Malpositioned UAC used for glucose infusion • Postexchange transfusion • Sepsis • Hypothermia • Large-for-gestational age infants	• Prematurity with limited hepatic glycogen stores • IUGR • Decreased caloric intake • Inborn errors of carbohydrate, amino acid, and fatty acid metabolism • Hormone deficiencies (growth hormone, ACTH thyroid, glucagon, and cortisol deficiencies or unresponsiveness) • Midline central nervous system deformities • Pituitary and hypothalamus deformities • Perinatal stress and/or asphyxia

IUFD-intrauterine fetal demise; RDS-respiratory distress syndrome; IUGR-intrauterine growth restriction; UAC-umbilical artery catheter; ACTH-adrenocorticotropic hormone

    c. Treatment for symptomatic infants or those who have a serum glucose concentration < 25mg/dL:

        (1) Feed infants every 2 to 4 hours as tolerated and/or administer IV dextrose: **D10W bolus (2 mL/kg) via IV** followed by a **continuous IV solution of D10W (6–8 mg/kg/min ≈ 85–110 mL/kg/day of D10W)**

        (2) IV solutions > 12.5% dextrose should be administered through a central catheter.

    d. Severe or unremitting hypoglycemia:

        (1) Diazoxide, epinephrine, or growth hormone

        (2) Glucagon: 0.1–0.3 mg/kg; intramuscular (IM), IV, or subcutaneously (SC); every 6 hours; maximum dose = 1 mg/dose; contraindicated in small-for-gestational-age infants.

        (3) Hydrocortisone: 5 mg/kg/day; IV; divided every 6 to 8 hours; decreases peripheral glucose use; increases gluconeogenesis; and increases the effects of glucagon.

  D. Hyperglycemia (Polk, 1998): blood glucose > 125 mg/dL

    1. Etiology of hyperglycemia: increased glucose intake; sepsis; medications (eg, steroid, phenytoin, and, occasionally, methylxanthine administration); stress; and transient neonatal diabetes mellitus (DM)

2. Clinical manifestations of hyperglycemia: osmotic diuresis with resultant dehydration, acidemia, and ketosis; intraventricular hemorrhage

3. Treatment for hyperglycemia:
   a. Decrease the amount of dextrose the infant is receiving.
   b. Regular insulin: (0.05–0.1 unit/kg; SQ; every 6 hours) *or* (0.01–0.1 units/kg/hour via continuous IV administration)
   c. If possible, discontinue the administration of phenytoin and caffeine.
   d. IV dextrose concentrations < 4.7% are hypo-osmolar and may lead to hemolysis with resultant hyperkalemia.

II. Protein

A. Calories:
   1. 10% to 15% of total daily calories should be from protein.
   2. Protein = 4 kcal/g
   3. Administering > 3 g/kg/day via hyperalimentation can lead to hyperammonemia and acidosis.

B. Calculations:
   1. Formula to determine % amino acid in hyperalimentation:
      a. $\% \text{ amino acids} = \dfrac{\text{desired g/kg/day} \times \text{weight (kg)}}{\text{total cc/day}} \times 100$
      b. Example: $\dfrac{3 \text{ g/kg/day} \times 3 \text{ kg}}{240 \text{ mL/day}} \times 100 = 3.75\%$ amino acids
   2. Formula to determine the amount of g/kg/day received from hyperalimentation:
      a. $\text{g/kg/day} = \dfrac{\text{total cc/day} \times \% \text{ amino acids (expressed as decimal)}}{\text{weight (kg)}}$
      b. Example: $\dfrac{240 \text{ mL/day} \times 0.0375}{3 \text{ kg}} = 3 \text{ g/kg/day}$
   3. Formula to calculate the total calories/day from protein:
      a. Total calories/day = total mL/day × % amino acid (expressed as decimal) × 4 (calories/g)
      b. Example: 240 mL/day × 0.0375 × 4 = 36 calories/day from protein

III. Fat

A. Calories:
   1. < 50% total daily calories should be from fat.
   2. Oral intake = 9 calories/g
   3. IV preparation (with glycerol additive) = 11 calories/g; intralipids are an emulsion of soybean oil and egg yolk phospholipids supplying triglycerides and long-chain fatty acids (Koletzko, 1997); intralipids 20% = 20 g/100 mL (0.2 g/mL) and 2.2 calories/mL; intralipids 10% = 10 g/100 mL (0.1 g/mL) and 1.1 calories/mL.

B. Calculations:
   1. Formula to calculate the amount of lipids (cc/day) to administer:

    a. mL/day $= \dfrac{\text{weight (kg)} \times \text{desired g/kg/day}}{\text{g/mL (eg 20\% IL)}}$

    b. Example: $\dfrac{3 \text{ kg} \times 3 \text{ g/kg/day}}{0.2 \text{ g/mL}} = 45$ mL/day of 20% intralipids

  2. Formula to calculate amount of g/kg/day that are received from intralipids:

    a. g/kg/day $= \dfrac{\text{total volume/day} \times \text{g/mL}}{\text{weight (kg)}}$

    b. Example: $\dfrac{45 \text{ mL/day} \times 0.2 \text{ g/mL}}{3 \text{ kg}} = 3$ g/kg/day

  3. Formula to calculate total calories/day from fat:

    a. calories/day = total volume/day × calories/mL

    b. Example: 45 mL/day × 2.2 calories/mL = 99 calories/day from fat

C. Intralipid administration: begin with 0.5–1.5 g/kg/day dependent upon gestation and weight. Increase in increments of 0.5–1.5 g/kg/day to a maximum of approximately 3 mg/kg/day. Administration of 0.5–1 g/kg/day is sufficient to prevent essential fatty acid deficiency (Zenk, Sills, & Koeppel, 2000).

IV. Vitamins and trace elements

A. Water-soluble vitamins: there is no evidence of toxic levels because of high renal clearance.

  1. B_1 (thiamine): involved in carbohydrate metabolism and essential for nerve function

  2. B_2 (riboflavin): coenzyme in cellular metabolism; functional for normal vision

  3. B_3 (niacin): helps synthesize fatty acids and cholesterol; converts phenylalanine to tyrosine.

  4. B_6 (pyridoxine): coenzyme in metabolism of proteins; aids formation of neurotransmitters.

  5. Pantothenic acid: essential to the formation of coenzyme A that is involved in synthesis and breakdown of fatty acids

  6. Biotin: functions as a coenzyme in synthesis of amino acids and fatty acids.

  7. Folate (folic acid): deficiency leads to growth retardation, megaloblastosis, and anemia.

  8. Vitamin B_{12} (cobalamin): essential for red blood cell formation

  9. Vitamin C (ascorbic acid): has a role in synthesis of neurotransmitters; positively affects the absorption of iron.

B. Fat-soluble vitamins: there is a potential for toxicity because they are stored in tissues.

  1. Vitamin A (retinol): important in cell differentiation and immune function

  2. Vitamin D (calciferol): considered a hormone produced in the skin when exposed to sunlight; important in the metabolism of calcium and phosphorous

  3. Vitamin E (α-tocopherol): has antioxidant activity as a free radical scavenger.

  4. Vitamin K: involved in clotting cascade

C. Requirements of water- and fat-soluble vitamins (MVI Pediatrica [Astra Pharmaceutical Products]) based on weight for parenteral administration (Table 8.3):
  1. < 1 kg: 1.5 mL of MVI/24 hour
  2. 1 to 3 kg: 3.25 mL of MVI/24 hour
  3. > 3 kg: 5 mL of MVI/24 hour
D. Requirements for water- and fat-soluble vitamins for enterally fed infants:
  1. For feedings of human breast milk without human milk fortifier (HMF) supplementation: 1 mL/day of Poly-vi-sol Infant Drops or Vi-Daylin MV Drops
  2. For infants on full feeds (150 mL/kg/day) of premature infant formula, no additional vitamin supplementation is needed (Cloherty & Stark, 1998).
  3. Vitamin E:
     a. Limited studies on actual requirements for premature infants on either breast milk or premature formula: no proven benefit regarding retinopathy of prematurity (ROP), intraventricular hemorrhage (IVH), or bronchopulmonary dysplasia (BPD) outcome
     b. Recommended dose: 25 IU PO once a day until 36 weeks' postconceptual age. Do not give vitamin E supplement until infant is tolerating full feeds secondary to high osmolality.
E. Trace elements:
  1. Zinc: essential for growth and development; there is better absorption from human breast milk than from formula.
  2. Copper: essential part of many enzymes, particularly oxidative enzymes; do not add to hyperalimentation (HAL) for infants with cholestasis.
  3. Manganese: functions in metabolic processes; manganese is

 TABLE 8.3 Vitamin Requirement and Availability

Vitamin	Requirement kg/d	Amount in 5 cc Multivitamin Infusion
A	280–500 μg	700 μg
E	2.8 μg	7 μg
K	100 μg	200 μg
D	4 μg	10 μg
C	25 mg	80 mg
Thiamine	350 μg	1.2 mg
Riboflavin	150 μg	1.4 mg
Pyridoxine	180 μg	1 mg
Niacin	6.8 mg	17 mg
Pantothenate	2 mg	5 mg (pantothenic acid)
Biotin	6 μg	20 μg
Folate	56 μg	140 μg (folic acid)
B_{12}	0.3 μg	1 μg

Adapted from Zenk, K. E., Sills, J. H., & Koeppel, R. M. (2000). *Neonatal medications & nutrition: A comprehensive guide* (2nd ed.). Santa Rosa, CA: NICU Ink.

excreted via bile; therefore, a reduced amount is required in HAL for infants with cholestasis.

4. Chromium: plays a role in preventing glucose intolerance; remove from HAL for infants with compromised urine output since chromium is eliminated via the kidneys.

5. Selenium: antioxidant activity and involved in thyroid function; breast milk is sufficient in selenium.

6. Fluoride: decreases incidence of dental caries; no requirement for first 6 months of age.

7. Molybdenum: recommended for infants on long-term HAL

8. Iron (Zenk, 2000): essential mineral found in various enzymes and hemoglobin
   a. Supplementation at birth does not prevent physiologic anemia.
   b. Goal of supplementation is to prevent iron-deficiency anemia.
      (1) Term infants receiving iron-fortified formula need no supplements.
      (2) Term breastfeeding infants need no supplements until 6 months.
      (3) Preterm infants: supplementation is recommended until 12 months of age (begin supplementing premature infants at 1 month of age *or* when tolerating full feeds with Fer-In-Sol, 0.1–0.2 mL/day [2.5–5 mg of elemental iron], PO.
   c. Iron supplements affect vitamin E absorption; therefore, do not give simultaneously.

9. Carnitine (Zenk, 2000): element with essential role in fatty acid oxidation for energy; neonates have limited stores of carnitine; therefore, supplement 10 mg/kg/day in HAL.

10. Parenteral trace element administration (Table 8.4):
    a. Standard dose for both term and preterm infants is 0.2 mL/kg/day.
    b. Decrease copper and manganese for infants with cholestasis.
    c. Eliminate chromium for infants with renal dysfunction.

 TABLE 8.4 Trace Elements Requirement and Availability for Parental Nutrition

Trace Elements	Preterm Requirements (μg/kg/day)	Term Requirements (μg/kg/day)	Amount in Neotrace (μg/mL)
Zinc	400	< 3 mo: 250 > 3 mo: 100	500–1,500
Copper	15–20	15–20	100
Manganese	1	1	25–30
Chromium	0.2	0.2	0.85–1

Adapted from Zenk, K. E., Sills, J. H., & Koeppel, R. M. (2000). *Neonatal medications & nutrition: A comprehensive guide* (2nd ed.). Santa Rosa, CA: NICU Ink.

F. Calorie content of formulas and nutritional supplements:
  1. Formulas: 20 cal/oz (0.67 cal/mL); 22 cal/oz (0.73 cal/mL); 24 cal/oz (0.8 cal/mL); 27 cal/oz (0.9 cal/mL)
  2. Nutritional supplements:
     a. Medium chain triglyceride (MCT oil): 7.7 cal/mL
     b. Vegetable oil: 8 cal/mL
     c. Human milk fortifier: 2 packs/50 mL breast milk increases the caloric content by 4 cal/oz.
     d. Polycose: 2 cal/mL
     e. Rice cereal: 15 cal/tbsp
     f. Microlipid: 4.4 cal/mL

▼ References

Atkinson, S. A., & Zlotkin, S. (1997). Recognizing deficiencies and excesses of zinc, copper and other trace elements. In R. C. Tsang, S. H. Zlotkin, B. L. Nichols, & J. W. Hansen (Eds.), *Nutrition during infancy: Principles and practice* (2nd ed., pp. 209–232). Cincinnati, OH: Digital Educational Publishing.

Brooks, C. (1997). Neonatal hypoglycemia. *Neonatal Network, 16.* 15–22.

Butte, N. F. (1997). Meeting energy needs. In R. C. Tsang, S. Zlotkin, B. L. Nichols, & J. W. Hansen (Eds.), *Nutrition during infancy: Principles and practice* (2nd ed., pp. 57–82). Cincinnati, OH: Digital Educational Publishing.

Cloharty, J. P., & Stark, A. R. (Eds.). (1998). *Manual of neonatal care* (4th ed, pp. 545–546). Philadelphia: Lippincott-Raven.

Gomella, T. L., Cunningham. M.D., Eyal, F.G., & Zenk, K.E. (Eds.). (1999). *Neonatology: Management, procedures, on-call problems, diseases, and drugs* (4th ed.). Norwalk, CT: Appleton & Lange.

Groh-Wargo, S., Thompson, M., & Cox, J.H. (2000). *Nutritional care for high risk newborns* (3rd ed.). Chicago: Precept Press.

Gross, S. J. (1993). Vitamin E. In R. C. Tsang, A. Lucas, R. Uauy, & S. Zlotkin (Eds.), *Nutritional needs of the preterm infant: Scientific basis and practical guidelines* (pp. 101–109). Pawling, NY: Williams & Wilkins.

Heird, W. C., & Gomez, M. C., (1993). Parenteral nutrition. In R.C. Tsang, A. Lucas, R. Uauy, & S. Zlotkin (Eds.), *Nutritional needs of the preterm infant: Scientific basis and practical guidelines* (pp. 225–242). Pawling, NY: Williams & Wilkins.

Koletzko, B. (1997). Importance of dietary lipids. In R. C. Tsang, S. H. Zlotkin, B. L. Nichols, & J. W., Hansen (Eds.), *Nutrition during infancy, principles and practice* (2nd ed.). Cincinnati, OH: Digital Education Publishing, Inc.

Ogata, E. S. (1999). Carbohydrate homeostasis. In G. B. Avery, M. A. Fletcher, & M. G. MacDonald (Eds.), *Neonatology: Pathophysiology and management of the newborn* (5th ed., pp. 699–714). Philadelphia: Lippincott Williams & Wilkins.

Polk, D. H. (1998). Disorders of carbohydrate metabolism. In H. W. Taeusch & R. A. Ballard (Eds.), *Avery's diseases of the newborn* (7th ed., pp. 1235–1241). Philadelphia: WB Saunders.

Reifen, R. M., & Zlotkin, S. (1993). Microminerals. In R. C. Tsang, A. Lucas, R. Uauy, & S. Zlotkin (Eds.), *Nutritional needs of the preterm infant: Scientific basis and practical guidelines* (pp. 195–207). Pawling, NY: Williams & Wilkins.

Schanler, R. J. (1997). Who needs water-soluble vitamins? In R. C. Tsang, S. H. Zlotkin, B. L. Nichols & J. W. Hansen (Eds.), *Nutrition during infancy: Principles and practice* (2nd ed., pp. 255–284). Cincinnati, OH: Digital Educational Publishing.

Sun, Y., Awetwant, L., Collier, S. B., Gallagher, L. M., Olsen, I. E., & Stewart, J. E. (1998). Nutrition. In J. P. Cloharty, & A. R. Stark (Eds.), *Manual of neonatal care* (4th ed., pp. 101–134). Philadelphia, PA: Lippincott-Raven.

Thureen, P. J. (1999). Early aggressive nutrition in the neonate. *NeoReviews*, 45–55.

Zenk, K. E., Sills, J. H., & Koeppel, R. M. (2000). *Neonatal medications & nutrition: A comprehensive guide* (2nd ed.). Santa Rosa, CA: NICU Ink.

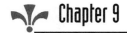 **Chapter 9**

Drug Infusion Calculations and Procedures

Paulette S. Haws, MSN, RNC, NNP

I. Drug infusion calculations
    A. μg/kg/minute (or Rule of 6s) (Tables 9.1 and 9.2)
    B. μg, mg, or unit/kg/hour (Table 9.3)
II. Body surface area (BSA) (m²) calculations
    A. Mosteller's formula (Briars & Bailey, 1994):

$$\text{BSA (m}^2) = \frac{\sqrt{\text{height (cm)} \times \text{weight (kg)}}}{3{,}600}$$

 TABLE 9.1 Drug Infusion Calculations in μg/kg/min (Rule of 6s)

Formula: $\dfrac{6 \times \text{weight (kg)} \times \text{desired μg/kg/min}}{\text{desired mL/h}} = \dfrac{\text{amount of drug (mg) added to}}{\text{IVF to make 100 mL}}$

Medication	Dosage (Young & Mangum, 2001)	Calculations	
Dopamine	2–20 μg/kg/min	$\dfrac{6 \times \text{weight (kg)} \times 10 \text{ μg/kg/min}}{1 \text{ mL/h}} =$	mg added to make 100 mL
Dobutamine	5–25 μg/kg/min	*1 mL/h = 10 μg/kg/min	
Nitroprusside	0.25–2 μg/kg/min		
Example: Infuse dopamine at 5 μg/kg/min for a 2-kg infant and run at 0.5 mL/h		$\dfrac{6 \times 2 \text{ kg} \times 5 \text{ μg/kg/min}}{0.5 \text{ mL/h}} =$	120 mg added to make 100 mL
		Dopamine 120 mg (40 mg/mL) =	3 mL drug + 97 mL IVF
Epinephrine	0.1–1 μg/kg/min	$\dfrac{6 \times \text{weight (kg)} \times 0.1 \text{ μg/kg/min}}{1 \text{ mL/h}} =$	mg added to make 100 mL
Isoproterenol	0.05–0.5 μg/kg/min	*1 mL/h = 0.1 μg/kg/min	
PGE₁	0.01–0.1 μg/kg/min		
Lidocaine	10–50 μg/kg/min	$\dfrac{6 \times \text{weight (kg)} \times 100 \text{ μg/kg/min}}{1 \text{ mL/h}} =$	mg added to make 100 mL
		*1 mL/h = 100 μg/kg/min	

IVF = intravenous fluid; PGE₁, = Prostaglandin E₂.

TABLE 9.2 Alternate Formula for PGE₁

PGE₁ formulas (Example: Infuse PGE₁ at 0.01 µg/kg/min for a 2-kg infant)

Rule of 6s	$\dfrac{6 \times \text{weight (kg)} \times \text{desired µg/kg/min}}{\text{desired mL/h}} = \dfrac{\text{amount of drug (mg) added to}}{\text{make 100 mL intravenous fluid}}$
	Example: $\dfrac{6 \times 2 \text{ kg} \times 0.01 \text{ µg/kg/min}}{1 \text{ mL/h}} = 0.12$ mg added to 100 mL
Alternate formula	*Add 500 µg of PGE₁ to 50 mL D5W (10 µg/mL)
	$\dfrac{\text{weight (kg)} \times \text{desired µg/kg/min} \times 60}{10} = \text{rate to set intravenous pump}$
	Example: $\dfrac{2 \text{ kg} \times 0.01 \text{ µg/kg/min} \times 60}{10} = 0.12$ mL/h

PGE₁, = Prostaglandin E₂

Example: $m^2 = \sqrt{\dfrac{50 \text{ cm} \times 3 \text{ kg}}{3,600}} = 0.204$

B. Body surface nomogram (Figure 9.1)

III. Procedures

Wash hands before and after each procedure. Use the appropriate personal safety protection devices (gloves, eye protection, gown, mask, and cap) required for each procedure.

  A. Arterial catheterization:

   1. Umbilical cord usually contains two arteries (small-diameter thick-walled muscular vessels located inferior to the vein) and one vein (large-diameter thin-walled vessel usually located superior to the arteries) surrounded by clear Wharton's jelly. Two vessel cords (one artery and a vein) occur in approximately 1% of the population and may be associated with congenital cardiovascular or renal abnormalities (Conner, 1993).

   2. Umbilical artery catheterization (UAC) (Gomella, 1999; MacDonald, 1993):

   a. Indications: invasive blood pressure monitoring; frequent blood sampling; cardiac catheterization; and exchange transfusion

   b. Catheter size: 3.5 FR to 5 FR

   c. Calculation for approximate insertion distance (low-lying UAC):

   (1) (distance [cm] between umbilicus and shoulder ÷ 2/3) + 1 cm

   (2) BW [kg] + 7 cm = distance in cm

   d. Calculation for approximate insertion distance (high-lying UAC):

   (1) (3 × BW [kg]) + 9 = distance in cm

   (2) See Figure 9.2.

   e. Procedure:

TABLE 9.3 Drug Infusion Calculations in μg, mg, or unit/kg/h

Ratio and proportion formula (two steps):

A. **Desired** μg*/kg/h × **weight** (kg) = **amount** μg*/h

B. Use ratio and proportion to calculate amount to add to intravenous fluid (IVF) eg, amount μg*/h :IV rate :: x μg*:total IVF

or

$$\frac{\text{Desired (amount/h)}}{\text{Have (IV rate)}} \times \text{Volume (total IVF)} = \text{Amount of drug to add to IVF}$$

A. **Desired** μg*/kg/h × **weight** (kg) = **amount** μg*/h

B. $\dfrac{\textbf{Amount } \mu g*/h}{\textbf{IV rate}}$ × **total IVF** in buretrol/syringe = amount of drug to add to IVF

---

*insert appropriate unit of measurement

Medication	Examples

Fentanyl   Infuse fentanyl at 2 μg/kg/h for a 2-kg infant and run at 1 mL/h.

Ratio and Proportion formula

A. **2** μg/kg/h × **2** kg = **4** μg/h

B. $\dfrac{4 \ \mu g/h}{1 \ mL/h}$ ∷ $\dfrac{\times \ \mu g}{50 \ mL \ IVF}$ = 200 μg added to make 50 mL IVF

or

$\dfrac{\text{Desired}}{\text{Have}}$ × Volume = Amount of drug to add to IVF

A. **2** μg/kg/h × **2** kg = **4** μg/h

B. $\dfrac{4 \ \mu g}{1 \ mL/h}$ × 50 mL IVF = 200 μg added to make 50 mL IVF

Insulin   Infuse regular insulin at 0.05 units/kg/h for a 2-kg infant and run at 1 mL/h.

Ratio and Proportion formula

A. **0.05** units/kg/h × **2** kg = **0.1** units/h

B. $\dfrac{0.1 \ \text{units/h}}{1 \ mL/h}$ ∷ $\dfrac{x \ \text{units}}{50 \ mL \ IVF}$ = 5 units added to make 50 mL IVF

or

$\dfrac{\text{Desired}}{\text{Have}}$ × Volume = Amount of drug to add to IVF

A. **0.05** units/kg/h × **2** kg = **0.1** units/h

B. $\dfrac{0.1 \ \text{units/h}}{1 \ mL/h}$ × 50 mL IVF = 5 units added to make 50 mL IVF

---

(1) Clean cord and surrounding skin with antimicrobial solution and drape the area.

(2) Tie umbilical tape around the base of the cord for hemostasis and cut the cord with a scalpel approximately 1 cm above the skin.

(3) Identify the appropriate vessel, carefully dilate it, and gently insert the catheter.

Nomogram for estimating surface area of infants and young children. To determine the surface area of the patient, draw a straight line between the point representing the height on the left vertical scale and the point representing the weight on the right vertical scale. The point at which this line intersects the middle vertical scale represents the patient's surface area in square meters. (Courtesy of Abbott Laboratories.)

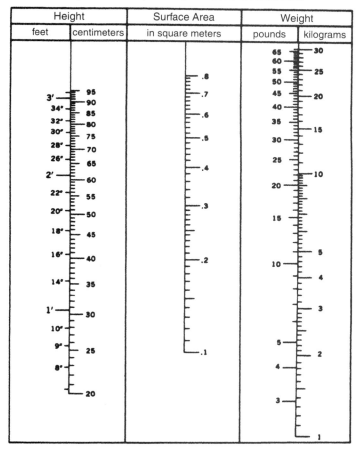

Figure 9.1. Body surface area nomogram. From Karch, A. (2003). *2003 Lippincott's nursing drug guide.* Philadelphia: Lippincott Williams & Wilkins.

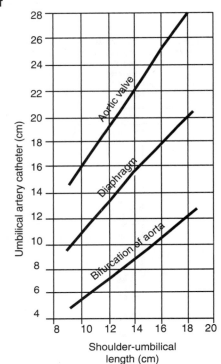

Figure 9.2. Umbilical artery catheter length. Used with permission from Siberry, G. K., & Iannone, R. (2000). *The Harriet Lane handbook.* (15th ed.). St. Louis: Mosby.

(4) Secure the catheter with suture and/or tape.

(5) Confirm proper catheter placement: aspirate blood from catheter; x-ray confirmation (UAC will enter the abdomen, dip down toward the legs, and then turn up toward to chest); *low placement* (tip of the catheter in the abdominal aorta at approximately *L 3-5*, ie, below the level of the mesenteric and renal arteries); and *high placement* (tip of the catheter in the descending aorta between *T 6-9*)

  f. Precautions:

(1) Do not use hyperosmolar solutions in the UAC.

(2) Add heparin (0.5–1 U/mL) to the intravenous fluid (IVF).

(3) After the sterile field is broken and the UAC secured, do not advance the catheter.

(4) Do not insert a UAC with documented omphalitis or suspected necrotizing enterocolitis or bowel hypoperfusion.

  g. Complications:

(1) Arterial compromise of lower extremities, bowel, or kidneys: cyanotic lower extremity or toes (warm the opposite leg; if the color remains cyanotic or the extremity

blanches, then remove the catheter); blanched lower extremity or toes (remove the catheter)

  (2) Hemorrhage secondary to arterial puncture or discon-nected tubing; thromboembolic accidents

  (3) Infection

3. Peripheral arterial catheterization (PAL):

  a. Indications: frequent blood sampling and continuous blood pressure (BP) monitoring

  b. Sites:

   (1) Radial artery (brachial artery should not be used sec-ondary to minimal collateral circulation and potential damage to the median nerve). Confirm intact ulnar artery by performing Allen's test before inserting catheter into radial artery (occlude radial and ulnar arteries until hand blanches; release pressure from ulnar artery; adequate collateral circulation is present when entire hand becomes pink in < 10 seconds).

   (2) Posterior tibial artery (reserve the femoral artery for use during emergencies)

  c. Procedure:

   (1) Locate the artery by either palpating or transilluminating the vessel.

   (2) Clean the area with antimicrobial solution.

   (3) Enter the artery at a 30° to 45° angle with a 22- or 24-gauge angiocatheter.

   (4) When blood return is noted, remove the stylet, flush the catheter, and secure with suture or tape.

   (5) Attach to continuous fluid infusion (eg, 0.45NSS with heparin 0.5–1 U/mL).

  d. Complications: arterial compromise to fingers or toes; thromboembolic accidents; hemorrhage secondary to discon-nected tubing; and an arterial blood gas (ABG) sample that contains too much heparin may falsely lower the pH and/or PCO_2 values.

B. Venous catheterization:

1. Umbilical venous catheterization (UVC) (Gomella, 1999; Roberts, 2000):

  a. Indications: emergency administration of medications and/or volume replacement; fluid administration; exchange transfu-sion; and central venous pressure monitoring

  b. Catheter size: 5 FR to 8 FR (single or double lumen); micro-premies may need 3.5 FR.

  c. Calculation for approximate insertion distance (Figure 9.3):

   (1) **(distance [cm] between umbilicus and shoulder ÷ 2/3) + 1 cm**

   (2) One half of the distance in cm of a high-lying UAC + 1 = distance in cm

  d. Procedure:

   (1) Clean cord and surrounding skin with antimicrobial solu-tion and drape the area.

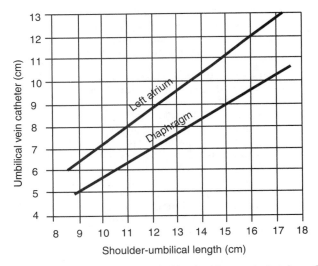

Figure 9.3. Umbilical vein catheter length. Used with permission from Siberry, G. K., & Iannone, R. (2000). *The Harriet Lane handbook.* (15th ed.). St. Louis: Mosby.

(2) Apply umbilical tape around the base of the cord for hemostasis and cut the cord with a scalpel approximately 1 cm above the skin.

(3) Identify the appropriate vessel, carefully dilate it, and gently insert the catheter. If the catheter "bounces" in the liver and cannot be advanced, attempt any one *or* all of the following: advance the catheter through the ductus venosus while flushing it with fluid; pass a second, smaller catheter (3.5 FR) over the first catheter while the first remains positioned in the liver; or apply gentle pressure over the right upper quadrant while advancing the catheter.

(4) Secure the UVC with suture and/or tape and obtain x-ray confirmation.

(5) Confirm proper catheter placement: easy blood withdrawal from catheter; chest and abdominal x-ray (the catheter will course straight into the abdomen and then up toward the chest); the tip of the catheter should be in the inferior vena cava approximately 0.5–1 cm above the diaphragm (~T9), ie, between the diaphragm and right atrium.

e. Complications: infection; thromboembolic accidents; hepatic damage; hemorrhage secondary to punctured vessel or disconnected catheters; and cardiac dysrhythmias secondary to misplaced catheters

2. Percutaneously inserted central catheter (PICC) (Gomella, 1999):

    a. Indications: long-term IV access for hyperalimentation or antimicrobial administration

    b. Procedure:

        (1) Locate a suitable vein (eg, cephalic and basilic veins in the arm or saphenous vein in the leg).

        (2) Measure the distance from the insertion site to the desired tip location (eg, superior vena cava for arm veins or inferior vena cava for leg veins).

        (3) Select the appropriate size catheter (length and gauge) for the size of the neonate.

        (4) Clean the skin with antimicrobial solution and drape the area.

        (5) Insert the introducer needle into the vein, confirm blood return, release the tourniquet, and advance the catheter through the introducer.

        (6) Remove the introducer from the vein, separate it in half, and insert the rest of the catheter.

        (7) Secure the catheter in place with a sterile dressing.

        (8) Remove the stylet wire from the catheter and infuse IV fluid.

        (9) Obtain x-ray confirmation.

    c. Precautions:

        (1) Use of hypertonic solutions is not recommended if the tip of the catheter is not centrally located.

        (2) Use 3-mL syringe to flush the line.

        (3) BP measurements on the extremity with the PICC line may occlude or damage the catheter.

        (4) Infusion of blood products through a small-gauge PICC may occlude the catheter.

        (5) Catheter removal: if the catheter does not come out readily, apply a warm compress to the area along the catheter tract, and then slowly withdraw the catheter; inspect and measure the catheter after removal to insure that the catheter is intact.

    d. Complications: infiltration (assess for swelling in the area where the tip of the catheter is supposed to be located); occlusion; infection; and air embolism

3. Intraosseous catheter placement (Gomella, 1999; Revenis, 1993; Roberts, 2000)

    a. Indications: vascular access via bone marrow cavity during emergencies when IV access is unavailable; infusion of IVF, blood products, and medications.

    b. Preferred sites:

        (1) Proximal anterior tibia approximately 2 cm below and 1–2 cm medial to the tibial tuberosity

        (2) Distal medial tibia approximately 1–2 cm above the medial malleolus

        (3) Distal anterior femur approximately 1–3 cm above the lateral condyle

    c. Needle sizes: bone marrow aspiration needle (18 gauge); short spinal needle (18–20 gauge); short hypodermic needle (18–20 gauge); or butterfly needle (16–19 gauge)

     d. Procedure:

       (1) Clean the area with antimicrobial solution.

       (2) Anesthetize the area down to the periosteum with 1% lidocaine.

       (3) Insert the needle and, at an angle that is slightly less than perpendicular to the skin and with the tip pointing away from the growth plate and/or joint, advance approximately 1 cm. (Do not advance the catheter if a sudden decrease in resistance is felt.)

       (4) Remove the stylet and tape securely in place.

     e. Confirmation of placement: needle stands upright without support; bone marrow aspiration (may not be possible with smaller bore needles); no detectable subcutaneous infiltration when the needle is flushed with normal saline solution (NSS)

     f. Precautions: dilute hypertonic or alkaline solutions (1:2) with NSS; to decrease the possibility of infection use this method for < 4 hours.

     g. Complications: fat embolism; fracture; infiltration of fluid into the subcutaneous tissue or subperiosteum; osteomyelitis, cellulitis; and subcutaneous abscess

   4. Saphenous venipuncture (Short, 1993):

     a. Indications: blood collection for diagnostic studies

     b. Site: medial aspect of the thigh

     c. Needle size: 23- or 25-gauge butterfly

     d. Procedure:

       (1) Clean the area with antimicrobial solution.

       (2) Place the infant supine with the leg flexed at the knee and hip flexed and abducted (frog-leg position). Locate and palpate the groove between the medial border of the sartorius muscle and the lateral border of adductor longus muscle. The insertion site is approximately halfway up the thigh from the knee.

       (3) Enter the skin at a 60° to 90° angle and gently advance the needle while applying suction until blood return is obtained.

       (4) Remove needle and apply pressure for several minutes.

     e. Precautions:

       (1) Avoid venipuncture if there is a local infection.

       (2) Do not proceed if there is a coagulopathy.

     f. Complications: deep vein thrombosis; hemorrhage; and femoral artery laceration

C. Thoracentesis (needle aspiration) and chest tube placement (thoracostomy drainage) (Fletcher & Eichelberger, 1993; Gomella, 1999; Roberts, 2000):

   1. Indications: relief of pneumothorax that is contributing to respiratory compromise and/or cardiovascular collapse; drain pleural effusion (eg, hemothorax, chylothorax, or empyema); pleural drainage after surgical intervention (eg, thoracic, cardiac, esophageal, or vascular problems); or obtain fluid for diagnostic studies.

2. Insertion sites:
   a. Anterior tubes inserted at the first to third anterior midclavicular intercostal space evacuate free air.
   b. Posterior tubes inserted at the fourth to sixth mid to anterior axillary intercostal space evacuate pleural fluid. **(Nipple is located approximately at the fourth intercostal space.)**
3. Drainage devices:
   a. 23-gauge butterfly or 22-gauge angiocatheter for thoracentesis
   b. 8-FR to 12-FR chest tube for thoracostomy drainage
4. Procedure:
   a. Document the need for needle aspiration and/or chest tube insertion with a chest x-ray (anteroposterior [AP] *and* cross-table lateral or left lateral decubitus view).
   b. Needle aspiration of a tension pneumothorax:
      (1) Place infant in supine position.
      (2) Clean the skin with antimicrobial solution.
      (3) Insert a 23-gauge butterfly or 22-gauge angiocatheter (attached to a stopcock and 10–20 mL syringe) at the second intercostal midclavicular space.
      (4) Aspirate free air.
      (5) *Chest tube insertion may still be necessary in the presence of persistent lung disease and/or positive pressure ventilation.*
   c. Chest tube insertion:
      (1) Place the infant in the appropriate position (supine for anterior chest tube placement *or* lateral decubitus with affected side up and arm extended above the head for posterior chest tube placement).
      (2) Clean the skin with antimicrobial solution and drape the area.
      (3) Anesthetize the area down to the level of the pleura with 0.5% to 1% lidocaine.
      (4) Make a small incision with a scalpel blade (approximately the width of the chest tube) one intercostal space below the desired insertion site.
      (5) Spread the tissues with a curved hemostat down to the level of the rib.
      (6) Puncture the pleura with the hemostats or trocar *over the top of the rib* at the desired intercostal space and carefully slide chest tube into the pleural space (listen for a rush of air as the pleural cavity is entered).
      (7) Suture chest tube in place and apply an occlusive dressing.
      (8) Attach the chest tube to negative-pressure vacuum drainage (−10- to −30-cm H_2O seal).
      (9) Confirm placement with AP and lateral chest x-rays.
5. Complications: infection; bleeding; intercostal nerve damage; parenchymal lung damage; and punctured diaphragm, liver, or spleen

D. Lumbar puncture (LP) (Gomella, 1999; Marban, 1993):

1. Indications: diagnose central nervous system (CNS) infection (eg, meningitis), subarachnoid hemorrhage, or malignancy; administration of intrathecal antimicrobial or chemotherapeutic medications; evaluation of the efficacy of pharmacotherapy for CNS infection; and serial LPs for drainage of cerebrospinal fluid (CSF) in the treatment of hydrocephalus

2. Contraindications: anomalous lumbosacral region; bleeding diathesis (eg, platelet count < 50,000); cardiorespiratory instability; documented or suspected infection around the puncture site; and increased intracranial pressure (ICP)

3. Insertion sites:
   a. Use L4-L5 and L3-L4 interspaces. **(L4 vertebral body is located along a line drawn between the iliac crests.)**
   b. To avoid spinal cord damage, **do not use interspaces above L3**.

4. Needle size: short, 22-gauge spinal needle (with stylet)

5. Procedure:
   a. Position infant in a lateral recumbent *or* sitting position with spine flexed.
   b. Clean the skin with an antimicrobial solution and drape the area.
   c. Anesthetize the area with 1% lidocaine.
   d. Insert needle midline, just below the palpated spinous process, and direct the needle cephalad toward the umbilicus (a "pop" may be felt as the needle punctures the dura).
   e. Remove the stylet and collect CSF (~ 1 mL for each tube) for the appropriate diagnostic studies.
   (1) Tube 1—culture and gram stain.
   (2) Tube 2—glucose and protein.
   (3) Tube 3—cell count and differential.
   (4) Tube 4—optional.
   f. Replace the stylet and remove spinal needle.

6. Complications: infection or bleeding; herniation through the foramen magnum secondary to ICP; and epidermal spinal cord tumor

E. Pericardiocentesis (Fletcher and Eichelberger, 1993; Gomella, 1999):

1. Indications: relief of cardiac tamponade secondary to pericardial effusion or pneumopericardium **(signs of tamponade include distant heart sounds, bradycardia, hypotension, decreased electrocardiogram [ECG] voltage, and "halo" around heart on transillumination or x-ray);** obtaining pericardial fluid for diagnostic studies

2. Insertion site: ~ 0.5 cm to the left or below the xiphoid process

3. Needle size: 20- to 24-gauge catheter (with stylet) with stopcock and syringe

4. Procedure:
   a. Place infant in supine.
   b. Clean skin with antimicrobial solution and drape the area.
   c. Anesthetize the area with 1% lidocaine.

  d. Insert the catheter at a 30° to 45° angle to the skin, pointing the tip toward the left scapula (apply constant suction to the attached syringe during the insertion).

  e. Remove the stylet from the catheter and aspirate fluid or air until vital signs stabilize.

  f. Remove catheter *or*, for short-term continuous pericardial drainage, tape in place and attach to continuous suction.

  g. Obtain chest x-ray to confirm placement.

  5. Complications: punctured heart, lung, and liver; pneumothorax, pneumopericardium, or hemopericardium; and infection

F. Paracentesis (Gomella, 1999; Roberts, 2000):

  1. Indications: peritoneal fluid removal for diagnostic studies and/or to improve ventilation

  2. Site: "lateral to the rectus muscle in the right or left lower quadrants, a few centimeters above the inguinal ligament" (Roberts, 2000, p. 62)

  3. Needle size: 22- to 25-gauge angiocatheter

  4. Procedure:

  a. Position infant supine and restrain the legs.

  b. Clean the skin with antimicrobial solution and drape the area.

  c. Insert the catheter (Z-track fashion) in the appropriate site and apply continuous suction to the attached syringe while advancing the catheter.

  d. When fluid is noted, remove the stylet, reattach the syringe, and slowly withdraw the amount required for studies and/or to improve ventilation.

  e. Remove the catheter and cover with a sterile dressing.

  5. Complications: hypotension secondary to rapid or excessive fluid withdrawal; bowel perforation; bladder perforation; and peritoneal fluid leak from insertion site

G. Suprapubic tap:

  1. Indications: urine collection for urinalysis or culture when bladder catheterization is not possible

  2. Puncture site: "~ 0.5–1 cm above the pubic symphysis, in the midline of the lower abdomen" (Gomella, 1999, p. 156)

  3. Needle size: 22- to 25-gauge × 1-inch butterfly

  4. Procedure:

  a. Place infant supine with legs in frog-leg position.

  b. Clean the skin with antimicrobial solution.

  c. Insert needle at a 90° angle and aspirate while advancing the needle.

  d. Withdraw urine and send for appropriate diagnostic studies.

  e. Remove needle and apply pressure to the puncture site.

  5. Complications: puncture of the posterior bladder wall; bleeding (rare and usually transient) (do not perform procedure if there is a low platelet count); and bowel perforation if landmarks are not properly identified

▼ References

Briars, G. L., & Bailey, B. J. R. (1994). Surface area estimation: Pocket calculator v. nomogram. *Archives of Disease in Childhood, 70*(3), 246–247.

Conner, G. K. (1993). Abdomen assessment. In E. P. Tappero & M. E. Honeyfield (Eds.), *Physical assessment of the newborn: A comprehensive approach to the art of physical examination* (pp. 81–90). Petaluma, CA: NICU Ink.

Fletcher, M. A., & Eichelberger, M. R. (1993). Thoracostomy tubes. In M. A. Fletcher & M. G. MacDonald (Eds.), *Atlas of procedures in neonatology* (2nd ed., pp. 309–333). Philadelphia: Lippincott.

Gomella, T. L. (1999). Section II: Procedures. In T. L. Gomella, M. D. Cunningham, F. G. Eyal, & K. E. Zenk (Eds.), *Neonatology: Management, procedures, on-call problems, diseases, drugs* (4th ed., pp. 148–190). Stamford, CT: Appleton & Lange.

MacDonald, M. (1993). Umbilical artery catheterization. In M. A. Fletcher & M. G. MacDonald (Eds.), *Atlas of procedures in neonatology* (2nd ed., pp. 155–174). Philadelphia: Lippincott.

Marban, S. L. (1993). Lumbar puncture. In M. A. Fletcher & M. G. Macdonald (Eds.), *Atlas of procedures in neonatology* (2nd ed., pp. 109–114). Philadelphia: Lippincott.

Revenis, M. E. (1993). Intraosseous infusions. In M. A. Fletcher & M. G. MacDonald (Eds.), *Atlas of procedures in neonatology* (2nd ed., pp. 398–401). Philadelphia: Lippincott.

Roberts, W. B. (2000). Procedures. In G. K. Siberry & R. Iannone (Eds.), *The Harriet Lane handbook* (15th ed., pp. 43–71.). St. Louis: Mosby.

Short, B. L. (1993). Venipuncture. In M. A. Fletcher & M. G. MacDonald (Eds.), *Atlas of procedures in neonatology* (2nd ed., pp. 87–91). Philadelphia: Lippincott.

Young, T. E., & Mangum, B. (Eds.), (2001). *Neofax, 2001* (14th ed). Raleigh, NC: Acorn Publishing.

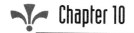

Chapter 10

Infectious Diseases

Cynthia J. Kelley, MSN, RNC, NNP

Infection in the neonatal period may be acquired congenitally, perinatally, and/or nosocomially. **Handwashing by health care personnel *before* and *after* contact with patients is the single most important measure in the prevention of infection.**

I. **Congenital infections** (Gonik, 1994; Remington & Klein, 2001):
- A. Modes of transmission:
  1. Ascending infection from the cervix
  2. Transplacental passage of blood-borne pathogens from the mother's bloodstream
  3. Spread of local infection from nearby tissues and organs such as the peritoneum, gastrointestinal (GI) tract, or fallopian tubes
  4. Invasive procedures for diagnosis and fetal therapy may introduce organisms that infect the fetus.
  5. Before membranes rupture, organisms can invade via microscopic defects in the membranes.
- B. Take a careful maternal history that elicits the following information (Gonik, 1994):
  1. Recent or current flu-like symptoms (eg, arthralgia, rash, and fever) or swollen lymph nodes?
  2. Exposure to chickenpox or exanthematous illnesses (eg, fifth disease)?
  3. Place of employment (eg, cytomegalovirus [CMV] exposure is common among daycare workers)?
  4. Does mother eat raw meat, own a cat, or work at gardening?
  5. Is there an illicit drug history?
  6. Maternal rubella titer?
- C. Common congenital infections (listed alphabetically) (Table 10.1).
  1. *Chlamydia trachomatis* (obligate intracellular bacteria) (Fanaroff & Martin, 2002; Remington & Klein, 2001):
     - a. Transmission: sexual contact; vertical transmission during vaginal delivery; small risk for infants born by cesarean section, unless there is rupture of membranes; incubation period is 5 to 14 days.
     - b. Clinical manifestations:
       - (1) Neonatal conjunctivitis (with persistent conjunctivitis, neovascularization of the cornea and scarring ensues): presents after the first week of life, up to 3 weeks of age; watery discharge that becomes purulent; swollen eyelids; and red thickened conjunctiva; pseudomembrane of the conjunctiva

TABLE 10.1 TORCHES: Acroynm for Congenital Infections

Acronym Letter	Infection
T	*Toxoplasma gondii*
O	Other: AIDS/HIV, chickenpox (varicella-zoster virus), Chlamydia, Gonorrhea, hepatitis B, Parvovirus B19, and Ureaplasma
R	Rubella
C	Cytomegalovirus
H	Herpes simplex virus
E	Echoviruses
S	Syphilis (*Treponema pallidum*)

(2) Pneumonia (occurs with or without conjunctivitis): presents 4 to 11 weeks after birth; nasal congestion and obstruction, paroxysmal staccato cough, rales, tachypnea, apnea, bilateral infiltrates on x-ray, and abnormal arterial blood gas (ABG) (mild to moderate hypoxemia); and increased eosinophil count

c. Diagnosis:
  (1) Conjunctivitis: giemsa-stained conjunctival scrapings of the lower conjunctiva to obtain cells with inclusion bodies diagnostic of chlamydial infection; and chlamydial antigen detection (direct fluorescent antibody [DFA] method). Be aware of the possibility of a double infection (eg, *Neisseria gonorrhoeae*, herpes simplex, and pyogenic conjunctivitis).
  (2) Pneumonia: culture or DFA of tracheal secretions or nasopharyngeal aspirate; significant increase in IgM antibody levels

d. Interventions:
  (1) Conjunctivitis: 2 weeks of oral erythromycin 50 mg/kg/day (Remington & Klein, 2001)
  (2) Pneumonia: erythromycin 50 mg/kg/day orally in divided doses; supportive therapy
  (3) The infant's mother and sexual partner should be treated.

e. Outcome:
  (1) Conjunctivitis: untreated cases may clear without complications; superficial corneal vascularization and conjunctival scarring possible if left untreated
  (2) Pneumonia: more serious and prolonged illness if untreated; higher risk of developing chronic respiratory problems

2. Chickenpox (varicella-zoster) (a member of the herpesvirus family) (Gonik, 1994; Pickering, 2000; Remington & Klein, 2001):
  a. Transmission:
    (1) Transplacental passage during maternal varicella infection; droplet and airborne transmission of infected nasopharyngeal secretions from one individual to another

onto the nasal, oral, or conjunctival mucosa; and direct contact with infected vesicular fluid.

(2) Individuals are most contagious for 1 to 2 days before and shortly after the rash presents. Contagion persists until the lesions crust over. The incubation period is usually 14 to 16 days. Neonates born to mothers with active infection; varicella can develop between 1 and 16 days of life. There is typically a 9- to 15-day interval from outbreak of rash in a mother to onset in her infant.

b. Congenital varicella syndrome (Gonik, 1994; Long, Pickering, & Prober, 1997): the timing of the initial infection affects the spectrum of congenital defects seen. Most cases occur in infants infected between 8 and 20 weeks' gestation. Clinical manifestations include:

(1) Skin: cutaneous defects, cicatricial scars, hypopigmentation, and bullous lesions

(2) Extremities: hypoplastic limb, muscular atrophy and denervation, joint abnormalities, and absent or malformed digits

(3) Eye: chorioretinitis, microphthalmia, and anisocoria

(4) Central nervous system (CNS): intrauterine encephalitis with cortical atrophy, seizures, and mental retardation

(5) Urinary tract: hydronephrosis/hydroureter

(6) GI: esophageal dilation/reflux

c. Neonatal varicella (up to 25% mortality rate): greatest risk of infection in infants born to mothers exposed to varicella or with clinical manifestations of disease within 2 weeks of delivery; severity of neonatal illness correlates with the development of maternal IgG and passive transfer of antibody protection; varicella immune globulin administration within 1 day of life improves neonatal disease and reduces infant mortality for those infants born to mothers with active infection. Clinical manifestations include:

(1) Fever may develop within the first days of life followed by vesicular eruption.

(2) Disseminated cutaneous disease and/or visceral involvement may occur.

(3) Rash may become confluent and hemorrhagic.

(4) Pulmonary involvement with cyanosis and hypoxia

d. Diagnosis: tissue culture from vesicle; DFA of vesicle scraping—scraping must include epithelial cells from the base of a newly formed vesicle; serum IgM, IgG (detectable within 3 days in most patients and increases during recovery period); and polymerase chain reaction (PCR) of body fluid or tissue

e. Interventions:

(1) VZIG (varicella-zoster immunoglobulin) for neonates whose mothers develop varicella ≤ 4 days before delivery or 2 days after delivery

(2) Delay delivery, if possible, in cases of late gestational maternal varicella infection to allow transfer of maternal IgG antibodies.

      (3) Isolate infant from other patients to prevent nosocomial spread.

      (4) Isolate infant from the mother until mother's lesions have crusted over to prevent neonatal infection.

      (5) Acyclovir intravenous (IV) therapy

3. CMV (member of the herpes family of DNA viruses) (Gonik, 1994; Remington & Klein, 2001):

    a. Transmission: transplacental passage any time during pregnancy; more likely to occur and to cause fetal injury with primary maternal infection than with recurrent infections

    b. Clinical manifestations: > 90% CMV infections in normal healthy individuals are asymptomatic. Symptoms include: intrauterine growth restriction (IUGR); hepatic damage (jaundice [direct hyperbilirubinemia] and abnormal liver function studies; petechiae or purpura; and thrombocytopenia); pneumonia; and CNS effects (lethargy, poor feeding, microcephaly, intracranial calcifications, chorioretinitis, deafness, and seizures)

    c. Diagnosis: rapid immunofluorescent assay of urine

    d. Interventions:

      (1) Head ultrasound, ophthalmologic examination, and hearing test

      (2) Pharmacotherapy: Ganciclovir and Foscavir have been evaluated in clinical trials and may be considered for use in select patients.

    e. Outcome:

      (1) 85% of infants are asymptomatic at birth; 17% of these infants suffer sequelae that include hearing loss and neurodevelopmental problems.

      (2) CMV is the most common cause of mental retardation and nonhereditary sensorineural deafness. Most symptomatic infants will have mild to severe handicaps.

      (3) The risk of sequelae is much less for infants born after recurrent maternal infection.

4. Enteroviruses (small single-stranded RNA virus) (Gonik, 1994; Pickering, 2000; Remington & Klein, 2001):

    a. Non-polio enteroviral infections (group A and B coxsackieviruses, echoviruses, and enteroviruses)

    b. Transmission: transplacental spread is rare but may occur with significant maternal viremia. Infant may acquire infection during vaginal delivery from a colonized colon or cervix; severity of infant's illness depends upon the amount of antiviral antibody acquired transplacentally or from breast milk; the incubation period is 3 to 6 days.

    c. Clinical manifestations:

      (1) General: presents with sepsis "picture" (difficult to distinguish from bacterial infection).

      (2) Cardiac, respiratory, and hepatic function may be affected in severe cases.

      (3) Effects associated with specific viral strains: group A coxsackievirus (generally benign); group B coxsackievirus (small risk of cardiac or GI anomalies); echovirus (most serious infection, especially if it occurs immediately before delivery [known cause of stillbirth])

d. Diagnosis:

(1) Clinical history: history of maternal illness and symptoms; consider season of the year, geographic location, exposure, incubation period, and clinical symptoms.

(2) Laboratory: viral cultures (nose, throat, stool, blood, urine, cerebrospinal fluid [CSF], and other body fluids); rapid identification using polymerase chain reaction (PCR) methods

e. Interventions:

(1) No specific therapy for the treatment of enteroviruses

(2) IVIG may be of some benefit in immunosuppressed patients.

(3) Supportive measures

5. Hepatitis B (HBV) (small DNA virus) (Gonik, 1994; Pickering 2000; Remington & Klein, 2001):

a. Transmission:

(1) Contact with infected blood or body fluids (eg, semen, saliva)

(2) Maternal-fetal (transplacental or at the time of birth)

(3) Acute HBV infection: most infants become infected by transmission in the third trimester or near the time of delivery.

(4) Interpersonal contact over extended periods

(5) Transmission of perinatal HBV infection is preventable in 95% of cases by early active and passive immunization of infants.

(6) Incubation period is 1 to 6 months. The virus can survive at ambient room temperatures on household surfaces for 1 week or longer.

(7) Mothers positive for both hepatitis B surface antigen (HBsAG) and hepatitis B e antigen (HBeAG) are at greatest risk for transmitting the virus.

b. Clinical manifestations: usually a benign disease in neonates although fulminant fatal neonatal hepatitis has been described

c. Maternal screening and neonatal diagnosis is made on serologic testing (Pickering, 2000):

(1) *HBsAG* positive: indicates HBV is present; patient is infectious; earliest marker; antigen used in hepatitis B vaccine

(2) *HBeAG* positive: infectious (high degree of infectivity); generally persists 3 to 6 weeks; beyond 10 weeks is indicative of a carrier state.

(3) Hepatitis B antibody to surface antigen (*anti-HBs*) positive: indicates immunity to HBV; occurs from infection or vaccine; usually not present in carriers

(4) Hepatitis B core antibody (*Anti-HBc*) positive: indicates past or current HBV infection; does not develop in response to vaccine.

(5) IgM antibody to core antigen (*IgM Anti-HBc*): indicates acute or recent HBV infection (including HBsAG-negative persons during "window" phase of infection).

(6) Antibody to HBe (*Anti-Hbe*): identifies HBsAG carriers; low infectivity.

d. Interventions (Pickering, 2000):

(1) HBV-positive mothers: treat infant (term and preterm) with hepatitis B vaccine (recombinant) **and** hepatitis B immunoglobulin (HBIG) within 12 hours of life; in preterm infants this initial dose should *not* be counted in the required 3-dose vaccine series.

(2) HBV-unknown mothers:

(a) Term infants: give hepatitis B vaccine within 12 hours of life. If the mother's status is determined to be HBsAG positive, HBIG should be given as soon as possible, but not after 7 days of life.

(b) Preterm infants: < 2 kg (give hepatitis B vaccine within 12 hours of life and **HBIG within 12 hours of life** if the mother's status cannot be determined within this time period); > 2 kg (give hepatitis B vaccine within 12 hours of life and **HBIG within 7 days of birth** only if the mother's status is determined to be positive)

(3) HBV-negative mothers: routine immunization for all infants—refer to American Academy of Pediatrics (AAP)/Advisory Committee on Immunization Practices (ACIP) immunization schedule. Preterm infants should receive their first hepatitis B vaccine when they are ≥ 2 kg.

(4) Other measures to reduce vertical transmission: elective cesarean section in HBeAg-positive pregnant HBsAg carrier; gentle resuscitation to eliminate trauma that would create a portal of entry; gastric aspiration to remove infected fluid; avoidance of breastfeeding (it is essential to weigh the risk:benefit ratio); avoid the use of fetal scalp electrodes; screen for HBsAG in pregnant women; and standard precautions for hospitalized patients

(5) Infants born to HBsAG-positive mothers and receive hepatitis B vaccine and HBIG should be tested for anti-HBs and HBsAG 1 to 3 months after completion of the immunization series.

e. Outcome: the risk of chronic infection for a child infected in the newborn period, in the absence of immunoprophylaxis, is 70% to 90% (Gonik, 1994); 25% to 30% of carriers ultimately die as a result of long-term sequelae of HBV (eg, primary hepatocellular carcinoma; cirrhosis; chronic active hepatitis).

6. Herpes simplex virus (HSV) (large double-stranded DNA virus) (Remington & Klein, 2001):

a. Transmission:

(1) Intrapartum (85% to 90% of cases): exposure to active lesions during delivery

(2) In utero: transplacental or ascending infection (premature rupture of membranes [PROM] increases the risk for ascending infection)

(3) Postnatal exposure to persons with active orolabial herpes and transmitted by respiratory droplets or direct contact

(4) Primary maternal HSV infection: 50% infection rate in the neonate

(5) The transmission rate is 2% to 5% for recurrent infection or asymptomatic shedding of HSV during pregnancy.

b. Clinical manifestations:

(1) Usually present in the first 1 to 2 weeks of life; ranges from 24 hours after birth to 4 to 6 weeks postnatally.

(2) Symptoms are usually nonspecific; may involve multiple organ systems and mimic enteroviral disease or bacterial sepsis. Initial symptoms include irritability, seizures, respiratory distress, jaundice, bleeding diathesis, and shock. May or may not have skin lesions.

(3) Classification of neonatal HSV infection: localized disease (15%) (skin, eye, or mouth disease); encephalitis (15%) with/without skin, eyes, and/or mouth involvement (fatal in 50% of cases when untreated); disseminated disease (70%) (involves multiple organs); asymptomatic infection (rare in newborns)

c. Diagnosis: direct immunofluorescent stain of lesion scrapings for rapid identification; viral cultures of skin lesions (obtain cells from the base of the lesion; PCR of spinal fluid to detect viral DNA; virus may also be isolated from stool, urine, throat, nasopharynx, and conjunctivae; and platelet counts, CSF analysis, and liver function tests aid in determining a disease classification.

d. Interventions (Pickering, 2000):

(1) Supportive care

(2) Pharmacotherapy: Acyclovir 60 mg/kg/day, IV, divided every 8 hours for 14 to 21 days depending upon disease classification

(3) Topical ophthalmic drug for ocular involvement (in addition to IV acyclovir)

(4) Isolation of affected infant to prevent nosocomial transmission

e. Outcome:

(1) Kerato-conjunctivitis can progress to chorioretinitis, cataracts, and retinal detachment.

(2) Neurologic impairment (even for localized disease); spastic quadriplegia; microcephaly; blindness; porencephalic cysts; hydranencephaly; hearing loss

(3) Recurrent skin lesions

7. HIV (human RNA retroviruses, HIV type-1 and HIV type-2 [less common]) (Fanaroff & Martin 2002; Pickering, 2000; Remington & Klein, 2001; Young & Magnum, 2002):

a. Transmission:

(1) Through contact with infected blood, semen, cervical secretions, and human milk; vertical transmission before or around the time of birth; breastfeeding; and percutaneous or mucous membrane exposure to contaminated blood or body fluids

(2) Increased risk for perinatally acquired infection with the following: mothers who seroconvert during pregnancy or postpartum and are breastfeeding; advanced maternal HIV disease; first-born twin who is delivered vaginally; prolonged rupture of membranes (ROM); and operative delivery (eg, forceps, vacuum)

(3) The median age for onset of symptoms is 12 to 18 months for untreated perinatally infected infants.

b. Clinical manifestations (Pickering, 2000; Remington & Klein, 2001): most infants are asymptomatic at birth (signs and symptoms begin to appear within the first 1 to 2 years of life; *rapid progressors* who have very high viral loads early in life become symptomatic within a month or 2 after delivery); preterm delivery; growth delay, failure to thrive, and developmental delays; and infections that are serious and/or life-threatening and are recurrent (bacterial, viral, fungal, and protozoal)

c. Diagnosis: HIV testing for pregnant women to identify at-risk population. Recommended evaluation for asymptomatic infants born to HIV-positive mothers (or mothers who are in a high-risk category) includes:

(1) Complete blood count (CBC), serum chemistry, and liver function studies

(2) HIV DNA PCR during the first 48 hours of life (do not perform on cord blood due to potential contamination with maternal blood). Repeat test at 1 to 2 months and again at 3 to 6 months of age.

(3) Positive tests should be repeated to confirm the diagnosis; two separate positive samples are indicative of congenital infection.

(4) Urine for CMV (refer to the *American Academy of Pediatrics Red Book* for information on specific diagnostic criteria and categorization of HIV infection)

d. Interventions:

(1) Care of the mother: follow Centers for Disease Control (CDC) guidelines for gestational antiretroviral prophylaxis to lower the maternal viral load and reduce the risk of vertical transmission.

(2) Care of the neonate exposed to HIV in utero: begin a 6-week course of prophylactic zidovudine (refer to a neonatal medication manual for dosing); monitor CBC during zidovudine therapy for anemia, thrombocytopenia, and neutropenia; at 4 to 6 weeks of life begin prophylaxis for pneumocystis carinii pneumonia (PCP) and continue for 1 year; trimethoprim-sulfamethoxazole 75 mg/m^2/dose, twice a day, 3 days a week (Fanaroff & Martin, 2002); rou-

tine immunization schedule (**use killed injectable polio vaccine [IPV] in place of live attenuated oral preparation [OPV]**)

  e. Outcome: believed to be uniformly fatal; median survival of infected children is 8 to 13 years.

8. *N. gonorrhea* (GC) (gram-negative diplococcus) (Fanaroff & Martin, 2002; Pickering, 2000; Remington & Klein, 2001):

  a. Transmission: neonatal infection usually occurs during passage through the birth canal; may occur in utero after rupture of membranes; 2- to 7-day incubation period.

  b. Clinical manifestations:

   (1) May be asymptomatic in pregnant women.

   (2) Gonococcal ophthalmia neonatorum (can result in blindness if untreated)

   (3) Mucosal disease: vaginitis (rare) and urethritis (rare); anorectal; rhinitis; umbilical cord infection (funisitis); scalp abscess

   (4) Septic arthritis: onset 1 to 4 weeks after delivery; polyarticular involvement; decreased limb movement (pseudoparalysis)

   (5) Systemic disease is rare except for septic arthritis.

   (6) Preterm delivery

  c. Diagnosis: routine prenatal screening; gram stain and culture of conjunctival exudate; cultures of oropharynx and anal canal if gram-stain of conjunctival exudate suspicious for gonorrhea; evaluate for other sexually transmitted diseases (STDs).

  d. Interventions:

   (1) Infants born to GC-positive mother (Remington & Klein, 2001): single dose of ceftriaxone (50 mg/kg IV or intramuscularly [IM], not to exceed 125 mg); give with caution to infants with elevated bilirubin, especially preterm infants.

   (2) Infants *with* gonococcal infection (Remington & Klein, 2001):

    (a) Gonococcal ophthalmia: irrigate eyes with saline to eliminate discharge; ceftriaxone 25–50 mg/kg/day IV or IM once daily × 7 days *or* cefotaxime 25 mg/kg IV or IM every 12 hours × 7 days

    (b) Disseminated infection (arthritis and septicemia): evaluate for disseminated infection (blood and CSF cultures); ceftriaxone

   (3) Ophthalmic prophylaxis immediately postpartum (within 1 hour of birth) with one of the following: 1% silver nitrate in a single-dose ampule; 0.5% erythromycin ophthalmic ointment in single-use tubes; 1% tetracycline ophthalmic ointment in single-use tubes

9. Parvovirus B19 (erythema infectiosum or fifth disease) (small single-stranded DNA virus) (Gonik, 1994; Fanaroff & Martin, 2002; Remington & Klein, 2001):

  a. Transmission: transplacental passage

   b. Clinical manifestations:
      (1) Fetal death rate of < 10% (most often when < 20 weeks' gestation at time of infection)
      (2) Prematurity; small for gestational age (SGA)
      (3) Nonimmune hydrops secondary to either severe aplastic anemia and/or myocarditis as a fetus. Intrauterine transfusions to correct anemia may improve survival. One third of cases resolve spontaneously, resulting in a healthy infant.
      (4) Severe anemia and thrombocytopenia; altered hepatic function; extramedullary hematopoiesis
      (5) Hypoxic injury; high-output heart failure; myocarditis; ascites; organomegaly
      (6) Respiratory distress
   c. Diagnosis: history of a rash illness or arthropathy during pregnancy (often asymptomatic); (antibody assays [anti-B19 IgM and IgG] and B19 DNA detection by PCR)
   d. Interventions: supportive therapy based on infant's clinical presentation
10. Rubella virus (German measles) (single-stranded RNA virus) (Gonik, 1994; Remington & Klein, 2001):
   a. Transmission: transplacental passage highest during the first and third trimesters but can occur at any time during pregnancy. Incubation period from 14 to 21 days. More severe disease in the fetus/newborn when acquired before 8 weeks' gestation; minimal risk of congenital anomalies if infection occurs after 17 weeks.
   b. Clinical manifestations:
      (1) Hepatosplenomegaly; hepatitis; jaundice; thrombocytopenia with petechiae and purpura; dermal erythropoiesis (**"blueberry-muffin" lesions**); hemolytic anemia; chronic rash
      (2) Adenopathy; meningoencephalitis; large anterior fontanel; cloudy cornea
      (3) Interstitial pneumonia; myocarditis; diarrhea; disturbances in bone growth
   c. Diagnosis: serologic testing
   d. Interventions:
      (1) No medication available to decrease transplacental transmission
      (2) Prevention with appropriate vaccination following established guidelines
      (3) Long-term follow-up recommended for infants exposed after 12 weeks' gestation to detect subtle late-appearing abnormalities (eg, hearing loss, mental impairment)
   e. Fetal/neonatal outcomes:
      (1) Bilateral sensorineural deafness
      (2) Microcephaly, mental and motor retardation, and IUGR
      (3) Cardiac anomalies: patent ductus arteriosus (PDA), pulmonary artery stenosis, and pulmonary valve stenosis

    (4) Ocular anomalies: cataracts, retinopathy, and microphthalmia

11. Syphilis (*Treponema pallidum*) (spirochete) (Long, Pickering, & Prober, 1997; Pickering, 2000; Remington & Klein, 2001)

    a. Transmission: transplacental passage any time during pregnancy or at birth

    b. Early-onset disease (transplacental transmission):

        (1) 60% of infected infants are asymptomatic at birth; symptoms can appear anytime in the first 2 years of life.

        (2) Infections are typically widespread, causing an inflammatory response with fibrosis of organ tissues.

        (3) No primary or chancre stage occurs with congenitally acquired syphilis.

        (4) Presenting symptoms include: prematurity; IUGR; pneumonia; nonimmune hydrops fetalis; lymphadenopathy; clear nasal discharge (very infectious); hepatosplenomegaly and elevated liver enzymes; skeletal abnormality (symmetric; involves long bones; osteochondritis; pseudoparalysis due to pain); skin involvement (maculopapular rash that changes from erythematous to coppery color; vesiculobullous lesions; petechiae); CNS (abnormal CSF; abnormal neurologic symptoms not usually present); and hematologic (anemia; elevated white blood cell [WBC] with monocytosis; thrombocytopenia)

    c. Late-onset disease: seen in patients over 2 years of age and not contagious; symptoms result from growth disturbances in organs and chronic inflammation.

    d. Diagnosis:

        (1) Screening test on mother early in pregnancy and at delivery (rapid plasma reagin [RPR], Venereal Disease Research Laboratory [VDRL]). Repeat screen in third trimester in high-risk population (those recently infected may not test positive).

        (2) **A careful review of the mother's history and the infant's physical examination is vital to diagnosis.**

        (3) Infant quantitative serologic test (RPR, VDRL) if born to mother with positive test. If nontreponemal test (RPR, VDRL) is reactive, a treponemal test (fluorescent treponemal antibody absorption [FTA-ABS] or microhemagglutination-Treponema pallidum [MHA-TP]) is usually done. Infant titer two- to fourfold greater than that of the mother is indicative of infection. A titer equal to or less than that of mother does not exclude infection.

        (4) Work-up for infant suspected of having congenital syphilis: x-rays of long bones; CSF analysis; VDRL (if positive, obtain serum treponemal test); examination of placenta and amniotic fluid if possible

        (5) To assure that all possible cases are evaluated and treated, the following **CDC definitions of congenital syphilis** should be followed: **confirmed case** (presence of spirochetes *or* the infant's serologic titer is fourfold greater than the mother); **presumed case** (symptomatic or asymptomatic): mother with positive serology was (1) not treated, (2) inadequately treated, (3) treated late in pregnancy (within the month before birth), or (4) the infant has physical signs, abnormal CSF, or radiograph changes.

   e. Interventions:

   (1) For infants with proven or probable disease (refer to your institution's neonatal medication manual): aqueous crystalline penicillin G, IV, for 10 to 14 days; procaine penicillin G, IM, for 10 days; **if more than 1 day of treatment is missed the course must be restarted.**

   (2) Benzathine penicillin G, IM × 1 dose, with the following conditions: maternal therapy was adequate but given < 1 month before delivery; fourfold decrease in maternal titer was not demonstrated after treatment; mother treated with erythromycin.

   (3) Follow-up: treated infants should be evaluated at 1, 2, 3, 6, and 12 months of age; RPR done at 3, 6, and 12 months after treatment or until results become nonreactive; CSF evaluation at 6 months for infants treated with congenital neurosyphilis; and retreatment as necessary based on findings at time of follow-up evaluation

   f. Outcome: depends on the amount of damage done up until the time of treatment; late treatment does not reverse the effects of congenital syphilis.

12. *Toxoplasma gondii* (protozoan parasite) (Gonik, 1994; Remington & Klein, 2001):

   a. Transmission is transplacental passage following parasitemia in the mother who contracts the illness after ingestion of infective oocysts from contaminated soil or uncooked meat.

   b. Clinical manifestations: vary in severity and range from normal appearance at birth to erythroblastosis, hydrops fetalis, and the classic triad (*hydrocephalus, chorioretinitis, and intracranial calcifications*); may have multiple organ involvement.

   c. Diagnosis (Pickering 2000): isolation of the organism from cultures of the placenta, umbilical cord, or infant's blood; PCR of blood, CSF, and amniotic fluid; serologic IgM or IgA assay (positive within first 6 months of life)

   d. Interventions:

   (1) Ophthalmologic examination, hearing test, head ultrasound, and spinal tap

   (2) Pharmacotherapy (Pickering, 2000; Remington & Klein, 2001): pyrimethamine and sulfadiazine given in combination act synergistically against organism. Treatment lasts for a full year. Folinic acid supplementation is required during sulfadiazine therapy.

   (3) Biweekly CBCs to monitor possible neutropenia, anemia, and platelet depression

    e. Outcome: sensorineural hearing loss; visual impairment and relapsing chorioretinitis; cognitive impairment, neurologic deficits, and seizures

13. Ureaplasma urealyticum (UU) (member of the Mycoplasmataceae family, smallest free-living organisms, no cell wall) (Long, Pickering, & Prober, 1997; Pickering 2000; Remington and Klein, 2001):

    a. Transmission:

        (1) Venereal: major route of transmission for adults; found in the vagina of 40% to 80% of sexually mature asymptomatic women

        (2) Transplacental passage and ascending transmission during passage through a colonized birth canal

        (3) Mode of delivery does not affect rate of transmission.

        (4) Increased in the presence of chorioamnionitis or amniotic fluid infection

    b. Clinical manifestations: prematurity; pneumonia (congenital and neonatal); some evidence that UU contributes to chronic lung disease in preterm infants; CNS infection with variable clinical findings; and neonates are frequently colonized.

    c. Diagnosis: culture (specimen collection requires specific transport medium, should go directly to laboratory for processing; bacteria lose viability at room temperature); PCR testing available

    d. Interventions:

        (1) Therapy is not indicated if the patient is asymptomatic.

        (2) Erythromycin is the drug of choice for respiratory infections.

        (3) A drug with better blood-brain barrier penetration should be used if CNS infection is suspected.

II. Infections of the newborn

  A. Neonatal sepsis (Fanaroff & Martin, 2002; Remington & Klein, 2001):

    1. Early-onset sepsis: sepsis occurs in the first 7 days of life.

      a. Characteristics: source of organism is mother's genital tract and/or amniotic fluid; usually fulminant with higher mortality rate

      b. Common offending organisms (those found in vaginal flora): group B β-hemolytic streptococci (GBS); *Escherichia coli*; *Listeria monocytogenes* (can be acquired transplacentally); *Haemophilus influenzae*; staphylococcus

    2. Late-onset/nosocomial sepsis: infections that occur after the first week of life and are acquired from the postnatal environment

      a. Characteristics: acquired from direct and indirect contact with organisms found in the nursery environment; colonization may occur long before or immediately before infection; frequently complicated by meningitis

      b. Common offending organisms (Box 10.1)

    3. Risk factors for sepsis (Fanaroff & Martin, 2002)

      a. Early-onset sepsis:

▼ **BOX 10.1** | **Common Organisms for Neonatal Sepsis**

Bacteria
- *Staphylococcus aureus* (coagulase positive)
- Methicillin-resistant *S. aureus*
- *Staphylococcus epidermidis* (coagulase negative)
- Enterobacteriaceae (gram-negative enteric rods):
  Escherichia coli
  Klebsiella
  Serratia marcescens
  Enterobacter
  Citrobacter
  Proteus
  Salmonella and Shigella
- Vancomycin-resistant enterococcus
- *Pseudomonas aeruginosa* (gram negative)

Fungus
- *Candida albicans* (ovoid budding yeast)
- *Malassezia furfur* (lipophilic yeast)

Virus
- Respiratory syncytial virus
- Rotavirus
- Enteroviruses
- Cytomegalo-virus

---

(1) Maternal colonization with GBS; untreated or incompletely treated focal infections of the mother (eg, urinary tract infection [UTI], vaginal or cervical infection) or systemic infections; maternal fever; chorioamnionitis; ROM for more than 24 hours; use of fetal scalp electrodes; perinatal asphyxia in the presence of PROM

(2) Malnutrition in the mother

(3) Prematurity; low birth weight

(4) Male gender

   b. Nosocomial infection:

(1) Low birth weight; limitations of immune defense

(2) Total parenteral nutrition; tube feedings

(3) Antibiotic administration (superinfections and infections due to resistant organisms); corticosteroid use; histamine H2-receptor antagonists

(4) Surgery; environment

B. Clinical presentation (symptoms are often subtle and nonspecific):

   1. Respiratory: apnea, tachypnea, grunting, nasal flaring, retractions, decreased oxygen saturation, and acidosis

   2. Cardiovascular: bradycardia, tachycardia, decreased cardiac output, hypotension, and decreased perfusion

   3. CNS: temperature instability, lethargy, hypotonia, irritability, and seizures

4. GI: feeding intolerance, abdominal distention, vomiting, and diarrhea
5. Skin: jaundice and pallor
6. Hematologic: neutropenia, bandemia, thrombocytopenia, and petechiae
7. Abnormal blood studies: hypoglycemia/hyperglycemia and metabolic acidosis

C. Diagnosis:
1. Cultures: blood, CSF, urine, and other (eg, wound drainage)
2. Laboratory studies:
   a. CBC with differential: evaluate platelet count (may be low or decreasing with infection); Dohle bodies, toxic granulation, or neutrophil vacuolization on smear; increased lymphocyte count with acute viral infections
   b. Disseminated intravascular coagulopathy (DIC) screen
   c. Analysis of CSF (color, cell count, protein, glucose) (Table 10.2)
   d. Blood chemistries (ABG, electrolytes, and blood glucose)
3. Consider other disease processes that present with sepsis-like "picture" (eg, inborn error of metabolism, congenital heart disease).
4. Calculations (ANC and I:T ratio) evaluate the WBC differential (Lott, 1994) and assist in identifying the presence of infection and/or predicting an infant's ability to mount an adequate response to infection (Table 10.3).
5. Radiographic/imaging studies as indicated (based on clinical presentation and offending organism): chest x-ray; abdominal x-ray (assess for septic ileus, NEC, perforation); bone scan (S*taphylococcus aureus* is the predominant cause of osteomyelitis);

 TABLE 10.2 Normal Values for Cerebrospinal Fluid Analysis

WBC count	Preterm mean (range) 9 (0–25 WBCs/mm^3) 57% polymorphonuclear lymphocytes (PMNs) Term mean (range) 8 (0–22 WBCs/mm^3) 61% PMNs
Predicted WBC	Formula: CSF RBC $\times \dfrac{\text{Peripheral blood WBC}}{\text{Peripheral blood RBC}}$ For traumatic taps there should be a similar ratio of WBC:RBC in both the CSF and peripheral blood. For CSF pleocytosis (before a traumatic tap), the CSF ratio WBC:RBC should exceed the peripheral ratio WBC:RBC.
Glucose	Preterm mean (range) 50 (24–63 mg/dL) Term mean (range) 52 (34–119 mg/dL)
Protein	Preterm mean (range) 115 (65–150 mg/dL) Term mean (range) 90 (20–170 mg/dL)
Color	Clear or xanthochromic

Adapted from Siberry, G. K., & Iannone, R. (Eds.), *Harriet Lane handbook* (15th ed., pp. 119–130). St. Louis: Mosby; and Bonadio, W. A. (1992). Interpreting the traumatic lumbar puncture. *Contemporary Pediatrics,* February, 23–32.

TABLE 10.3 ANC and I:T Ratio Calculations

	Formula
Absolute neutrophil count (ANC) :	ANC = WBC × (% neutrophils + % immature cells)
ANC < 500 indicates a decreased ability to mount a response to infection.	Example: WBC 1,200, 12% neutrophils, 40% bands 1,200 × (12% + 40%) = 1,200 × 52% = 624
Immature:total (I:T) ratio: I:T ratio ≥ 0.2 constitutes a 'left shift' and is suggestive of infection.	$$I{:}T = \frac{\text{Total immature neutrophils*}}{\text{Total (neutrophils* + immature)}}$$ Example: 12 neutrophils; 40 bands; 2 metamyelocytes
Immature neutrophils include bands, myelocytes, metamyelocytes, and promyelocytes.	$$\frac{40 \text{ bands} + 2 \text{ metas}}{12 \text{ neutrophils} + (40 \text{ bands} + 2 \text{ metas})} = \frac{42}{54} = 0.77$$
Neutrophils (polymorphonuclear leukocytes) are also known as segs, PMNs, and polys.	

echocardiogram (assess for endocarditis); renal ultrasound (assess for renal candidiasis); and brain imaging (brain abscess commonly occurs with *Citrobacter* sepsis but can occur with other organisms)

D. Interventions (Baltimore, 1998; Cavaliere, 1995; Payne, 1994):

  1. Pharmacotherapy:

    a. Initiate *empiric* antimicrobial therapy until offending organism is identified. Broad-spectrum antibiotics cover potential organisms. Gram stains of cultured specimens can guide initial antibiotic therapy.

    b. Change to *definitive* antimicrobial therapy directed at eradicating specific organisms after culture identification.

    c. Consider CSF penetrance when selecting antimicrobials.

  2. Drugs listed are those *commonly* used in the initial treatment of suspected sepsis in neonates:

    a. Antimicrobials (refer to a neonatal medication manual for dosing, interval, and monitoring of therapeutic peak and trough levels for specific drugs)

      (1) Broad-spectrum coverage for *early-onset* sepsis: ampicillin

      (2) Gram-positive organism coverage for *late-onset* sepsis: vancomycin

      (3) Gram-positive organism coverage: penicillins and first-generation cephalosporins (eg, cefazolin)

(4) Gram-negative organism coverage: aminoglycosides (eg, gentamicin) and third-generation cephalosporins (eg, ceftriaxone, ceftazidime, and cefotaxime)

(5) **Peak levels affect the dosage** (eg, high peak level → decrease the dose).

(6) **Trough levels will affect time interval** (eg, high trough level → lengthen the interval between doses).

   b. Antifungals: fluconazole and amphotericin B

   c. Antivirals: acyclovir

3. Bacterial organisms (Table 10.4)

4. Supportive therapy based on the infant's clinical presentation/course may include: oxygen therapy, respiratory support, and vasoactive drugs.

5. Prevention includes:

   a. **Diligent hand washing**

   b. Screen visitors and health care personnel for viral diseases.

   c. Appropriate immunization of individuals having contact with patients

   d. Isolation of infected patients as appropriate to prevent spread

TABLE 10.4 **Bacterial Organisms**

Organism	Gram Positive	Gram Negative

Cocci
Pairs: streptococcus
  or staphylococcus
 	
Clusters: staphylococcus
Chains: streptococcus
	Streptococcus: group A, B, D
	Staphylococcus: aureus
	  (coagulase positive) epidermis
	  (coagulase negative)
		Neisseria: gonorrhea
		  (diplococcal)
		  meningitis

Rods
Short, pleomorphic,
  club shaped
	Aerobic
	Listeria
	
	Anaerobic
	Clostridia:
	  difficile
	  perfringens
	  botulinum
	  tetani
		Aerobic
		Enterobacter:
		  Escherichia coli
		  Klebsiella
		  Proteus
		  Salmonella
		  Serratia
		  Shigella
		  Haemophilus influenzae
		  Pseudomonas
		Anaerobic
		Bacteroides fragilis

Adapted from Lott, J. W., Kenner, C., & Polak, J. D. (1994). General evaluation for suspected infection. In J. W. Lott (Ed.), *Neonatal infection: Assessment, diagnosis, and management* (pp. 23–36). Petaluma, CA: NICU Ink.

▼ References

Baltimore, R. S. (1998). Neonatal nosocomial infections. *Seminars in Perinatology, 22* (1); 25–32.

Bonadio, W. A. (1992). Interpreting the traumatic lumbar puncture. *Contemporary Pediatrics*, pp. 23–32.

Cavaliere, T. A. (1995). Pharmacologic treatment of neonatal sepsis: Antimicrobial agents and immunotherapy. *JOGNN, 24*(7), 647–658.

Fanaroff, A. A., & Martin, R. J. (2002). *Neonatal-perinatal medicine: Diseases of the fetus and infant* (7th ed.). St. Louis: Mosby.

Gonik, B. (Ed.). (1994). *Viral diseases in pregnancy*. Springer-Verlag: New York.

Jarvis, W. R. (1996). The epidemiology of colonization. *Infection Control and Hospital Epidemiology, 17*(1), 47–52.

Long, S. S., Pickering, L. K., & Prober, C. G. (1997). *Principles and practice of pediatric infectious diseases*. New York: Churchill Livingstone.

Lott, J. W., Kenner, C., & Polak, J. D. (1994). General evaluation for suspected infection. In J. W. Lott (Ed.), *Neonatal infection: Assessment, diagnosis, and management* (pp. 23–36). Petaluma, CA: NICU INK.

Payne, N. R., Schilling, C. G., & Steinberg, S. (1994). Selecting antibiotics for nosocomial bacterial infections in patients requiring neonatal intensive care. *Neonatal Network, 13*(3), 41–51.

Pickering, L. K. (Ed.). *2000 Red book: Report of the committee on infectious diseases* (25th ed.). Elk Grove Village, IL.

Remington, J. S., & Klein, J. O. (2001). *Infectious diseases of the fetus and newborn infant* (5th ed.). Philadelphia: W.B. Saunders.

Siberry, G. K., & Iannone, R. (Eds.), *Harriet Lane handbook* (15th ed., pp. 43–71.). St. Louis: Mosby.

Young, T. E., & Mangum, B. (Eds.). (2002). *Neofax 2002* (15th ed.). Raleigh, NC: Acorn Publishing.

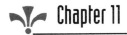 **Chapter 11**

Hematology

Susan E. Cheeseman, MSN, RNC, NNP

I. Hematopoiesis (Christensen, 2000; Phipps & Shannon, 1993; Yoder, 2000)
   A. Definition: formation, production, and maintenance of blood cells. Pluripotent cells develop into committed unipotent stem cells (colony-forming units), which evolve into specific cell lines. It begins in the yolk sac (16 days' gestation), migrates to the liver (peaks at 4 to 5 months' gestation), and finally establishes itself as medullary (bone marrow) hematopoiesis (after 22 weeks' gestation). Sites of extramedullary hematopoiesis (spleen, lymph nodes, thymus, kidneys) aid production of cells during fetal life when long bones are small (Figure 11.1).
II. Erythrocytes (red blood cells [RBCs]) (Christensen, 2000; Ohls, 2000; Yoder, 2000)
   A. Description: a blood cell arising from the proerythroblast cell line; anucleate biconcave disc (7 nm in diameter) containing high concentrations of hemoglobin in its cytoplasm
   B. RBC function: tissue oxygenation by hemoglobin transport; carbon dioxide removal through reaction with carbonic anhydrase; and hemoglobin serves as a buffer to maintain acid-base balance.
   C. Erythropoietin (EPO): the hormone that regulates erythropoiesis and synthesis of hemoglobin. EPO is produced postnatally in the kidneys; during fetal life, extrarenal sites (liver and submandibular glands) predominate. EPO production is increased in response to anemia and low oxygen availability to tissues and decreased in response to hypertransfusion.
   D. Erythropoiesis: production of erythrocytes. Erythroid precursors mature in the bone marrow through the normoblast and reticulocyte stages.
      1. Reticulocytes, in the absence of stress, mature 1 to 2 days in the bone marrow and then another day in the circulation before maturing to erythrocytes.
         a. Reticulocyte count: assesses the level of reticulocyte production. High counts signify increased erythropoiesis.
         b. Reticulocyte percentage: reports percentage of erythrocytes that stain as reticulocytes and does not account for differences in absolute number of erythrocytes between anemic and nonanemic infants (Table 11.1).
         c. Corrected reticulocyte count: correction is made for Hct, adjusting to a standard Hct (usually 45% [0.45]) (Christensen, 2000).

   Infant's reticulocyte *count* (%) × $\dfrac{\text{infant's Hct}}{0.45}$

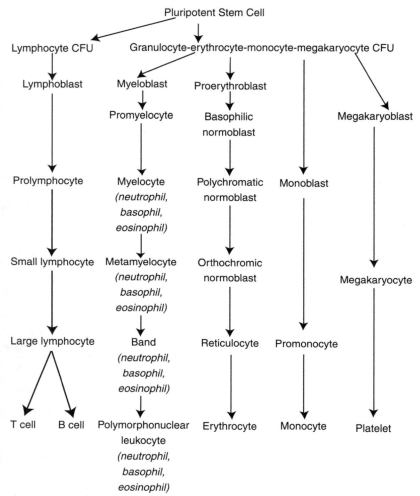

CFU=colony-forming unit.

Figure 11-1. Maturation of Blood Cell Components. From Christensen, R. D. (2000). Expected hematologic values for term and preterm neonates. In R. D. Christensen (Ed.), *Hematologic problems of the neonate* (pp. 117–136). Philadelphia: Saunders; and Phipps, R. H., & Shannon, K. M. (1993). Hematologic problems. In M. Klaus & A. A. Fanaroff (Eds.), *Care of the high-risk neonate* (4th ed., pp. 397–425). Philadelphia: Saunders.

TABLE 11.1 Normal Hematologic Values

	Age						
Value	28 Weeks' Gestation	34 Weeks' Gestation	Full-Term Cord Blood	1 Day	3 Days	7 Days	14 Days
Hemoglobin (g/dL)	14.5	15	16.8	18.4	17.8	17.0	16.8
Hematocrit (%)	45	47	53	58	55	54	52
Red blood cells (10⁶/mm³)	4.0	4.4	5.25	5.8	5.6	5.2	5.1
MCV (μm³)	120	118	107	108	99	98	96
MCH (pg)	40	38	34	35	33	32.5	31.5
MCHC (%)	31	32	31.7	32.5	33	33	33
Reticulocytes (%)	5–10	3–10	3–7	3–7	1–3	0–1	0–1
Platelets (K/mm³)			290	192	213	248	252

MCH = mean corpuscular hemoglobin; MCHC = mean corpuscular hemoglobin concentration; MCV = mean corpuscular volume. From Klaus, M. H., & Fanaroff, A. A. (2001). *Care of the high-risk neonate* (5th ed., pp. 574, 577). Philadelphia: WB Saunders.

    d. Reticulocyte count is inversely proportional to gestational age; falls markedly during the first few days of life. *Persistent reticulocytosis may indicate chronic blood loss or hemolysis.*

   2. Nucleated RBC: circulating immature (prereticulocyte) RBC. Number is inversely proportional to gestational age and declines rapidly in the first week. Increase may indicate hemolysis, acute blood loss, hypoxemia, congenital heart disease, or infection.

   3. Spherocyte: small spherical doughnut-shaped RBC lacking central pallor. It is observed in neonates (up to 40% spherocytes) with clinically significant ABO hemolytic disease; not commonly found in Rh disease. Hereditary spherocytosis (HS) is a congenital hemolytic anemia due to defects in the erythrocyte membrane. Anemia is the most common finding in neonates, as well as jaundice and splenomegaly.

   4. Schistocyte: RBC with an irregular shape resulting from mechanical fragmentation associated with the following disorders: macroangiopathic anemia (mechanical intravascular hemolysis within large blood vessels) and microangiopathic anemia (mechanical intravascular hemolysis within small blood vessels)

  E. RBC values:

   1. In the newborn period the erythrocyte values (hemoglobin concentration, Hct and erythrocyte count) vary based on: gestational age; time of sampling relative to delivery; specific illness and level of support needed; and method for obtaining blood samples (peripheral capillary samples yield higher RBC concentrations than samples obtained by arterial or venipuncture or from an

indwelling arterial or venous catheter; warming the extremity
can result in better correlation between capillary and venous erythrocyte values).

2. Hb: major iron-containing component of the RBC; it delivers
oxygen from lungs to tissue cells through the circulation. Fetal
hemoglobin (Hb F) is the major component of the RBCs by 10
weeks' gestation; at birth RBCs contain 70% to 90% Hb F; transition to adult hemoglobin (Hb A) begins at the end of fetal life.
Hemoglobin binds with 2, 3-diphosphoglycerate (2,3-DPG) to
release an oxygen molecule; Hb F has far less affinity for 2,3-
DPG than Hb A; levels of 2,3-DPG are directly proportional to
gestational age. Hb F has a greater affinity for oxygen than Hb A,
resulting in decreased oxygen release to the tissues.

3. Hct: measurement of the proportion of a blood sample occupied
by erythrocytes expressed as a percentage. Values rise immediately after birth and then decline to cord levels in the first week.

4. Erythrocyte (RBC) count: number of circulating mature RBCs
per cubic millimeter (mm³). RBC lifespan: preterm infant (35 to
50 days); term infant (60 to 70 days)

5. RBC indices: measure of RBC size and Hb content used for des-
ignation of anemias (Christensen, 2000)

   a. Mean corpuscular volume (MCV): measure of the average size
   of the circulating RBCs, expressed in femtoliter (fL, 10^{-15} L);
   increased MCV (macrocytes); decreased MCV (microcytes).
   Preterm infants have larger MCV values than term infants;
   MCV decreases as gestation progresses; decrease continues
   after birth to adult size by 4 to 5 years. Consider α-thalassemia or iron deficiency with MCV < 94 fL.

   b. Mean corpuscular hemoglobin (MCH): measure of the
   amount of Hb in an average circulating RBC; increased MCH
   (hyperchromic cells); decreased MCH (hypochromic cells).
   MCH decreases as gestation progresses; decrease continues
   after birth to adult size by 4 to 5 years.

   c. Mean corpuscular hemoglobin concentration (MCHC): a measure of the concentration of Hb in an average circulating
   RBC, expressed in units of grams of Hb per deciliter of
   packed RBCs (PRBCs) (g/dL); increased MCHC (hyperchromic cells); decreased MCHC (hypochromic cells). Adults,
   preterm, and term neonates share the same MCHC range.

F. RBC disorders:

   1. Physiologic anemia (Kling, Schmidt, Roberts, & Widness, 1996;
   Ohls, 2000): normal decrease in Hb concentration reflecting a
   natural adaptation to the extrauterine environment (or physiologic nadir). Term infants: improved oxygenation after birth
   results in decreased erythrocyte production; Hb concentration
   decreases during the first 2 to 3 months of life, remains stable
   during the next several weeks, and then slowly rises in the fourth
   to sixth months of life.

   2. Anemia of prematurity: considered physiologic because it is
   characteristic of healthy preterm infants; rate of decline and
   nadir are inversely proportional to gestational age; low iron con-

centration secondary to decreased blood volume and decreased concentration of circulating hemoglobin iron; diminished EPO production in response to anemia; shortened red cell life span; and growth causes dilutional anemia as a result of decreased Hb concentration with expanding blood volume.

3. Pathologic anemia (Christensen, 2000; Manco-Johnson, Rodden, & Collins, 2002): inability of the circulating erythrocytes to meet the oxygen demands of the tissues secondary to low Hb concentration and/or decreased number of RBCs. Etiology includes increased loss (hemorrhagic); increased destruction of red cells (hemolytic); and inadequate production of red cells (hypoplastic).

4. **Hemorrhage** (Cunningham, 2001; Manco-Johnson, et al., 2002; Ohls, 2000): most common cause of anemia in neonates; blood loss can occur before birth, during, and after delivery (Table 11.2).

   a. Internal hemorrhage should be suspected in the first 24 to 72 hours when a decreased Hct is not associated with signs of external blood loss or hyperbilirubinemia (Doyle, Schmidt, Blanchette, & Zipursky, 1999; Ross, 1999).

   b. Adrenal hemorrhage: hemorrhage into the adrenal gland
      (1) Risk factors include: traumatic delivery; sepsis; asphyxia; defect in hemostasis; large-for-gestational-age infant; and infant of a diabetic mother (IDM) or prediabetic mother.
      (2) Clinical manifestations: occurs most often on the right; symptoms usually develop on days of life (DOL) 1 through 7 (ranges from anemia and jaundice to marked anemia and shock, flank mass with bluish discoloration of the overlying skin); azotemia, proteinuria, and hematuria; signs of adrenal insufficiency may be subtle and/or delayed; hypoglycemia is more common than hyponatremia.
      (3) Diagnosis: adrenal enlargement on renal ultrasound
      (4) Interventions: differentiate from renal vein thromboses; hematuria is less pronounced in adrenal hemorrhage; blood and volume replacement; treat adrenal insufficiency with glucocorticoid and mineralocorticoid steroids; adrenal calcification may be seen within 3 to 4 weeks after an acute event.

   c. Hepatic hemorrhage: clinical manifestations include abdominal distention and discoloration; scrotal swelling; pallor; and peritoneal effusion without free air.

   d. Splenic rupture can result from birth trauma or from distention by extramedullary hematopoiesis, such as that seen in erythroblastosis fetalis.

   e. Pulmonary hemorrhage: mortality rate > 75%; common in sick preterm infants requiring mechanical ventilation presenting usually in the first week of life. Clinical manifestations include: gross bleeding usually seen in the endotracheal tube; sudden onset pallor, shock, apnea, bradycardia, and cyanosis;

TABLE 11.2 Causes of Hemorrhage in the Neonate

Before Delivery	During Delivery	During/After Delivery
Fetomaternal hemorrhage	Placental disorders: abruption, previa, malformation, trauma, or incision at Cesarean-section	Intracranial/subperiosteal hemorrhage
Twin-to-twin transfusion		Internal hemorrhage:
Hemorrhage after percutaneous umbilical blood sampling	Umbilical cord disorders: velamentous cord insertion, malformation, cord accident, vasa previa, nuchal cord, early or delayed cord clamping	Adrenal, hepatic, splenic
		Retroperitoneal
		Pulmonary
Traumatic amniocentesis		Gastrointestinal
Maternal trauma		Defects in hemostasis: congenital or consumptive coagulopathy latrogenic blood loss:
Trauma after external cephalic version		Phlebotomy
		Central line accidents
		Arterial line accidents

Adapted from Ohls, R. K. (2000). Evaluation and treatment of anemia in the neonate. In R. D. Christensen (Ed.), *Hematologic problems of the neonate* (pp. 137-169). Philadelphia: Saunders; and Manco-Johnson, M. Rodden, D. J., & Collins, S. (2002). Newborn hematology. In G. B. Merenstein & S. L. Gardner (Eds.), *Handbook of neonatal intensive care* (5th ed., pp. 419-422). St. Louis: Mosby.

and hypoxia, severe retractions, and increased work of breathing.

f. Gastrointestinal (GI) hemorrhage. Etiology includes: peptic ulcer; enterocolitis; nasogastric catheter; and hemangiomas of the GI tract. Maternal blood swallowed from delivery or breast may be confused with GI bleeding. The Apt test is used to distinguish swallowed maternal blood from neonatal blood and is based upon alkali resistance of fetal hemoglobin (Apt, 1955).

g. Iatrogenic blood loss from phlebotomy or arterial/central line accidents; symptoms may develop if a loss of ≥ 20% occurs within a 48-hour period.

5. Hemolytic anemia: results from increased rate of erythrocyte destruction (Bussel, Zabusky, Berkowitz, & McFarland, 1997; Cohen & Manno, 1999; Doyle, et al., 1999; Manco-Johnson, et al., 2002; Ohls, 2000; Phibbs & Shannon, 1993).

a. Etiology (Box 11.1)

b. Clinical manifestations: jaundice presenting within the first 24 hours of life; pallor; *direct hyperbilirubinemia; hepatosplenomegaly*; petechiae and purpura secondary to thrombocytopenia and disturbances in hemostasis; and hydrops fetalis (severe anemia, congestive heart failure [CHF], and diffuse edema)

c. Common hematologic findings include: *anemia* (degree reflects the severity of the hemolytic process); *reticulocytosis* or reticulocytopenia; increased nucleated RBCs; polychromasia; anisocytosis; spherocytosis (ABO incompatibility); cell fragmentation (disseminated intravascular coagulopathy [DIC]); neutropenia; neutrophilia; thrombocytopenia (with/without DIC); increased or decreased serum EPO concentration; and positive Direct Coombs with Rh disease.

d. Interventions: blood product and volume replacement; exchange transfusion (for Rh disease); phototherapy; and respiratory support

e. Isoimmune-mediated hemolysis: fetal cells bearing antigens of paternal origin enter the maternal circulation through transplacental hemorrhage and stimulate production of immunoglobulin G (IgG) antibodies. IgG antibodies are transferred across the placenta and destroy the fetal red cells. Predisposing factors include: previous pregnancy; rupture of ectopic pregnancy; spontaneous or therapeutic abortion; fetomaternal transfusion; maternal blood transfusion; amniocentesis; chorionic villi sampling; placental abruption; manual removal of placenta; and pregnancy-induced hypertension (PIH).

(1) Rh incompatibility or erythroblastosis fetalis: occurs in second and subsequent pregnancies.

(2) ABO incompatibility: more common and less severe than Rh disease; may occur during the first pregnancy because A and B antigens are ubiquitous in foods and bacteria, causing sensitization. It is most often seen in mothers with O blood type (absence of antigen) carrying fetus with A or B blood type.

▼ **BOX 11.1** | **Etiology of Hemolytic Anemia in the Neonate**

Isoimmune-mediated hemolysis

Rh incompatibility (anti-D antibody) and ABO incompatibility

Minor blood group incompatibility (c, C, e, G, FGya [Duffy], Kell group, jka, MNS, Vw)

Drug-induced hemolytic anemia (penicillin, α-methyl 3, 4-dihydroxyphenylalanine, cephalothin)

Infection

Bacterial sepsis (*Echerichia coli,* Group B streptococcus)

Congenital TORCH (toxoplasmosis, other [viruses], rubella, cytomegalovirus, herpes [simplex viruses]) infections

Congenital syphilis

Congenital malaria

Parvovirus B19

Metabolic disorders

Galactosemia

Organic aciduria; orotic aciduria

Prolonged or recurrent acidosis

Congenital red cell membrane disorders

Hereditary spherocytosis, elliptocytosis, poikilocytosis, pyropoikilocytosis, and stomatocytosis

Infantile pyknocytosis

Congenital red cell enzyme disorders

Glucose-6-phosphate dehydrogenase deficiency

Pyruvate kinase deficiency

Glucose phosphate isomerase deficiency

Congenital hemoglobinopathies

α-Thalassemia syndromes; α-chain structural abnormalities

γ-Thalassemia syndromes; γ-chain structural abnormalities

Nutritional deficiencies

Vitamin E deficiency

Macroangiopathic and microangiopathic

Disseminated intravascular coagulation

Cavernous hemangioma

Renal vein thrombosis; renal artery stenosis

Large vessel thrombi

Severe coarctation of aorta

Modified from Ohls, R. K. (2000). Evaluation and treatment of anemia in the neonate. In R. D. Christensen (Ed.), *Hematologic problems of the neonate* (pp. 137–169). Philadelphia: Saunders; and Manco-Johnson, M., Rodden, D. J., & Collins, S. (2002). Newborn hematology. In G. B. Merenstein & S. L. Gardner (Eds.), *Handbook of neonatal intensive care* (5th ed., pp. 419–442). St. Louis: Mosby.

(3) Minor blood group incompatibility (c, anti-Kell, and E are most common)

f. Infection: may cause hemolytic anemia and bone marrow suppression with reticulocytopenia; microspherocytes may be prominent. Cytomegalovirus (CMV) is the most common TORCH infection leading to hemolytic anemia. Parvovirus B19 may lead to hydrops fetalis, especially with first and second trimester exposure.

g. Metabolic diseases can present as hemolytic disease in the newborn infant.

h. Congenital disorders of the red cell membrane are usually autosomal dominant and lead to lifelong hemolytic anemia. Hyperbilirubinemia and anemia in the neonate are pronounced. Hereditary spherocytosis commonly presents with jaundice and, less often, with anemia. Hereditary elliptocytosis rarely presents in the newborn infant. Congenital red cell membrane enzyme deficiencies:

    (1) Glucose-6-phosphate dehydrogenase deficiency: enzyme deficiency that alters the production of nicotinamide-adenine dinucleotide phosphate (NADPH) (needed to break down free radicals [oxidants] in the cells); most common inherited disorder; X-linked recessive

        (a) Clinical manifestations: hyperbilirubinemia with/without hemolysis, may be severe; low Hct and high reticulocyte count; peripheral smear: pincer cells, RBC fragments, and pyknocytes

        (b) Interventions: suspect G6PD deficiency in male infants with jaundice, acute hemolytic anemia, and a negative Coombs test; G6PD screen; phototherapy and possible exchange transfusion; avoid drug and chemicals reported to produce hemolysis in patients with G6PD deficiency; be aware of an increased risk for late-onset neonatal sepsis.

    (2) Pyruvate kinase deficiency: enzyme deficiency that leads to decreased adenosine triphosphate (ATP) production, decreased intracellular K^+ and H_2O, and increased intracellular Ca^{++}, resulting in abnormal RBC shape and membrane rigidity; autosomal recessive. Clinical manifestations include hyperbilirubinemia, and a peripheral blood smear that shows macrocytes, speculated red cells, target cells, spherocytes, and (less often) acanthocytes.

i. Congenital hemoglobinopathies: inherited disorders resulting in defects in the quantity or function of the Hb proteins. The clinical expression of a hemoglobinopathy is dependent upon affected globin chain, developmental state of globin synthesis, and amount and function of alternate hemoglobins. Hemoglobinopathies presenting at birth affect either the α or γ chains of Hb.

    (1) The thalassemias are disorders manifested by absence or decrease of specific globin proteins, resulting in production of hemoglobins with decreased oxygen affinity. Infants will have lower Hb without signs of tissue hypoxia.

(2) β chains of Hb are not produced until 3 months' postnatal age; therefore, β thalassemia and sickle cell anemia rarely present in the nursery.

j. Vitamin E deficiency: occurs with chronic malabsorption.

(1) Clinical manifestations include: hemolytic anemia with reticulocytosis and thrombocytosis; and lower extremity edema. Normal serum vitamin E level is 5–10 mg/dL.

(2) Interventions: be aware that diets high in polyunsaturated fatty acids and iron increase requirement for vitamin E. Infant formulas contain vitamin E but some infants < 1,500 g may benefit from oral supplementation of water-soluble α-tocopherol (vitamin E): 25–50 IU/24 hours (Hirshfeld, Getachew, & Sessions, 2000).

k. Macroangiopathic and microangiopathic hemolytic anemias: sluggish blood flow predisposes the activation of the coagulation system with consumption of platelets and fibrinogen resulting in bleeding (Phibbs & Shannon, 1993).

6. **Hypoplastic anemia**: diminished RBC production is manifested by a decreased Hct, decreased reticulocyte count, and normal bilirubin level (Cohen & Manno, 1999).

a. Neonatal leukemia: rare; may present with leukocytosis, thrombocytopenia, and anemia as the bone marrow is replaced with leukemic blasts.

b. Diamond Blackfan syndrome (congenital hypoplastic anemia): congenital failure of red cell production; autosomal recessive and dominant; mostly sporadic

(1) Clinical manifestations include: *thumb abnormalities*; web neck; cleft lip and/or palate; short stature; thrombosis; *anemia*; increased Hb F; pure red cell aplasia; and leukemia.

(2) Interventions: initial transfusion of PRBC is usually necessary and corticosteroid therapy.

c. Pearson syndrome (or refractory sideroblastic anemia with vacuolization of bone marrow precursors): deletion or rearrangement of mitochondrial deoxyribonucleic acid (DNA)

(1) Clinical manifestations include: pallor; macrocytic anemia presenting at birth; neutropenia; thrombocytopenia; pancreatic exocrine insufficiency; splenic atrophy; diabetes mellitus (DM); and lactic acidosis.

(2) Outcome: poor prognosis; median survival is 2 years.

d. Osteopetrosis: abnormally dense bone caused by osteoclast dysfunction compressing the marrow cavity and preventing normal intramedullary hematopoiesis. Hematologic findings: normochromic, normocytic anemia; reticulocytosis; increased nucleated RBCs; hepatosplenomegaly related to partial extramedullary compensation; and diminished RBC production in the bone marrow. Only bone marrow transplantation has offered long-term improvement.

7. Acute and chronic blood loss: clinical manifestations of anemia

depend upon the extent and duration of blood loss. The diagnosis depends upon whether the low Hb level is due to decreased red cell production, shortened red cell survival, or a combination of the two processes.

a. Physical examination (Ohls, 2000) (Table 11.3): cardiovascular function (tachycardia, murmur, gallop rhythm); level of activity; pallor; jaundice; skin lesions (petechiae and purpura); abdominal distention or mass, hepatosplenomegaly, adrenal or kidney rupture; lymphadenopathy; hydropic changes; and congenital malformations

b. Family history: bleeding, anemia, or splenectomy in other family members; unexplained jaundice, cholelithiasis, or splenectomy; ethnic and geographic origins; specific hereditary disorders or sibling who is affected

c. Obstetric history: maternal blood type; bleeding episodes before delivery (eg, placental previa, abruption, cord rupture); traumatic birth; multiple births

d. Infant history: infant's age when anemia is diagnosed (marked anemia at birth is associated with hemorrhage or severe isoimmunization; anemia during the first 48 hours of life is associated with external or internal hemorrhage; anemia after 48 hours of life is usually hemolytic and commonly associated with jaundice); gestational age and hospital course

e. Laboratory studies for infant: complete blood count (CBC) with differential; reticulocyte count; peripheral smear; blood type for infant and mother; bilirubin level (fractionated); direct antiglobulin test (Coombs test); studies for infection (TORCH [immunoglobulin M (IgM) levels; urine culture for CMV; eye examination] and blood and urine cultures); Apt test to distinguish swallowed maternal blood from neonatal blood; and ultrasound examination of the head or abdomen for occult blood loss

f. Tests for parents include CBC, peripheral smear, RBC indices, and RBC enzymes (G6PD, pyruvate kinase). Maternal blood smear for fetal erythrocytes (Kleihauer-Betke test)

g. Intrinsic RBC defect: RBC enzyme studies; analysis of the globin chain ratio; studies of RBC membrane

h. Interventions:

(1) Acute blood loss and shock: establish venous access (umbilical or peripheral vein); obtain CBC, type, and cross-match; without available cross-matched blood, infuse type O, Rh-negative PRBCs (10–20 mL/kg); administer normal saline (20 mL/kg bolus); repeat as needed. With acute blood loss, the infant will show dramatic improvement. Infants with internal hemorrhage, DIC, or subgaleal hemorrhage may remain limp and unresponsive. Evaluate infant's bleeding status and administer fresh frozen plasma and platelets as needed. Iron replacement should be started after the infant is stable.

TABLE 11.3 Acute Versus Chronic Blood Loss in the Neonate

Characteristic	Acute Blood Loss	Chronic Blood Loss
General appearance	Pale, hyperalert, "stunned" gaze	Pale, normal neurologic examination
Cardiovascular system	Tachycardia, weak pulses, low blood pressure	Normal; rarely may have congestive heart failure with hepatomegaly; normal or increased blood pressure
Respiratory system	Tachypnea, no supplemental O_2 requirement	Normal; may be tachypneic (rare), requiring supplemental O_2 if congestive heart failure is present
Hematologic system		
Hemoglobin	May be normal; ↓ over 24 h	Low at birth
Morphology	Macrocytic normochromic (normal)	Microcytic; hypochromic
Iron	Normal	Low
Course	Promptly treat hypovolemia; may need rapid volume expansion to prevent shock, disseminated intravascular coagulation, and death	Usually uneventful hospital course; may need treatment for congestive heart failure and hydrops
Treatment	Volume expansion with isotonic fluid and PRBCs, FFP, and platelets; iron therapy later; EPO therapy may be appropriate to enhance erythropoiesis	Initiate iron therapy; PRBC transfusion rarely needed; EPO therapy may be appropriate to enhance erythropoiesis

PRBC = packed red blood cells; FFP = fresh frozen plasma; EPO = erythropoietin
From Ohls, R. K. (2000). Evaluation and treatment of anemia in the neonate. In R. D. Christensen (Ed.), *Hematologic problems of the neonate* (pp. 137–169). Philadelphia: Saunders.

      (2) Chronic blood loss: asymptomatic (treatment focuses on diagnostic work-up; iron replacement should be initiated [ferrous sulfate 6 mg/kg/day, oral preparation]); CHF and hydrops (support cardiac function with vasopressors and diuretics; thoracentesis to relieve significant pleural effusions and improve pulmonary function, and maintain oxygen delivery to tissues)
  G. Polycythemia (Linderman & Haga, 2000; Shaw, 1998): peripheral venous Hct > 65%
    1. Primary polycythemia: results from increased fetal production of EPO, leading to an increased RBC mass. Risk factors include: intrauterine hypoxia (PIH, intrauterine growth restriction [IUGR], maternal renal disease, heart disease, severe DM,

maternal smoking); neonatal thyrotoxicosis; congenital adrenal hyperplasia; high-altitude conditions; postmaturity; chromosome abnormalities (eg, trisomies 13, 18, and 21); hyperplastic visceromegaly (Beckwith-Wiedemann syndrome); and decreased erythrocyte deformability.

2. Secondary polycythemia: results from the transfer of erythrocytes to the fetus during delivery or in utero through twin-twin transfusion or maternal fetal transfusion.

3. Clinical manifestations include: weak suck (feeding difficulties); vomiting; plethora; rubeosis-like cyanosis; jaundice; lethargy; difficult to arouse; hypotonia; tremulousness; irritable when aroused; easily startled; myoclonic jerks; cardiomegaly (heart murmur); hepatomegaly; and tachypnea.

4. Laboratory findings: hypoglycemia; hypocalcemia; elevated Hct; and thrombocytopenia

5. Complications associated with polycythemia: respiratory distress syndrome (RDS), CHF; abnormal electroencephalographic pattern; convulsions; peripheral gangrene; priapism; necrotizing enterocolitis; ileus; and acute renal failure

6. Interventions: partial exchange transfusion with fresh frozen plasma or normal saline (lowers the Hct to approximately 60%; reverses clinical symptoms and increases capillary perfusion, cerebral blood flow, and cardiac function); correct glucose and electrolyte imbalances; improve oxygenation.

III. Thrombocytes (platelets) (Arnett, 1998; Doyle, et al., 1999; Manco-Johnson, et al., 2002; Sola, DelVecchio, & Rimsza, 2000; Sola & Christensen, 2000)

A. Description: small non-nucleated disc-shaped cells derived from megakaryocytes in the bone marrow (Figure 11.1)

B. Platelet function: aids in hemostasis (coagulation and thrombus formation); in the absence of injury, circulate freely for 7 to 10 days without wall adhesion or aggregation with other platelets until removal by the spleen. Normal range: 100,000–300,000 mm³ in term and preterm infants

C. Thrombocytopenia: platelet count < 150,000 mm³; < 50,000 mm³ is severe thrombocytopenia and may be associated with clinical bleeding.

1. Etiology includes: immune mediated (neonatal alloimmune and autoimmune); infectious (bacterial, viral, and fungal); genetic causes; drug related; DIC; and miscellaneous.

2. Clinical manifestations include: petechiae (small, flat hemorrhages in the skin that do not blanch; usually more concentrated in skin creases of the neck, axilla, and around tourniquet site; can be scattered over the entire body); ecchymosis (over presenting part); cephalhematoma; and bleeding (mucous membranes, GI tract, genitourinary system, umbilical cord, puncture sites, superficial cuts, or abrasions).

3. Interventions: determine the etiology and treat the underlying disorder.

a. Obtain family and obstetric history: previous siblings with thrombocytopenia; maternal platelet count; medications;

autoimmune disorders (PIH; DM; chorioamnionitis); placental insufficiency; asphyxia

b. Infant history: age of onset of thrombocytopenia (early onset [within the first 72 hours of life]—consider maternal reasons; late onset—consider nosocomial infection, necrotizing enterocolitis [NEC], thrombosis, or medications); asymptomatic versus symptomatic presentation; infant medications

c. Physical examination: signs of clinical manifestations (see previous Clinical manifestations section); jaundice; IUGR, microcephaly, and hepatosplenomegaly with infectious cause (absent with immune etiology); and congenital anomalies consistent with syndromes

d. Appropriate diagnostic testing: coagulation screen and platelet count (for infants with active bleeding); platelet count; peripheral blood smear (identifies immature forms and size of platelets); prothrombin time (PT); partial thromboplastin time (PTT); fibrinogen

e. Platelet transfusions are indicated for the following:

(1) Active bleeding with any degree of thrombocytopenia

(2) Term infant: platelet count < 20,000 to 30,000 without active bleeding

(3) Preterm infant: platelet count < 50,000 without active bleeding; platelet count < 100,000, weight < 1,500 g, and critically ill

(4) Transfuse standard platelet suspension, irradiated, CMV negative platelets; 10–20 mL/kg over 1 to 2 hours. Repeat platelet count after transfusion: failure to achieve or sustain a rise in platelet count suggests a destructive process.

4. Immune-mediated thrombocytopenia:

a. Neonatal alloimmune (or isoimmune) thrombocytopenia (NAIT): platelet antigen incompatibility between the mother and the fetus. Maternal IgG antibodies are produced against specific paternally derived antigens (most commonly PLA-1) on the infant's platelets. Maternal antibodies attach to and destroy fetal and neonatal platelets. First pregnancy can produce an infant who is affected; subsequent siblings have more severe disease.

(1) Clinical manifestations: maternal platelet level is normal; severe thrombocytopenia in an otherwise healthy infant; platelet count continues to fall during the first days of life and finally increases within 1 to 4 weeks. Intracranial hemorrhage (ICH) is a complication: occurs in 10% to 25% of infants; half of these ICHs occur in utero; increased risk for newborns with a sibling who is affected who had an antenatal ICH

(2) Interventions: washed (to remove the antibody), irradiated (to prevent graft-versus-host disease), *maternal platelets* when possible *or* type-specific donor platelets, irradiated, CMV negative; 10–20 mL/kg; infuse over 1 to 2 hours. Intravenous γ-globulin (IVIG) and corticosteroids

(Prednisone) were typically used for these neonates before the availability of IVIG.

(3) Obtain head ultrasound for infants with platelet counts < 50,000 mm³.

(4) Test maternal blood for human platelet antigen (HPA) type and the presence of platelet specific antibodies. Platelet antigen typing of mother, father, and infant can be obtained and aid in the management of future pregnancies. In subsequent pregnancies: fetal blood sampling at 18 to 26 weeks' gestation to determine fetal thrombocytopenia. Treatment includes maternal IVIG administration, maternal steroid administration, fetal platelet transfusions, and delivery by cesarean section for fetal platelet count < 50,000 mm³.

b. Autoimmune thrombocytopenia: mediated by the transplacental passage of maternal antiplatelet antibodies. Unlike NAIT, the antibody binds to maternal and fetal platelets, thereby affecting both mother and neonate.

(1) Underlying maternal disease: idiopathic thrombocytopenic purpura (ITP); systemic lupus erythematosus (SLE); lymphoproliferation disorders; hyperthyroidism

(2) Clinical manifestations: *maternal platelet level is low or normal; thrombocytopenia in the neonate* (not as severe as in NAIT); risk of bleeding is much less than in NAIT, especially ICH.

(3) Interventions: *random-donor*, irradiated, CMV-negative platelets; 10–20 cc/kg over 1 to 2 hours. Maternal IgG antibody has a broad spectrum against all platelets; platelet transfusions may be ineffective in raising the platelet count; donor platelets may survive long enough to contribute to hemostasis. IVIG and corticosteroids are more effective in treating autoimmune thrombocytopenia; some authors advocate starting IVIG and steroids for asymptomatic infants with platelet counts < 20,000 to 30,000 mm³.

5. Thrombocytopenia associated with infections:

a. Bacterial infections: duration of thrombocytopenia is variable. Principal mechanisms include: accelerated destruction secondary to endothelial damage with subsequent platelet adhesion and aggregation; platelet lysis or removal by the reticuloendothelial system; and decreased platelet production.

b. Fungal infections: thrombocytopenia may be the earliest laboratory finding; empiric antifungal treatment is indicated for susceptible infants while awaiting culture results.

c. Viral infections: TORCH, especially CMV, can cause thrombocytopenia. Coxsackievirus B can cause fulminant hepatitis and thrombocytopenia. Congenital parvovirus B19 is most commonly associated with hydrops and anemia, but thrombocytopenia can be part of the pathology. Congenital Epstein-Barr virus, mumps, and adenovirus infections may cause thrombocytopenia. Principal mechanism: combination of diminished production and accelerated destruction

6. Thrombocytopenia associated with genetic disorders:
   a. Thrombocytopenia-absent radius syndrome (TAR): autosomal recessive congenital syndrome frequently associated with hemorrhagic anemia in the newborn
      (1) Clinical manifestations: severe thrombocytopenia (platelet counts < 10,000 to 30,000 mm³) in 59% at birth or before 1 week of age, and 90% by 2 months of age; bilateral absent radii; thumbs and digits are always present; heart defects (Tetralogy of Fallot and atrial septal defect)
      (2) Outcome: 25% of the affected individuals die in the first year of life, particularly in the first 4 months from intracranial hemorrhage. Thrombocytopenia resolves by school age for the majority.
   b. Fanconi's anemia: autosomal recessive with marked variability in the clinical phenotype
      (1) Clinical manifestations: *radial defects* (49% of infants); *underdevelopment or absent thumbs*; *supernumerary thumbs*; thrombocytopenia and leukopenia, progressing to pancytopenia that does not usually present until childhood; short stature; microcephaly; eye anomalies; renal and urinary tract anomalies; and brownish pigmentation of the skin (café-au-lait spots)
      (2) Outcome: tendency to develop myeloid leukemia or myelodysplastic syndrome
   c. Congenital megakaryocytic hypoplasia: rare disorder characterized by moderate to severe thrombocytopenia with the absence of physical abnormalities; frequently diagnosed as NAIT initially, until maternal alloantibodies cannot be demonstrated
   d. Wiskott-Aldrich syndrome: X-linked immunodeficiency disease associated with severe bleeding, thrombocytopenia, and eczema. Clinical manifestations include GI bleeding or excessive bleeding from circumcision and thrombocytopenia with small platelets that have impaired function.
   e. Noonan's syndrome: rare autosomal-dominant disorder characterized by facial anomalies, congenital heart disease, skeletal abnormalities, genital malformations, and mild mental retardation
   f. Alport's syndrome: characterized by hereditary nephritis and nerve deafness; thrombocytopenia with large platelets (macrothrombocytopenia)
   g. Inherited metabolic disorders
   h. Chromosomal abnormalities: trisomies 13, 18, and 21; Turner's syndrome

7. Drug-induced thrombocytopenia:
   a. Maternal medications: meperidine (Demerol); promethazine (Phenergan); aspirin; quinine; quinidine; thiazides; hydralazine; sulfonamides; tolbutamide

    b. Neonatal medications: indomethacin; aspirin; nitric oxide; ampicillin; furosemide; theophylline; heparin

8. DIC

9. Miscellaneous causes of thrombocytopenia: thrombosis (renal vein, intracardiac, and vascular); giant hemangioma syndrome (Kasabach-Merritt); NEC; IUGR; PIH; asphyxia; idiopathic

D. Thrombocytosis: moderately elevated platelet count (450,000 to 600,000 mm³)

    1. Etiology includes: physiologic (preterm infants' platelet counts can increase to 600,000 mm³ by 4 weeks of age); reactive (variety of conditions characterized by infection and inflammation); iron deficiency; medications (antibiotics [eg, cephalosporins, ceftriaxone, and ceftizoxime] and methadone [platelet count may reach 1,000,000 mm³]); asplenia syndrome; Down syndrome; cerebral ischemia; vitamin E deficiency; congenital neoplasms; congenital adrenal hyperplasia; and recombinant thrombopoietin administration.

    2. Clinical presentation: infants rarely manifest signs of thrombocytosis.

    3. Interventions: correct the underlying cause.

E. Inherited and acquired bleeding disorders (defects in hemostasis): hemostasis is the arrest of bleeding by the biochemical and physiologic properties of coagulation and vasoconstriction. This process involves the interaction of the blood vessel, platelets, and the factors of coagulation and fibrinolysis and their inhibitors. Inherited or acquired defects in any of these components can lead to bleeding or abnormal thrombus formation (Edstrom, Christensen, & Andrew, 2000; Manco-Johnson, et al., 2002; Rivlin & Bussel, 1999) (Box 11.2).

    1. Clinical features of inherited bleeding disorders:

        a. Bleeding in a well-appearing neonate is associated with thrombocytopenia, disorders of the hemostatic system, vitamin K deficiency, or less commonly severe congenital coagulation factor deficiencies.

        b. Bleeding in a sick neonate most often results from DIC, liver failure, or underlying congenital coagulation deficiencies. Other common causes include hypoxia, shock, NEC, and thrombosis.

        c. Deficiencies of factor II, V, VII, XI, XII, and XIII are rare autosomal-inherited disorders; deficiencies of factors VIII and IX are X-linked recessive disorders and the most common inherited causes of bleeding in neonates; combined deficiencies are rare but do present in the neonatal period.

        d. Tests for hemostasis (Table 11.4)

    2. Factor VII deficiency: most neonates with severe factor VII deficiency present with ICH and bleeding; associated with Dubin-Johnson and Gilbert syndromes; prenatal diagnosis and in utero factor VII replacement are possible; intervention involves replacement of factor VII concentrate.

    3. Factor VIII deficiency (hemophilia A): severity of factor VIII deficiency is defined by plasma concentrations: mild (5% to 50%); moderate (1% to 5%); severe (< 1%). Severe factor VIII defi-

---

▼ **BOX 11.2** | **Etiology for Defects of Hemostasis**

Inherited bleeding disorders
Factor II (prothrombin) deficiency
Factor V deficiency
Factor VII deficiency
Hemophilia A-factor VIII deficiency
Hemophilia B-factor IX deficiency
Factor X deficiency
Factor XI deficiency
Factor XIII deficiency
Von Willebrand's disease
Familial multiple factor deficiencies
Fibrinogen disorders
Acquired bleeding disorders
Vitamin K deficiency or hemorrhagic disease of the newborn
   (vitamin K is needed for synthesis of coagulation factors II, VII, IX,
   X, XI, and XII)
Disseminated intravascular coagulopathy
Liver disease
Inherited thrombotic tendencies
Factor V Leiden
Prothrombin G20210A
Protein C deficiency
Protein S deficiency
Antithrombin deficiency
Abnormal plasminogen
Dysfibrinogenemias
Acquired thrombotic tendencies
Renal vein and renal artery thromboses
Thromboses related to indwelling catheters
Thromboses related to surgery
Thromboses related to extracorporeal membrane oxygenation

---

ciency presents in male neonates with bleeding after circumcision or as ICH. Diagnosis is confirmed by measuring factor levels; prenatal diagnosis and in utero factor VIII replacement are possible. Intervention involves replacement of factor VIII concentrate.

4. Factor IX deficiency (hemophilia B or Christmas disease): severity of factor IX deficiency is defined by plasma concentration like factor VIII deficiency (see Factor VIII deficiency section); commonly presents with bleeding after circumcision or with ICH; bleeding from venipuncture sites and hematomas and umbilical bleeding also occur. Diagnosis is confirmed by measuring factor levels; prenatal

TABLE 11.4 Tests for Hemostasis

Tests	Description	Indications
Platelet count	Assesses platelet number	
Prothrombin time	Measures *extrinsic* and common portions of the coagulation cascade; requires fibrinogen, prothrombin, and factors V, VII, and X	May be prolonged in deficiencies of vitamin K-associated factors, malabsorption, liver disease, disseminated intravascular coagulation (DIC), and circulating inhibitors
Activated partial thromboplastin time	Measures *intrinsic* and common portions of the coagulation cascade; requires fibrinogen, prothrombin, and factors V, VIII, IX, X, XI, and XII	May be prolonged with heparin administration, hemophilia, von Willebrand's disease, disseminated intravascular coagulation (DIC), and the presence of circulating inhibitors (lupus anticoagulants or other antiphospholipid antibodies)
Fibrinogen	Circulating level of this protein substrate required for clot formation	
Fibrin split products or fibrin degradation products	Fibrinolytic activity	

diagnosis and in utero factor IX replacement are possible. Intervention involves replacement of factor IX concentrate.

5. Von Willebrand's disease: most common inherited bleeding disorder; autosomal dominant or recessive inheritance depending upon the specific variant, ie, deficiency of von Willebrand's factor *or* production of von Willebrand's factor with abnormal structure; rarely presents during the neonatal period because von Willebrand's factor is physiologically increased in neonates.

6. Vitamin K deficiency (or hemorrhagic disease of the newborn):
   a. Function of vitamin K: essential cofactor for coagulation factors II (prothrombin), VII, IX, X, and for the inhibitors protein S and protein C. Vitamin K deficiency results in reduced activity of vitamin K-dependent factors and inhibitors resulting in bleeding tendencies.
   b. Early onset (rare): hemorrhagic symptoms present during the first 24 hours of life. Etiology includes maternal intake of medications (eg, carbamazepine, phenytoin, barbiturates, certain cephalosporins, rifampin, isoniazid, and warfarin) that enter the placental/fetal circulation and affect neonatal vitamin K production.
   c. Classic (rare with the use of vitamin K prophylaxis): onset of hemorrhage occurs most often between 2 and 7 days of life in neonates who are breastfeeding and have inadequate intake.

    d. Late: occurs in neonates (male predominance) 2 weeks to 6 months after birth in association with conditions that affect vitamin K absorption (eg, chronic diarrhea, liver disease, and prolonged use of antibiotics). Incidence of ICH is > 59%; high mortality and long-term morbidity

    e. Clinical manifestations: GI bleeding; umbilical bleeding; bleeding after circumcision; bleeding from venipuncture sites; and intracranial bleeding

    f. Laboratory findings: PT prolonged due to decreased activity of vitamin K-dependent coagulation factors (diagnosis is confirmed when vitamin K administration results in bleeding cessation and a rapid decrease in PT values); fibrinogen (normal); antithrombin (normal); coagulation factor plasma concentrations (normal); and platelet count (normal)

    g. Interventions: subcutaneous or intravascular administration of vitamin K

  7. DIC: acquired hemorrhagic disorder associated with an underlying disease manifested as uncontrolled activation of coagulation and fibrinolysis. Consumption of clotting factors is probably initiated by release of thromboplastic material from damaged or diseased tissue into the circulation; fibrinogen converts to fibrin to form microthrombi.

    a. Predisposing factors: maternal (PIH, eclampsia, and placental abnormalities and abruption); intrapartal (fetal distress with hypoxia/acidosis, dead twin fetus, and traumatic delivery); neonatal (RDS, infection, thrombosis, severe Rh incompatibility, thrombocytopenia, tissue injury [birth trauma, breech crush injury], and conditions causing hypoxia, acidosis, hypotension, and shock)

    b. Clinical manifestations: *hemorrhage* (clotting factors and platelets are depleted; fibrinolysis is stimulated; endogenous thrombin and plasmin are formed); organ and tissue ischemia secondary to microvascular thrombosis by fibrin thrombi; and anemia (blood loss and red cell fragmentation by fibrin strands)

    c. Laboratory findings: thrombocytopenia; PT (prolonged); PTT (prolonged); fibrinogen (low); fibrin split products (FSP) (increased); D-dimers (increased); factors V and VIII (depleted); and thrombin/antithrombin complexes (increased)

    d. Interventions: accurate diagnosis and treatment of underlying disorders and plasma products for clinically significant bleeding

    e. Clinical goals: platelet count > 50,000 mm^3; fibrinogen concentrations > 1 g/L; and PT values within the physiologic range for postnatal or gestational age. Commonly used blood products (Table 11.5)

F. Thrombotic disorders (hypercoagulable states): present clinically as venous or arterial thrombosis. Etiology includes inherited or genetic (carefully assess family history for strokes, thrombosis, and spontaneous abortion).

  1. Factor V Leiden (activated protein C resistance): factor V Leiden mutation significantly reduces the inactivation of factor V by

TABLE 11.5 Commonly Used Blood Products

Blood Product	Description	Indications
Whole blood		Exchange transfusions Priming heart-lung oxygenators for extracorporeal membrane oxygenation
Packed red blood cells	Blood is spun to concentrate cells and allow the supernatant to be removed	Exchange transfusions Anemia
Washed red blood cells	Removes additional plasma, nonviable RBCs, WBCs, and metabolic wastes to reduce the possibility of graft-versus-host reaction	
Irradiated red blood cells	Prevents T-lymphocyte proliferation; when done in conjunction with washing removes up to 95% of T-lymphocytes	
Fresh frozen plasma	Rich source of coagulation factors containing 1 IU/mL of all clotting factors	10 to 15 mL/kg raises the overall level of clotting factor activity by 20% to 30%
Platelets		Thrombocytopenia Active bleeding
Granulocytes	Prepared from fresh donor blood through the process of plasmapheresis. WBCs are removed, but a large number of RBCs remain and unit needs to be typed and cross-matched. Usually irradiated to prevent graft-versus-host responses.	For septic infants with severe neutropenia
Cryoprecipitate	Plasma preparation rich in factor VIII, factor XIII, and fibrinogen. Single-donor preparation, decreased risk of infection compared to pooled substances	Treatment of hemophilia
Factor concentrations	Obtained from pooled plasma (risk of infection increases with the exposure to multiple donors)	Used as specific therapy for identified factor deficiencies

activated protein C; most common inherited venous thrombotic tendency in adults of European decent, resulting in lifelong hypercoagulable states with increased risks of venous (not arterial) thrombolic events (eg, stroke and catheter-related thromboses). Diagnosis is confirmed by specific polymerase chain reaction (PCR) analysis for factor V Leiden mutation.

2. Prothrombin G20210A mutation: genetic variation of the prothrombin gene, prothrombin G20210A; increased prothrombin

activity and increased prothrombin plasma concentrations, increased production of thrombin, resulting in increased risk for thromboses; second most common inherited disorder in adults of European descent, resulting in thrombolic tendencies. Diagnosis: specific PCR analysis for prothrombin G20210A

3. Protein C or protein S deficiency: autosomal dominant disorder. Homozygous form presents as purpura fulminans; heterozygous form as a threefold to sixfold increased risk for venous thrombosis. Diagnosis: consistently decreased or absent plasma levels

IV. Granulocytes (white blood cells [WBCs])

A. Definition: granulocytes are polymorphonuclear leukocytes (neutrophil, eosinophil, or basophil); neutrophils are the most numerous (55% to 70% of WBCs).

B. Neutrophil function includes: most accurate predictor of infection; function as phagocytes to ingest and destroy small particles such as bacteria, protozoa, cells and cellular debris, dust, and colloids. Neutrophils are increased at birth but decrease during the first week of life.

C. Neutropenia (Christensen, Calhoun, & Rimsza, 2000; Schibler, 2000): blood neutrophil concentration below the lower limit of values obtained for an age-defined population (Table 11.6)

1. Etiology: increased neutrophil destruction (*infection* [bacterial and fungal sepsis], isoimmunization [alloimmune] *and* autoimmune neonatal neutropenia, and chronic benign neutropenia); diminished neutrophil production (donor in twin-to-twin transfusion, drug or toxin induced, maternal hypertension [HTN]/PIH, neonatal chronic idiopathic, Rh hemolytic disease, severe combined immunodeficiency, viral infections [eg, rubella and CMV]); and excessive neutrophil margination (pseudoneutropenia and *endotoxemia*)

2. Clinical manifestations: associated physical and laboratory findings can suggest the specific underlying disorder.

3. Interventions: history and physical examination

a. For infants presenting with neutropenia early in the neonatal period consider the following: maternal peripartum infection

TABLE 11.6 WBC and Neutrophil Counts (10^3 cells/μL) for Term and Preterm Infants

Age (Days)	Total WBCs	Neutrophils	Bands/Metas
Term infant			
1	10–26	5–13	0.4–1.8
3	5–14.5	2–7	0.2–0.4
6	6–14.5	2–6	0.2–0.5
Preterm infant			
1	5–19	2–9	0.2–2.4
3	5–14	3–7	0.2–0.6
6	5.5–17.5	2–7	0.2–0.5

Adapted from Klaus, M. H., & Fanaroff, A. A. (2001). *Care of the high-risk neonate* (5th ed., pp. 574, 577). Philadelphia: WB Saunders.

(eg, chorioamnionitis, maternal fever and/or bacteruria, and prolonged or premature rupture of membranes; maternal HTN; antepartum fetal distress; birth depression; and multiple gestation with twin-to-twin transfusion.

b. Timing, duration, and severity should guide laboratory studies.

(1) Neutropenia accompanied by an immature-to-total (I:T) neutrophil ratio exceeding 0.3 to 0.5 often accompanies sepsis. Neutropenia persisting more than 2 to 3 days warrants additional evaluation. Neutropenia with I:T ratio < 0.2 *or* neutropenia in an infant with IUGR born to a mother with HTN usually resolves spontaneously. Neutropenia persisting > 5 days, particularly with a count < 500/μL, warrants additional evaluation.

(2) Laboratory studies include: CBC; peripheral blood smear to examine neutrophil morphology; consider CBC on the mother to evaluate her neutrophil concentration. Bone marrow aspiration or biopsy is performed in rare instances when neutropenia is severe (< 500/μL) and prolonged (> 5 days). To evaluate neonatal alloimmune neutropenia: perform neutrophil antigen typing and antineutrophil antibody screen on maternal blood. To evaluate neonatal isoimmune neutropenia: perform granulocyte agglutination assay and a granulocyte immunofluorescence assay on infant and maternal blood.

c. Antibiotic administration is indicated for neutropenia associated with bacterial sepsis.

d. IVIG administration: may raise neutrophil concentration in cases of immune-mediated neutropenia; use of IVIG is controversial for treatment of sepsis.

e. G-CSF is a commercially available product used to treat iatrogenic neutropenia and bone marrow failure syndromes; effective in correcting neutropenia associated with congenital neutropenia, Kostman's syndrome, and cyclic neutropenia

D. Neutrophilia: elevated neutrophil count (or granulocytosis). Etiology includes: infection; birth asphyxia and other causes of acute and chronic hypoxia can induce granulocytosis; and rarely due to intrinsic disorders of the bone marrow

V. Other blood cells

A. Howell-Jolly bodies: spherical or ovoid eccentrically located granules, observed in the stroma of circulating erythrocytes; their significance is not exactly known but occur most frequently in severe hemolytic anemia.

B. Heinz bodies: intracellular inclusions usually attached to the red cell membrane, composed of denatured Hb; they occur in thalassemia, enzymopathies, and hemoglobinopathies.

C. Dohle bodies: discrete round or oval bodies found in neutrophils. The presence of Dohle bodies is suggestive of infection.

D. Toxic granulation suggests infection.

E. Megathrombocytes or giant platelets may be increased in conditions of accelerated platelet production, compensating for increased destruction.

▼ References

Apt, L., & Downey, W. S. (1955). "Melena" neonatorum: The swallowed blood syndrome: A simple test for the differentiation of adult and fetal hemoglobin in bloody stools. *Journal of Pediatrics, 46*, 6–10.

Arnett, C. (1998). Thrombocytopenia in the newborn. *Neonatal Network, 17*(8), 27–32.

Bussel, J. B., Zabusky, M. R., Berkowitz, R. L., & McFarland, J. G. (1997) Fetal alloimmune thrombocytopenia. *New England Journal of Medicine, 337*, 22–26.

Christensen, R. D. (2000). Expected hematologic values for term and preterm neonates. In R. D. Christensen (Ed.), *Hematologic problems of the neonate* (pp. 117–136). Philadelphia: Saunders.

Christensen, R. D., Calhoun, D. A., & Rimsza, L. M. (2000). A practical approach to evaluating and treating neutropenia in the neonatal intensive care unit. *Clinics in Perinatology, 27*(3), 577–601.

Cohen, A., & Manno, C. S. (1999). Anemia. In A. R. Spitzer (Ed.), *Intensive care of the fetus and neonate* (pp. 1084–1097). St. Louis: Mosby.

Doyle, J. J., Schmidt, B., Blanchette, V., & Zipursky, A. (1999). Hematology. In G. B. Avery, M. A. Fletcher, & M. G. MacDonald (Eds.), *Neonatology: Pathophysiology & management of the newborn* (5th ed., pp 1045–1091). Philadelphia: Lippincott Williams & Wilkins.

Edstrom, C. S., Christensen, R. D., & Andrew, M. (2000). Developmental aspects of blood hemostasis and disorders of coagulation and fibrinolysis in the neonatal period. In R. D. Christensen (Ed.), *Hematologic problems of the neonate* (pp. 239–271). Philadelphia: Saunders.

Hirschfeld, A. B., Getachew, A., & Sessions, J. (2000). Drug doses. In G. K. Siberry & R. Iannone (Eds.), *The Johns Hopkins hospital, the Harriet Lane handbook* (5th ed., pp. 599–891). St. Louis: Mosby.

Klaus, M. H., & Fanaroff, A. A. (2001). *Care of the high-risk neonate* (5th ed., pp. 574 and 577). Philadelphia: WB Saunders.

Kling, P. J., Schmidt, R. L., Roberts, R. A., & Widness, J. A. (1996) Serum erythropoietin levels during infancy: Associations with erythropoiesis. *Journal of Pediatrics, 128*, 791–786.

Linderman, R., & Haga, P. (2000). Evaluation and treatment of polycythemia in the neonate. In R. D. Christensen (Ed.), *Hematologic problems of the neonate* (pp. 171–183). Philadelphia: Saunders.

Manco-Johnson, M., Rodden, D. J., & Collins, S. (2002). Newborn hematology. In G. B. Merenstein & S. L. Gardner (Eds.), *Handbook of neonatal intensive care* (5th ed., pp. 419–442). St. Louis: Mosby.

Ohls, R. K. (2000). Evaluation and treatment of anemia in the neonate. In R. D. Christensen (Ed.), *Hematologic problems of the neonate* (pp. 137–169). Philadelphia: Saunders.

Phipps, R. H., & Shannon, K. M. (1993). Hematologic problems. In M. Klaus & A. A. Fanaroff (Eds.), *Care of the high-risk neonate* (4th ed., pp 397–425) Philadelphia: Saunders.

Rivlin, K. A., & Bussel, J. B. (1999). Thrombosis and hemostasis. In A. R. Spitzer (Ed.), *Intensive care of the fetus and neonate* (pp. 1098–1111). St. Louis: Mosby.

Ross, L. R. (1999). Disorders of the adrenal cortex. In A. R. Spitzer (Ed.), *Intensive care of the fetus and neonate* (pp. 1084–1097). St. Louis: Mosby.

Schibler, K. (2000). Leukocyte development and disorders during the neonatal period. In R. D. Christensen (Ed.), *Hematologic problems of the neonate* (pp. 311–342). Philadelphia: Saunders.

Shaw, N. (1998). Assessment and management of hematologic dysfunction. In C. Kenner, J. W. Lott, & A. A. Flandermeyer (Eds.), *Comprehensive neonatal nursing: A physiologic perspective* (pp. 520–563). Philadelphia: W. B. Saunders.

Sola, M. C., & Christensen, R. D. (2000). Developmental aspects of platelets and disorders of platelets in the neonatal period. In R. D. Christensen (Ed.), *Hematologic problems of the neonate* (pp. 273–309). Philadelphia: Saunders.

Sola, M. C., DelVecchio, A., & Rimsza, L. M. (2000). Evaluation and treatment of thrombocytopenia in the neonatal intensive care unit. *Clinics in Perinatology, 27*(3), 655–679.

Yoder, M. C. (2000). Embryonic hematopoiesis. In R. D. Christensen (Ed.), *Hematologic problems of the neonate* (pp. 3–19). Philadelphia: Saunders.

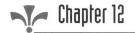 **Chapter 12**

Hepatic Diseases and Hyperbilirubinemia
Karen L. Williams, MSN, RNC, NNP

I. Hepatic diseases

The liver is the largest and most complex organ in the body. It is estimated that the liver performs more than 500 functions, including bile production; production and secretion of glucose, proteins, vitamins, fats, and other compounds; breakdown of hemoglobin; and conversion of ammonia to urea. Liver dysfunction in the infant can present with hepatomegaly, jaundice, and/or a bleeding disorder.

    A. Etiology of liver disease: the origin can be intrahepatic *or* extrahepatic, ie, within the biliary system (Balistreri, 1996; Bucuvalas & Balistreri, 1996).

        1. Intrahepatic disease processes result in: hepatocyte injury; injury to intrahepatic bile ducts and canaliculi; and injury to Kupffer cells (phagocytes lining the sinusoids of the liver).

        2. Extrahepatic diseases include those disorders that impair bile flow out of the liver: biliary atresia (congenital disorder in which the biliary structures are underdeveloped or absent); bile duct stenosis (narrowing of the distal portion of the common duct); biliary hypoplasia; choledochal cyst (rare congenital disorder characterized by cystic dilation of the common bile duct); abnormalities of the choledochopancreaticducatal junction (eg, congenital dilation of the biliary tree that leads to cyst formation); spontaneous perforation of the bile duct (commonly occurs at the junction of the cystic and common bile ducts); masses (eg, neoplasm or stone); and inspissated bile plug syndrome (the accumulation of bile or viscous mucus in the bile duct that leads to obstruction)

    B. Clinical manifestations of liver disease (Balistreri, 1996; Bucuvalas & Balistreri, 1996):

        1. Hepatomegaly: enlargement of the liver. Methods to determine liver size: palpation (the infant's liver edge can be felt 2 cm below the right costal margin; palpation of a liver edge $\geq$ 3.5 cm below the right costal margin is considered abnormal); percussion (the quality of the tone achieved during percussion will be "dull" compared to other abdominal organs); and imaging (radiographs and ultrasound)

        2. Jaundice: yellow discoloration of the skin and mucus membranes. It is the earliest symptom of liver dysfunction and *is visible when the indirect fraction is > 5 mg/dL.* New onset jaundice in an infant older than 2 weeks is abnormal. Total serum bilirubin values must be fractionated to determine the concentrations of unconjugated (indirect) and conjugated (direct) bilirubin.

        3. Cholestasis: pathologic condition that is the result of a prolonged elevation of direct (conjugated) bilirubin levels. It is evident when the direct serum bilirubin level comprises > 20% of the total serum bilirubin value (Gremse & Balistreri, 1989).

4. Bleeding diathesis (Balistreri, 1996): prolonged prothrombin time (PT) and partial thromboplastin time (PTT); petechiae and ecchymosis secondary to extramedullary hematopoiesis

C. Diagnostic testing (Balistreri, 1996; Bucuvalas & Balistreri, 1996; Novak, Suchy, & Balistreri, 1994; Slater, 1998):

1. Laboratory tests (serum, urine, and stool): it is important to test for potential causes of disease as well as determining liver function.

   a. Aspartate transaminase (AST, or SGOT): sensitive indicator of liver injury that is elevated with hepatocellular damage. AST is also present in heart and skeletal muscle, brain, and kidney. Therefore, elevated levels can be due to nonhepatic disorders. AST > alanine aminotransferase (ALT) in hemolytic disorders.

   b. ALT (or SGPT): found primarily in liver cells and highly specific for hepatocellular damage

   c. Alkaline phosphatase (Alk phos): present in liver and bone. Moderately elevated levels occur with most liver disease and extremely elevated levels are indicative of biliary tract disease (eg, obstruction and inflammation).

   d. γ-Glutamyltransferase (GGT): present in the liver, pancreas, and kidney. Moderately elevated levels are present in liver disease and higher levels are present with common bile duct obstruction.

   e. Lactic dehydrogenase (LDH): not a sensitive marker for hepatocellular damage. It is a better marker for hemolysis.

   f. Ammonia (NH_3) increases with urea cycle dysfunction, organic acidemia, and carnitine deficiency. Elevated levels are indicative of the liver's inability to detoxify ammonia.

   g. 5'-Nucleotidase increases with cholestasis and is specific in hepatobiliary disease.

   h. Bilirubin is the end-product of hemoglobin degradation and is formed in the reticuloendothelial system. Bilirubin circulates in two forms: conjugated (direct) and unconjugated (indirect). *Direct* bilirubin is that which has been *conjugated* in the liver to a *water-soluble* form. *Indirect (unconjugated)* bilirubin binds with albumin to form a *lipid-soluble* molecule. Elevated unconjugated bilirubin levels occur in severe hemolytic disease. Total bilirubin level is the sum of indirect and direct bilirubin levels.

   i. Evaluation for infection: complete blood cell count (CBC), reticulocyte count, and platelet count; TORCH complex and serology; Venereal Disease Research Laboratory (VDRL); and hepatitis B surface antigen (HBsAG) status of infant and mother.

   j. Immune studies: blood type and Coombs on mother and infant; immunoglobulin levels

   k. Proteins: albumin determines plasma oncotic pressure. Levels are decreased with moderate to severe liver disease; globulin levels are elevated with moderate to severe liver disease.

    l. Coagulation studies (refer to Chapter 11: Hematology): PT (may be prolonged with acute liver disease or vitamin K deficiency); PTT; fibrinogen levels and fibrin split products; and international normalized ratio (INR).

    m. Metabolic indicators: α_1-antitrypsin phenotype; serum amino acid profile; electrolytes contained in sweat; and thyroid studies (T_4 and thyroid-stimulating hormone [TSH])

    n. Urine studies: amino acid screen; reducing substances; and urobilinogen

    o. Stool samples: color; steatorrhea

2. Radiographic studies (Balistreri, 1996; Bucuvalas & Balistreri, 1996):

    a. Radiographs of the skull and long bones are important when evaluating for TORCH infection.

    b. Abdominal x-ray: may detect calcifications and gallstones in the biliary system

    c. Ultrasound: determines hepatic size, composition, and blood flow; visualizes choledochal cysts, gallstones, and bile duct dilation. Findings indicative of biliary atresia include small or absent gallbladder and the inability to visualize the common bile duct.

    d. Computed tomography (CT) scan: identifies infiltrates, tumors, and bile duct dilation and characterizes the density of the liver parenchyma.

    e. Cholescintigraphy: radionuclide imaging studies trace the intrahepatic and extrahepatic flow of bile after the administration of a technetium-99 labeled iminodiacetic acid (IDA) derivative. The scan helps to differentiate biliary atresia from other nonobstructive causes of cholestasis.

    f. Magnetic resonance imaging (MRI): scans an image in multiple planes that allows for tissue differentiation and identification of tumors or parenchymal lesions, as well as the quality of blood flow through vessels.

    g. Liver biopsy: histologic examination of liver cells (Balistreri, 1996; Bucuvalas & Balistreri, 1996; Halamek & Stevenson, 1997).

        (1) Histologic findings associated with *intrahepatic* disease: cholestasis; giant cells; minimal fibrosis; rare bile duct alteration; steatosis; and extramedullary hematopoiesis

        (2) Histologic findings associated with *extrahepatic* disease: cholestasis; bile duct proliferation; portal fibrosis; bile lakes; normal lobular architecture; and rare giant cells

D. Interventions (Gremse & Balistreri, 1989; Novak, Suchy, & Balistreri, 1994):

    1. Treat the underlying cause of the liver disorder and prevent progressive liver damage that leads to failure.

    2. Provide adequate nutrition and address the causes of malnutrition associated with cholestasis and liver dysfunction.

        a. Malabsorption of long-chain triglycerides: use a formula containing medium-chain triglycerides (MCT); oral administration of MCT oil

    b. Fat-soluble vitamin deficiencies:

      (1) Vitamin A (Aquasol A): 10,000–15,000 IU/day

      (2) Vitamin D: 5,000–8,000 IU/day of D_2 *or* 3-5μg/kg/day of 25-hydroxycholecalciferol

      (3) Vitamin E (α-tocopherol): 50–400 IU/day

      (4) Vitamin K: 2.5–5 mg/day as water-soluble derivative of menadione

    c. Water-soluble vitamin deficiency: supplement twice the recommended daily allowance.

    d. Micronutrient deficiency: supplement with calcium, phosphate, or zinc.

    e. Trace element retention: avoid foods that are high in copper.

  3. Pharmacotherapy for the retention of biliary components (bile acids, cholesterol):

    a. Bile acid binder: cholestyramine, 8–16 g/day

    b. Choleretics: phenobarbital, 3–5 mg/kg/day

    c. Rifampin, 10 mg/kg/day

    d. Ursodeoxycholic, 15 mg/kg/day

  4. Surgical correction: infants with extrahepatic biliary atresia may undergo the Kasai procedure, which involves resection of the extrahepatic bile ducts and creation of a channel for bile flow by using a piece of jejunum.

II. Hyperbilirubinemia

Bilirubin is the byproduct of the breakdown in the reticuloendothelial system of hemoglobin proteins. The majority of bilirubin is produced from the heme-containing protein in the red blood cell (RBC).

    Bilirubin exists in two forms: unconjugated (indirect) and conjugated (direct) bilirubin. When released into the circulation, bilirubin rapidly binds with albumin. Bound unconjugated bilirubin is converted in the liver's endoplasmic reticulum to the conjugated form by the enzyme *uridine diphosphate glucuronyl transferase* (UDPGT). Once converted, the water-soluble conjugated bilirubin enters the biliary tree, travels to the intestine, and is excreted in the stool (Halamek & Stevenson, 1997).

  A. Unconjugated (indirect) hyperbilirubinemia (Balistreri, 1996; Barsotti, 1999; Halamek & Stevenson, 1997; Oski, 1991; Schwoebel & Sakraida, 1997):

    1. Definition:

      a. Indirect serum bilirubin level ≥ 10 mg/dL for term infant *or* ≥ 4–5 mg/dL for preterm infants

      b. Physiologic jaundice: an increased concentration of serum unconjugated bilirubin during the first week of life that resolves spontaneously

      c. Pathologic jaundice: jaundice presenting before 24 hours of age and having a rate of rise that is > 0.5 mg/dL/hour

    2. Etiology:

      a. Increase in bilirubin production and enterohepatic circulation; decrease in bilirubin uptake into the liver

      b. Ethnic origin: those from Korea, China, and Japan and American Indians have higher bilirubin levels.

      c. Infants of diabetic mothers (IDM)

d. Increased RBC destruction:

  (1) Isoimmunization (refer to Chapter 3: High-Risk Pregnancies and Deliveries, ABO or Rh incompatibility): obtain the infant's blood type and Rh, Coombs', complete blood count (CBC), and reticulocyte count to determine the presence of hemolytic disease.

  (2) Defects in RBC metabolism: RBC enzyme defects impair erythrocyte function and shorten RBC life span (eg, G6PD deficiency; pyruvate kinase deficiency; hexokinase deficiency; and congenital erythropoietic porphyria).

  (3) Structural abnormalities of the RBC: abnormally shaped erythrocytes do not circulate well and sequester in the spleen resulting in increased destruction (eg, hereditary spherocytosis; hereditary elliptocytosis; and infantile pyknocytosis [a transient hemolytic disorder]).

  (4) Hemoglobinopathies: a group of diseases affecting erythrocytes due to the presence of one or more abnormally formed hemoglobin molecules (eg, sickle cell anemia and thalassemias)

e. Infection

f. Sequestration: hyperbilirubinemia occurs as the body metabolizes large collections of blood. Etiology includes birth trauma (eg, bruising, cephalohematoma, and subdural or subgaleal hematomas) and large hemangiomas (eg, Kasabach-Merritt syndrome)

g. Polycythemia secondary to: diabetes mellitus (DM); "milking" the umbilical cord; maternal-fetal transfusion; and fetal hypoxia

h. Disorders of bilirubin conjugation:

  (1) Hypothyroidism

  (2) Crigler-Najjar types I and II: disorders caused by a defect in the structure or inactivity of the UDPGT enzyme

  (3) Gilbert syndrome: defect in the hepatic uptake of bilirubin and decreased UDPGT function

  (4) Lucey-Driscoll syndrome: disorder caused by an unidentified inhibitor of glucuronyl transferase, resulting in a severe nonhemolytic unconjugated hyperbilirubinemia

i. Disorders of recirculation and excretion:

  (1) Intestinal obstruction: delayed passage of stool; structural (stenosis or atresia) or mechanical (ileus or meconium plug); pyloric stenosis; Hirschsprung disease; and cystic fibrosis

  (2) Breast milk jaundice: occurs after the fifth day of life and peaks by 3 weeks of life. It is believed to be the result of increased enterohepatic circulation of unconjugated bilirubin secondary to an unknown factor in breast milk.

3. Clinical manifestations and diagnosis:

  a. Hemolysis; hepatomegaly and/or splenomegaly; jaundice (progresses in a cephalocaudal direction)

    b. Umbilical cord blood bilirubin levels: an infant with a cord blood bilirubin level ≥ 4 mg/dL requires evaluation.

    c. Laboratory studies: mother and infant's ABO and Rh, direct antibody testing (DAT), total and direct bilirubin levels, reticulocyte count, CBC with differential and RBC smear, G6PD screen

4. Interventions:

    a. Track the "rate of rise." **Rapid rate of rise is > 0.5 mg/dL/hr or 5 mg/kg/day.**

    b. Hydration improves urine output, bile flow, and stool output.

    c. It is not necessary to stop breastfeeding unless the level is high enough to cause concern about the development of kernicterus (Halamek & Stevenson, 1997; Schwoebel & Sakraida, 1997).

    d. Phototherapy: bilirubin undergoes three types of photochemical reaction (photoisomerization, structural isomerization, or photo-oxidation) when exposed to light with a wavelength of 420–500 nm (blue light). Adverse effects of phototherapy include: retinal damage (**shield the infant's eyes with a light-occlusive covering**); increased body and environmental temperature; increased insensible and intestinal water loss; watery stools; skin rash; and "bronze baby syndrome" (the urine, serum, and skin become bronze when phototherapy is used to treat conjugated (direct) hyperbilirubinemia).

    e. Pharmacotherapy:

        (1) Phenobarbital (5 mg/kg/day): increases glucuronyl transferase activity.

        (2) Metalloporphyrins: tin and zinc protoporphyrins inhibit the activity of heme-oxygenase (the initial enzyme activated for the conversion of heme to bilirubin). This therapy is currently experimental.

    f. Exchange transfusion (Alexander & Robin, 2000; Ebel & Raffini, 2000; Halamek & Stevenson, 1997; Hinkes & Cloherty, 1998):

        (1) Indications: to correct anemia (eg, hydrops fetalis); for removal of hemolyzed and antibody coated RBCs (eg, Rh disease); for removal of bacterial toxins; to correct hyperbilirubinemia uncontrolled with phototherapy (double-volume exchange decreases plasma bilirubin levels to approximately one-half pre-exchange levels); and to decrease the infant's Hct (eg, polycythemia)

        (2) Mode of action: the goal is to remove approximately 63% (single-volume exchange) or 85% to 87% (double-volume exchange) of the infant's circulating blood volume and replace it with donor whole blood, packed red blood cells (PRBCs), or saline; double-volume exchange with whole blood is used to treat hyperbilirubinemia, DIC, and autoimmune thrombocytopenia; partial-volume exchange with normal saline (decreases Hct without decreasing blood volume [eg, polycythemia]) or PRBCs (increase Hct without increasing blood volume [eg, anemia associated with hydrops fetalis])

(3) Exchange transfusion calculations (Table 12.1)
(4) Procedure:
- **(a)** Pre-exchange blood work: CBC, reticulocyte count, peripheral smear, bilirubin, Ca^{++}, glucose, total protein, Rh, type, and Coombs'
- **(b)** Requires indwelling umbilical vein (UV) (double lumen) or UV and umbilical artery (UA) catheters in order to withdraw and replace blood.
- **(c)** Under sterile conditions small aliquots of blood (< 10% of the blood volume) are serially removed and replaced with donor blood or saline.
- **(d)** Postexchange blood studies: electrolytes, blood urea nitrogen [BUN], creatinine, Ca^{++}, glucose, CBC, platelets, bilirubin, and blood type
(5) Complications of exchange transfusion include: thrombocytopenia; portal vein thrombosis; perforation of the umbilical vein; necrotizing enterocolitis; cardiac arrhythmia; electrolyte disturbances (hypocalcemia, hypomagnesemia, and hypoglycemia); acidosis; graft versus host disease; and infection (eg, hepatitis B and C, HIV)

5. Outcome (Halamek & Stevenson, 1997; Hinkes & Cloherty, 1998):
   a. Severe anemia secondary to ongoing hemolysis in the presence of hemolytic disease. As maternal antibodies die there is a decrease in RBC destruction.
   b. Bilirubin-induced neurologic dysfunction, ie, adverse effects associated with elevated unconjugated bilirubin levels. These effects can be transient and reversible *or* permanent. The neurologic examination is significant for the following: lethargy; poor feeding or abnormal sucking pattern; alternating hypotonia and hypertonia; and abnormal BAER (brainstem auditory-evoked response), revealing auditory conduction abnormalities.

 TABLE 12.1 Exchange Transfusion Calculations

Partial exchange transfusion	Normal saline or fresh frozen plasma: $$\frac{EBV^* \times (\text{measured Hct} - \text{desired Hct})}{\text{measured Hct}}$$
	PRBCs: $$\frac{EBV \times (\text{desired Hct} - \text{measured Hct})}{(\text{PRBC Hct} - \text{measured Hct})}$$ *EBV = infant's weight (kg) × 80 cc
Double volume exchange transfusion	EBV × 2

EBV = estimated blood volume; Hct = hematocrit; PRBC = packed red blood cells.

    c. Kernicterus: irreversible brain injury characterized by yellow pigmentation deposited in specific areas of the brain, especially the basal ganglia and dentate nucleus of the cerebellum

      (1) Risk factors that contribute to a more permeable blood-brain barrier include systemic illness, prematurity, hypoxia, and acidosis.

      (2) Clinical manifestations include: seizures, opisthotonos, arching, alternating hypotonia and hypertonia, high-pitched cry, fever, and long-term effects (eg, asymmetric spasticity, upward gazing, hearing loss, and athetoid cerebral palsy).

B. Conjugated (direct) hyperbilirubinemia (Balistreri, 1996; Barsotti, 1999; Bucuvalas & Balistreri, 1996; Gremse & Balistreri, 1989; Hinkes & Cloherty, 1998):

    1. Definition: direct (conjugated) serum bilirubin ≥ 3 mg/dL *or* a fraction > 10% to 15% of the total serum bilirubin. It is due to a failure of conjugated bilirubin to be excreted from the liver (hepatocytes) into the duodenum because of deficient bile secretion or flow, thereby, causing liver cell injury.

    2. Etiology:

      a. Idiopathic: histologic changes within the liver without a confirmed etiology

      b. Hyperalimentation administration

      c. Intrahepatic disorders:

        (1) Bile duct paucity (hypoplasia): decreased number of bile ducts within the portal triad; syndromic (Alagille) paucity is characterized by a decreased number of intralobular bile ducts, cholestasis, and other congenital anomalies; nonsyndromic paucity has a decreased number of intralobular bile ducts without other abnormalities.

        (2) Byler's disease: a progressive hepatocellular disease of uncertain etiology

        (3) Defects in bile acid metabolism: Zellweger syndrome ([cerebrohepatorenal syndrome] an autosomal recessive disorder characterized by the absence of hepatic and renal peroxisomes); recurrent intrahepatic cholestasis (eg, familial benign recurrent cholestasis and hereditary cholestasis with lymphedema)

        (4) Anatomic defects: congenital hepatic fibrosis/infantile polycystic disease and Caroli disease (cystic dilation of intrahepatic ducts)

      d. Metabolic disorders:

        (1) Impaired amino acid and protein metabolism (eg, tyrosinemia)

        (2) Impaired lipid metabolism: Wolman disease ([autosomal recessive disorder] infants present with vomiting, diarrhea, failure to thrive, steatorrhea, and hepatosplenomegaly); Neimann-Pick disease ([autosomal recessive disorder] sphingomyelinase deficiency leading to an accumulation of sphingomyelin); Gaucher disease ([autosomal recessive disorder] glucocerebrosidase deficiency leading to an accumulation of glucosylceramide in the lysosomes of the reticuloendothelial cells of the liver); and cholesteryl ester storage disease

(3) Impaired carbohydrate metabolism: galactosemia ([autosomal recessive disorder] *infants are at increased risk for gram-negative sepsis*); fructosemia (hereditary intolerance to fructose); glucogenosis III and IV (enzyme deficiencies)

(4) Metal metabolism disorders: Wilson disease (disorder of copper metabolism); hemochromatosis ([neonatal iron storage disease] early-onset liver disease in the first 4 to 7 days, with increased iron deposition in liver, heart, pancreas, and endocrine organs)

(5) Other metabolic disorders: α_1-antitrypsin deficiency (autosomal recessive disorder); cystic fibrosis (infants may present with meconium ileus and cholestasis and progress to biliary obstruction secondary to excessive production of biliary mucus); erythropoietic protoporphyria ([autosomal dominant disorder] enzyme deficiency disorder characterized by hemolysis, splenomegaly, and pink-red urine that appears orange under ultraviolet light); familial erythrophagocytic lymphohistiocytosis (RBC hemolysis by phagocytic histiocytes); hypothyroidism; and hypopituitarism

  e. Genetic: trisomies 18 and 21 and Donahue syndrome (leprechaunism)

3. Clinical manifestations (Balistreri, 1996; Bucuvalas & Balistreri, 1996; Gremse & Balistreri, 1989): icterus, dark urine, acholic stools; hepatomegaly, splenomegaly; hepatitis secondary to infection (Box 12.1) or toxic exposure (eg, hyperalimentation, endotoxemia from infection, and medications.); petechiae; chorioretinitis; and microcephaly

4. Interventions (Balistreri, 1996; Barsotti, 1999; Bucuvalas & Balistreri, 1996; Gremse & Balistreri, 1989):

  a. Laboratory studies: CBC with differential and reticulocyte count; PT and PTT; liver function tests; TORCH work-up;

▼ **BOX 12.1** | **Infectious Causes of Hepatitis**

Bacterial	**Viral**
Listeria	Coxsackie
Syphilis	Cytomegalovirus
Tuberculosis	Echovirus
	Epstein-Barr
Parasitic	Hepatitis A, B, and C
Toxoplasmosis	Herpes
HIV	Parvovirus B19
	Rubella
	Varicella

α$_1$-antitrypsin; blood and urine cultures and urine-reducing substances

b. Treat cholestasis and the underlying cause of liver dysfunction either medically or surgically (eg, Kasai procedure for biliary atresia).

c. Provide adequate nutrition.

d. Address the causes of malnutrition associated with cholestasis and liver dysfunction (refer to "Interventions for hepatic diseases," section I, part D).

5. Outcome: depends upon the extent of parenchymal liver damage and whether the damage is irreparable.

▼ References

Alexander, D. C., & Robin, B. (2000). Neonatology. In G.K. Siberry & R. Iannone (Eds.), *The Harriett Lane handbook* (15th ed., pp. 417–438). St. Louis: Mosby.

Balistreri, W. F. (1996). Liver and biliary system: Development and function. In W. E. Nelson, R. E. Behrman, R. M. Kliegman, & A. M. Arvin (Eds.), *Nelson textbook of pediatrics* (15th ed., pp. 1125–1150). Philadelphia: WB Sanders.

Barsotti, M. (1999). Hyperbilirubinemia, direct (conjugated hyperbilirubinemia). In T. L. Gomella, M. D. Cunningham, F. G. Eyal, & K. E. Zenk (Eds.), *Neonatology: Management, procedures, on-call problems, diseases, drugs* (4th ed., pp. 230–232). Stamford, CT: Appleton & Lange.

Bucuvalas, J. C., & Balistreri, W. F. (1996) The liver and bile duct. In A. M. Rudolph, J. I. E. Hoffman, & C. D. Rudolph (Eds.), *Rudolph's pediatrics* (20th ed., pp. 1123–1150). Stamford, CT: Appleton & Lange.

Cunningham, M. D. (1999). Exchange transfusion. In T. L. Gomella, M. D. Cunningham, F. G. Eyal, & K. E. Zenk (Eds.), Neonatology: Management, procedures, on-call problems, diseases, drugs (4th ed., pp. 165–169). Stamford, CT: Appleton & Lange.

Ebel, B. E., & Raffini, L. (2000). Hematology. In G. K. Siberry & R. Iannone (Eds.), *The Harriett Lane handbook* (15th ed., pp. 307–331). St. Louis: Mosby.

Gremse, D. A., & Balistreri, W. F. (1989) Neonatal cholestasis. In E. Lebenthal (Ed.), *Textbook of gastroenterology and nutrition in infancy* (2nd ed., pp. 909–948). New York: Raven.

Halamek, L. P., & Stevenson, D. K. (1997). Neonatal jaundice and liver disease. In A. A. Fanaroff & R. J. Martin (Eds.), *Neonatal-perinatal medicine: Diseases of the newborn* (6th ed., pp. 1345–1383). St. Louis: Mosby.

Hinkes, M. T. & Cloherty, J. P. (1998). Neonatal hyperbilirubinemia. In J. P. Cloherty & A. R. Stark (Eds.), *Manual of neonatal care* (4th ed., pp. 175–209). Philadelphia: Lippincott-Raven.

Novak, D. A., Suchy, F. J., & Balistreri, W. F., (1994). Disorders of the liver and biliary system relevant to clinical practice. In F. A. Oski, C. D. DeAngelis, R. D. Feigin, J. A. McMillan, & J. B. Warshaw (Eds.), *Principles and practice of pediatrics* (2nd ed., pp. 910–1143). Philadelphia: JB Lippincott.

Oski, F. A. (1991). Disorders of bilirubin metabolism: General considerations. In H. W. Taeuch, R. A. Ballard, & M. E. Avery (Eds.), *Schaffer and Avery's diseases in the newborn* (6th ed., pp. 749–775). Philadelphia: WB Saunders.

Roy, C. C., Silverman, A., & Alagille, D. A. (1995). *Pediatric clinical gastroenterology* (4th ed., pp. 636–683). St. Louis: Mosby.

Schwoebel, A., & Sakraida, S. (1997). Hyperbilirubinemia: New approaches to an old problem. *Journal of Perinatal, Neonatal Nursing, 11*(3), 78–97.

Slater, R. (1998). Liver function tests in the newborn. *Neonatal Network, 17*(6), 75–78.

Sokol, R. J., & Narkewicz, M. R. (1997). Liver and pancreas. In W. M. Hays, J. R. Hayward, & M. J. Levin (Eds.), *Current pediatric diagnosis and treatment* (13th ed., pp. 568–600). Stamford. CT: Appleton & Lange.

Treem, W. R. (1990). Jaundice. In M. W. Schwartz, E. B., Charney, T. A. Curry, & S. Ludwig (Eds.), *Pediatric primary care: A problem oriented approach* (2nd ed., pp. 257–266). Chicago: Year Book Medical Publishers, Inc.

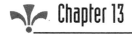 **Chapter 13**

Respiratory Disorders

Paulette S. Haws, MSN, RNC, NNP

Part A: **Respiratory Distress and Apnea**

I. Pulmonary versus nonpulmonary reasons for respiratory distress (Table 13.1)

II. Air leak syndromes

  A. All air leak syndromes result from overdistention of alveoli and terminal airways leading to uneven alveolar ventilation, air trapping, and eventual alveolar and/or terminal airway rupture. With this disruption of airway integrity there is movement of free air into the surrounding spaces of the pleural, pericardial, and/or peritoneal cavities (Casey, 1999; Pauly, 1999).

  B. Etiology: barotrauma secondary to mechanical ventilation; gas trapping secondary to a ball-valve effect in the presence of meconium, mucous, blood, and/or other material; intubation of right main stem bronchus; high opening distending pressures at birth; and lung compliance changes after surfactant therapy

  C. Pneumothorax: free air trapped between the visceral and parietal pleura

    1. Clinical manifestations:

      a. Infant may be asymptomatic; mild respiratory distress (eg, tachypnea, mild oxygen requirement)

      b. *Tension pneumothorax elicits classic signs of respiratory distress* (eg, tachypnea, grunting, retracting, flaring, decreased or absent breath sounds on the affected side, distant or shifted

 TABLE 13.1 Pulmonary Versus Nonpulmonary Reasons for Respiratory Distress Syndrome

Pulmonary	Nonpulmonary
Common: surfactant deficiency, transient tachypnea, aspiration (meconium, blood, amniotic fluid, formula), air leak syndromes, and pneumonia **Less common:** airway obstruction, pulmonary hemorrhage, pulmonary hypoplasia, rib-cage abnormalities, and space-occupying lesions (CDH, CAM)	**Metabolic:** acidosis, sepsis, hypoglycemia, hypothermia, and hypermagnesemia **Neuromuscular:** intracranial hemorrhage, maternal and neonatal drugs, neural tube defects, and phrenic nerve damage **Vascular:** PPHN, CHD, hypovolemia, anemia, and polycythemia

CDH = congenital diaphragmatic hernia; CAM = congenital adenomatoid malformation; PPHN = persistent pulmonary hypertension of the newborn; CHD = congenital heart disease.

heart sounds, cyanosis, oxygen requirement, respiratory acidosis, hypotension).

2. Diagnosis:
  a. Transillumination, a fiber-optic light placed on the infant's skin "lights up" the chest on the side of the suspected pneumothorax.
  b. Chest x-ray:
   (1) Anteroposterior view (AP): mediastinal shift away from the affected side; downward displacement of the diaphragm; lung tissue will be displaced away from the chest wall by free air.
   (2) Cross-table lateral view: rim of air will be seen around the lung.
   (3) Lateral decubitus view: pneumothorax may be detected when the infant is positioned with the suspected side up.

3. Interventions:
  a. Asymptomatic infants: usually resolves spontaneously.
  b. Mild respiratory distress: provide oxygen-rich environment (eg, 100% Oxy-Hood) to "facilitate nitrogen washout from blood and tissues and thus establish a difference in the gas tensions between the loculated gases in the chest and those in the blood. This diffusion gradient results in rapid resorption of the loculated gas, with resolution of the pneumothorax" (Pauly, 1999, p. 493).
  c. *Tension pneumothorax requires immediate evacuation* through needle aspiration and/or chest tube placement (second or third intercostal space along the midclavicular line for anterior placement; third, fourth, or fifth intercostal space along the anterior axillary line for posterior placement. **Nipple is located at approximately the fourth intercostal space**) (Gomella, 1999a).

D. Pneumomediastinum: free air in the mediastinum; often occurs during the first few breaths in term infants.
  1. Clinical manifestations (Casey, 1999; Pauly, 1999): usually asymptomatic unless accompanied by a pneumothorax; mild respiratory distress; increased anteroposterior diameter of the chest; and muffled heart sounds
  2. Diagnosis: AP chest x-ray shows a *"spinnaker sail sign"* indicating that the thymus is elevated off the heart and surrounded by air; cross-table lateral view shows an anterior collection of air.
  3. Interventions: usually resolves spontaneously without intervention; unless other air leak syndromes are present and require invasive intervention, simply provide an oxygen-rich environment to facilitate a nitrogen washout.

E. Pneumopericardium: free air travels along vascular sheaths and accumulates in the pericardial sac, often preceded by a pneumomediastinum.
  1. Clinical manifestations (Silverman, 1998):
   a. May be asymptomatic.
   b. *Signs of cardiac tamponade* (abrupt life-threatening event):

initial tachycardia with decreased pulse pressure followed by hypotension, bradycardia, and cyanosis

  c. *Shrinking QRS complex*, muffled or distant heart sounds, pericardial knock (Hamman sign), or millwheel-like murmur (bruit de moulin)

2. Diagnosis:

  a. *"Halo" of air completely surrounds heart* on all radiographic projections. The presence of air at the diaphragmatic cardiac (inferior) surface is diagnostic.

  b. Usually accompanied by pulmonary interstitial emphysema (PIE) or pneumothorax and often preceded by pneumomediastinum (Korones & Bada-Ellzey, 1993; Pauly, 1999)

3. Interventions: placement of a pericardial drain or pericardial tap is essential in the symptomatic infant with a cardiac tamponade.

F. PIE (Pauly, 1999; Silverman, 1998): air dissects into the perivascular tissues and travels around blood vessels, along lymphatics and bronchioles, or directly through the lung interstitium to the pleural surface. The extrapulmonary air may extend and cause a pneumothorax, pneumomediastinum, or pneumopericardium.

1. Clinical manifestations:

  a. Usually seen in infants with poor lung compliance who require continuous positive airway pressure or positive-pressure ventilation

  b. Hypoxia, hypercapnia, and acidosis. Slow deterioration in blood gas values, with apparent need for increased ventilatory support. *PIE may worsen with increased ventilatory support.*

  c. Bradycardia and hypotension

2. Diagnosis: chest x-rays demonstrate *radiolucencies* that are either *linear* (vary in length and do not branch; seen in periphery and medially and may be mistakenly interpreted as air bronchograms) or *cystic* (may be seen in one or both lungs). Lungs may appear hyperinflated with flattened diaphragm.

3. Interventions: minimize inflating pressures (peak inspiratory pressure [PIP] and positive-end expiratory pressure [PEEP]); shorten inspiratory time (IT); consider high-frequency ventilation; place the infant with affected side in dependent position; selectively intubate the unaffected or less affected lung.

G. Pneumoperitoneum (Gomella, 1999; Korones & Bada-Ellzey, 1993): abnormal collection of air in the peritoneal cavity secondary to gastrointestinal (GI) perforation, dissection of air through the diaphragmatic esophageal aperture, or iatrogenic reasons (eg, improperly placed suprapubic catheter)

1. Clinical manifestations: abdominal distention; respiratory distress with worsening blood gas values; and hypotension

2. Diagnosis:

  a. Determine the origin of the air leak: GI origin is suspected when there is abdominal abnormality on x-ray (eg, necrotizing enterocolitis [NEC]) and after abdominal surgery; respiratory origin is suspected with the presence of PIE, pneumothorax, or pneumomediastinum on x-ray.

      b. Radiographic studies:

        (1) AP chest and abdominal x-rays may demonstrate pleural air leaks, bowel gas patterns and intraluminal air, and/or air-fluid levels in the peritoneal cavity indicating an ileus.

        (2) Left lateral decubitus abdominal x-ray may demonstrate air rising anteriorly and accumulating over the liver.

    3. Interventions:

      a. Paracentesis may be required when diaphragmatic excursion is impeded secondary to extensive peritoneal air; nasogastric tube insertion

      b. Close observation with follow-up x-rays

      c. Possible abdominal laparotomy for GI perforation or NEC

III. Airway obstructions and anomalies

    A. Choanal atresia (Casey, 1999): bony or membranous protrusion into the nasal passage/s (unilateral or bilateral), producing partial or complete obstruction of the airway; may be present with other anomalies (eg, Treacher-Collins Syndrome, CHARGE Association, and TE fistula).

      1. Clinical manifestations:

        a. Bilateral obstruction (signs of respiratory failure); unilateral obstruction (intermittent respiratory distress)

        b. *Inability to pass a nasogastric tube is diagnostic.*

      2. Interventions: prone position with oral airway or intubation; surgical correction

    B. Cystic hygroma (Casey, 1999; Hartman, et al., 1999): benign congenital lymphangioma (watery cyst) that is usually multiloculated with poorly defined borders produced by abnormal prenatal lymphatic channel development. Most occur in the neck, posterior to the sternocleidomastoid muscle; they also occur in the groin, axilla, and mediastinum.

      1. Clinical manifestations: depend upon the size and location of the mass; distortion of the local anatomy; and respiratory distress secondary to airway compression

      2. Interventions: aspiration of the cyst to relieve airway compromise; surgical excision at 4 to 12 months of age if the patient is asymptomatic (multiple excisions are usually required to save vital nerve and vascular structures)

    C. Micrognathia (Casey, 1999): underdevelopment of the mandible; occurs with various syndromes (eg, Treacher-Collins syndrome, Pierre Robin sequence, cri-du-chat syndrome, and trisomy 18).

      1. Clinical manifestations: upper airway occlusion with resultant respiratory distress

      2. Interventions:

        a. Prone position; oral airway, intubation or tracheostomy

        b. Mandibular "catch up" growth occurs between 6 and 12 months of age

    D. Tracheomalacia (Casey, 1999; Desai, Statter, & Arensman, 1996; Hartman, et al., 1999): anterior-posterior collapse and obstruction of the trachea secondary to hypoplastic cartilage that inadequately supports the trachea during expiration

      1. Etiology: *primary* tracheomalacia is a self-limiting defect that usually resolves by 6 to 12 months of age (some sources state resolution occurs by 2 years of age); *secondary* tracheomalacia may be seen with certain defects, such as tracheoesophageal fistula or vascular compression or with patients who are ventilator dependent (eg, bronchopulmonary dysplasia [BPD]).

2. Clinical manifestations: expiratory stridor; wheezing; coughing; recurrent respiratory infections; chest x-ray shows diffuse overinflation.

3. Diagnosis: flexible bronchoscopy when the infant is having spontaneous respirations; computer tomography (CT) scan to demonstrate tracheal abnormalities

4. Interventions: tracheal intubation or tracheostomy with continuous positive airway pressure (CPAP) or PEEP

E. Tracheal stenosis (Desai, et al., 1996; Hansen & Corbet, 1998b; Hartman, et al., 1999): stenosis of a short area, or the entire trachea, often with absence of the tracheal cartilage

1. Etiology: laryngeal webs (may or may not have cartilaginous deformities); vascular rings; masses (eg, granulomas and polyps); or a complication of prolonged intubation leading to inflammation secondary to endotracheal tube manipulation and suctioning

2. Clinical manifestations:
   a. Stridor; wheezing; persistent cough; respiratory distress; symptoms worsen in the presence of upper airway infection; failure to maintain patent airway after extubation; chest x-ray demonstrates recurrent atelectasis and emphysema.
   b. Feeding difficulties

3. Diagnosis:
   a. Clinical history; radiographs; flexible bronchoscopy (at the bedside) or rigid bronchoscopy (in the operating room)

4. Interventions: tracheal dilation (eg, mucosal webs); short stenotic lesion may be repaired with an end-to-end anastomosis; long segment of stenotic trachea may require tracheostomy.

F. Vascular rings and slings (Desai, et al., 1996; Hansen & Corbet, 1998b; Hartman, et al., 1999): anomalous development of the great vessels that completely encircle the trachea *and* esophagus (**rings**) or pass around the trachea *or* esophagus without completely encircling them (**slings**)

1. Etiology is extensive. The more common anomalies include:
   a. Double aortic arch; right aortic arch with left ductus arteriosus or ligamentum arteriosum; left-sided origin of the innominate artery or right-sided origin of left common carotid artery; and an origin of the left pulmonary artery from the right pulmonary artery

2. Clinical manifestations:
   a. Inspiratory and expiratory stridor; barking cough; respiratory distress; apnea; infants position themselves with heads and necks hyperextended.
   b. Feeding difficulties often associated with regurgitation

3. Diagnosis:
   a. Chest x-ray: mild hyperinflation, right-sided aorta, narrowed trachea
   b. Barium swallow: indentation of the esophagus
   c. Endoscopy often shows a pulsatile mass at the carina.

       d. Magnetic resonance imaging (MRI) and echocardiogram demonstrate abnormalities.

    4. Interventions: surgical repair of the anomaly

IV. Parenchymal lung disease

  A. Hyaline membrane disease (HMD) (or respiratory distress syndrome [RDS] or surfactant deficiency): a developmental pulmonary disorder that begins at birth or shortly thereafter, persists for 48 to 96 hours, and resolves when initial diuresis commences. "The clinical course varies depending upon the gestational age of the infant, the severity of the disease, the presence of infection, the degree of shunting of blood through a PDA, and whether or not assisted ventilation was initiated" (Pauly, 1999, p. 503).

    1. Etiology:

      a. Surfactant deficiency; anatomical malformation (eg, congenital diaphragmatic hernia, congenital cystic adenomatoid malformation, and neuroblastoma); infection (eg, group B streptococcus, herpes simplex, and varicella); and aspiration (eg, meconium, blood, and amniotic fluid)

    2. Risk factors contributing to the development of HMD:

      a. Prematurity (increasing risk of HMD with decreasing gestational age and decreasing birth weight); male gender (2:1 male to female ratio)

      b. Maternal diabetes mellitus (DM); maternal chorioamnionitis; cesarean section without labor; and perinatal asphyxia

      c. Hypothermia; hypoglycemia; hydrops fetalis; and second twin

    3. Clinical manifestations:

      a. Increased work of breathing (grunting, retractions, nasal flaring, and paradoxical seesaw respirations); cyanosis secondary to hypoxemia; increasing oxygen requirement; respiratory acidosis

      b. Radiographic findings (classic triad): **air bronchograms**; **diffuse bilateral haziness**; and **small lung fields**

    4. Interventions:

      a. Ventilatory support (many practitioners maintain $PaCO_2$ between 45 and 60 mmHg and pH > 7.25) and supplemental oxygen to maintain PaO_2 > 50 mmHg

      b. Surfactant administration; antibiotic administration to treat suspected/actual infection

  B. BPD (or chronic lung disease [CLD]): a clinically useful definition of BPD is neonatal lung disease that follows a primary course of respiratory failure and is present in an infant who is oxygen dependent after 28 days of life and 36 weeks' postconceptual age and has an abnormal chest x-ray and physical examination (Casey, 1999; Zayek, 1999).

    1. Etiology is multifactorial (Zayek, 1999):

      a. *Lung injury* secondary to: surfactant deficiency; pulmonary edema; oxygen administration and oxygen toxicity with resultant endothelial and ciliary tissue injury and destruction, altered pulmonary lymphatic flow, altered surfactant synthesis, and decreased lung growth; mechanical ventilation leading to barotrauma; and inflammation with the presence of

neutrophils and the toxic substances associated with them (proteases, oxygen-free radicals, and mediators of inflammation)
   b. *Pathologic changes* after lung injury include: atelectasis leading to some alveolar areas filled with proteinaceous fluid whereas other areas are overexpanded; decreased airway epithelium and cilia and, in severe cases, necrotizing tracheobronchitis; and interstitial fibrosis, cystic dilation, interstitial edema, and lymphatic distention
2. Risk factors contributing to the development of BPD include (Zayek, 1999): prematurity (greater risk of lung damage in infants < 1,500 g); male gender; White race; severe RDS and mechanical ventilation lasting more than the first week of life; air leak syndromes; excessive fluid intake during the first few days of life; symptomatic PDA; nutritional deficiencies; and sepsis.
3. Clinical manifestations (Casey, 1999; Zayek, 1999):
   a. Increased work of breathing (tachypnea, retractions); abnormal breath sounds (rales, rhonchi, and wheezes); bronchospasm; abnormal blood gases (hypoxia, hypercapnia, and acidosis)
   b. Abnormal chest x-ray: lung findings are variable (diffuse haziness, areas of atelectasis and/or hyperinflation, streaky interstitial markings, and cystic changes).
   c. Cardiomegaly on chest x-ray; right ventricular hypertrophy and right axis deviation on ECG; cor pulmonale (enlarged right ventricle leading to right-sided congestive heart failure [CHF]); hepatomegaly secondary to right-sided heart failure
   d. Serum electrolyte imbalance (elevated serum bicarbonate) secondary to chronic carbon dioxide retention; fluid intolerance (excessive weight gain, edema, decreased urine output) without an increase in fluid intake
4. Complications:
   a. Prolonged ventilatory and oxygen support; tracheal malacia and tracheal stenosis; bronchospasm; BPD spells (irritable, agitated, cyanotic, hypoxia, increased work of breathing, and hypercapnia)
   b. Increased risk for infections (upper respiratory infections, otitis media, respiratory syncytial virus [RSV], pneumonia)
   c. Poor weight gain; poor nippling skills; gastroesophageal reflux
   d. Retinopathy of prematurity; developmental delays
   e. Increased risk for sudden infant death syndrome (SIDS)
5. Interventions:
   a. Ventilatory support (wean slowly from ventilator in order to allow time for the infant to compensate) and oxygen supplementation before and after extubation (to prevent hypoxia); maintain PaO_2 > 55 mmHg and pH > 7.25.
   b. Optimize nutrition to promote growth.
   c. Fluid restriction; diuretics for fluid management and control pulmonary edema.
   d. Bronchodilators; steroid administration (use varies among institutions and remains controversial)

C. Chronic pulmonary insufficiency of prematurity (CPIP) (or late-onset respiratory distress) (Casey, 1999; Hansen & Corbet, 1998a): occurs with premature infants who weigh < 1,500 g, have limited exposure to increased levels of supplemental oxygen, and have no significant underlying disease. They demonstrate recurrent apneic episodes and respiratory difficulties after the first few days of life.

1. Etiology: increased chest wall compliance, decreased intercostal muscle mass, and diaphragmatic fatigue lead to decreased minute volume and areas of atelectasis with resultant hypoxia, hypercapnia, and apnea.

2. Clinical manifestations:
   a. Chest x-ray demonstrates decreased lung volumes, areas of atelectasis, and diffuse haziness without cystic changes (within the first month of life).
   b. Increased need for supplemental oxygen and increased A-a gradient; transient cyanosis; increased work of breathing (retractions); hypercapnia; apnea and bradycardia
   c. Symptoms worsen for 2 to 6 weeks and then gradually resolve during the next several months.

3. Interventions: supplemental oxygen; nasal CPAP; methylxanthine administration (eg, caffeine, aminophylline, and theophylline); and optimize nutrition to promote growth.

D. Meconium aspiration syndrome (MAS) (Casey, 1999; Eichenwald, 1998; Pauly, 1999): meconium (contains epithelial cells, hair, mucus, and bile salts) is passed in utero as a result of asphyxia and hypercapnia and aspirated in the presence of gasping or deep fetal breathing movements. The meconium produces a chemical pneumonitis (secondary to the bile salts), partial or complete airway obstruction as a result of air trapping (secondary to a ball-valve effect), atelectasis, and hypoxia.

1. Risk factors:
   a. Post dates (rarely seen in infants < 36 weeks' gestation); chronic and/or severe asphyxia; and intrauterine growth restriction (IUGR)
   b. Maternal respiratory and cardiovascular disease; placental insufficiency; oligohydramnios; and maternal DM

2. Clinical manifestations:
   a. Green-stained amniotic fluid with or without particulate matter; yellowish-green discoloration of skin, nail beds, and umbilical cord
   b. Barrel-shaped chest with an increased AP chest diameter
   c. Mild to severe *respiratory distress*; abnormal blood gas results (*hypoxia even with elevated levels of supplemental oxygen, hypercapnia, and acidosis*)
   d. Chest x-ray: *white fluffy infiltrates,* hyperexpanded lung fields mixed with areas of atelectasis, and flattened diaphragms

3. Complications: *persistent pulmonary hypertension of the newborn (PPHN)*; *air leak syndromes*; hypoglycemia and hypocalcemia; and seizures (with severe asphyxia)

4. Interventions:

a. Delivery room management: suction nasopharynx and oropharynx with delivery of the head; endotracheal intubation and tracheal suctioning before the infant's first gasp

b. Respiratory support: *surfactant* administration (treats surfactant inactivation caused by the meconium); *hyperoxygenation* (dilates the pulmonary vasculature and closes the ductus arteriosus; monitor preductal and postductal pulse oximetry; maintain a PaO_2 > 80–90 mmHg); *hyperventilation* (induces respiratory alkalosis; short IT to decrease air trapping); *high-frequency* oscillatory (> 10 Hz increases the chance of air trapping) or jet ventilation; *NO* inhalation (decreases pulmonary vascular resistance and improves oxygenation); *extracorporeal membrane oxygenation* (ECMO) when conventional and high-frequency ventilation have failed

c. Prevent hypotension with fluids and vasopressors; antibiotic therapy

E. PPHN: (Alpan, 1999; Casey, 1999; Hansen & Corbet, 1998c; Van Marter,1998): PPHN occurs when there is a delay in the normal transition of the pulmonary and systemic circulations to separate; pulmonary vascular resistance (PVR) > systemic vascular resistance (SVR) causing a right-to-left shunt through the foramen ovale and ductus arteriosus with resultant hypoxemia and acidosis

1. Risk factors predisposing the newborn to PPHN:

   a. Pulmonary disorders: *air leak syndromes*, aspiration pneumonia (eg, *meconium aspiration*), *pulmonary hypoplasia*, RDS, space-occupying lesions, and abnormal development of the pulmonary vascular smooth muscles

   b. Congenital heart defects and prenatal closure of the PDA

   c. Metabolic disorders: *asphyxia* and *acidosis*, hypoglycemia and hypocalcemia, hypothermia, *hypovolemia*, hyperviscosity, *perinatal hypoxia*, and *sepsis*

   d. Central nervous system (CNS) disorders

2. Clinical manifestations:

   a. *Tachypnea* (initially) presents before 12 hours of age, *cyanosis* out of proportion to the amount of respiratory distress present, and *large A-a gradient* despite administering high oxygen concentrations

   b. Hypotension; systolic murmur; single loud second heart sound

3. Diagnostic studies:

   a. *Preductal and postductal oxygen saturation:* > 10% difference is indicative of right-to-left shunt at the ductal level.

   b. *Hyperventilation test* (when hyperventilating the infant [pH > 7.5 to 7.55, $PaCO_2$ < 25 mmHg] there is a significant increase in PaO_2 [> 30 mmHg] with PPHN; PaO_2 will not increase in the presence of cyanotic congenital heart disease); *hyperoxia test* (when providing 100% inspired oxygen a right-to-left shunt is present if the PaO_2 does not increase, indicating either PPHN or congestive heart disease [CHD]).

   c. Echocardiogram (dilated right ventricle, right-to-left shunt at the foramen and ductal levels, elevated pulmonary artery pressures); electrocardiogram (right axis deviation); chest x-ray (lungs may appear normal or demonstrate parenchymal disease; typically, *hyperlucency of lung fields with diminished pulmonary vascular markings*)

4. Interventions:
   a. Acute management: *immediate, vigorous delivery room resuscitation; be prepared to immediately treat air leak syndromes* with needle aspiration or chest tube insertion, assess for bilateral breath sounds; *maintain pulse oximetry at 98% to 100%; keep mean arterial pressure (which is volume dependent) elevated with volume replacement or vasopressors*
   b. Ongoing management: *correct hypovolemia and hypotension* (volume replacement, vasopressors); *correct hypoxemia and acidosis*; maintain adequate renal function.
5. Mechanical ventilation:
   a. Conventional mechanical ventilation or high-frequency jet and oscillatory ventilation
   b. Induce metabolic alkalosis (pH > 7.5) by means of hyperventilation or administrating *alkalizing agents (*eg, *sodium bicarbonate* or tromethamine) (institutional guidelines will vary); *hyperoxygenation* (PaO_2 > 90 mmHg) dilates the pulmonary vasculature; *hyperventilation* ($PaCO_2$ < 25 mmHg) decreases pulmonary vascular resistance.
   c. Inhaled nitric oxide (iNO) administration (a selective pulmonary vasodilator)
   d. ECMO for infants who fail conventional or high-frequency ventilation
6. Medications:
   a. Surfactant replacement for infants with parenchymal disease
   b. Muscle relaxants (to prevent the infant's own respiratory effort from interfering with the ventilator) (eg, *pancuronium*)
   c. Vasopressors (used to maintain systematic vascular pressure higher than pulmonary vascular pressure, thereby decreasing the right-to-left shunt) (eg, *dopamine, dobutamine*, and amrinone)
   d. Pulmonary vasodilators (eg, *iNO, isoproterenol*, and tolazoline [rarely used])
   e. Analgesics and sedatives (eg, *fentanyl* and *morphine*)
   f. Volume replacement (eg, *normal saline solution [NSS]* and blood products)

F. Transient tachypnea of the newborn (TTN) (or retained lung fluid, RDS Type II, and wet lung) (Casey, 1999; Gomella, 1999b; Whitsett et al., 1999): benign self-limited pulmonary disorder of the near-term, term, and large premature infant who has respiratory distress shortly after birth that usually resolves within 3 days
   1. Etiology: delayed clearance of fetal lung fluid; pulmonary immaturity; and mild surfactant deficiency
   2. Risk factors contributing to TTN:
      a. Birth asphyxia
      b. Breech delivery; precipitous delivery; prolonged labor; delayed cord clamping; cesarean section without labor
      c. Male sex; infant of a diabetic mother (IDM); macrosomia; polycythemia

    d. Maternal sedation; maternal asthma; fluid overload to mother

  3. Clinical manifestations: tachypnea, grunting, nasal flaring, and retractions; cyanosis (oxygen requirement does not usually exceed 40%); and barrel chest appearance secondary to increased AP diameter

  4. Diagnosis:

    a. Arterial blood gas (ABG) analysis: hypoxia and mild hypercapnia (usually $PaCO_2$ < 55 mmHg)

    b. Chest x-ray: hyperexpanded lung fields; diffuse haziness and streaky perihilar markings; flattened diaphragm; fluid present in the interlobar fissures

  5. Interventions:

    a. Oxygenation via hood or nasal cannula; ventilatory support (nasal continuous positive airway pressure [NCPAP] or intubation); and maintain normal blood gas values

    b. Adequate fluid intake and nutritional supplementation (consider hyperalimentation if tachypnea persists)

G. Pneumonia: fetal or newborn lung infection. The causative organism may be transmitted to the infant either transplacentally, during delivery, through aspiration of infected amniotic fluid, or during the newborn period as a nosocomial infection.

  1. Common causative agents:

    a. Viral (eg, *herpes*, rubella, cytomegalovirus [CMV], adenovirus, and varicella)

    b. Bacteria (eg, *group B streptococcus, Escherichia coli, Listeria*, Mycoplasma and Ureaplasma, Chlamydia, Klebsiella, Pseudomonas, Enterobacter, *Staphylococcus aureus*, and *Treponema pallidum*)

    c. Fungus (eg, *Candida*)

    d. Other (eg, *meconium*, amniotic fluid, blood, and formula)

  2. Maternal/fetal risk factors and intrapartum clinical manifestations: fetal tachycardia; loss of variability on fetal monitoring device; maternal fever and/or chorioamnionitis; foul-smelling or purulent amniotic fluid; preterm labor and delivery; and prolonged rupture of membranes (ROM) > 24 hours

  3. Clinical manifestations (neonatal) may include signs of uncomplicated RDS or systemic disease:

    a. Respiratory distress; hypoxia and acidosis; apnea and bradycardia

    b. Temperature instability; lethargy; poor tone; alteration in consciousness; seizures

    c. Fluctuations in serum glucose; poor feeding or feeding intolerance

    d. Hypotension and/or circulatory collapse

  4. Interventions:

    a. Provide oxygen supplementation and ventilatory support; maintain normal blood gas values; correct acidosis.

    b. Antibiotic therapy; maintain adequate fluid and electrolyte balance; maintain blood pressure.

    c. Provide neutral thermal environment; optimize nutrition.

V. Space-occupying lesions

A. Congenital adenomatoid malformation (CAM) (Casey, 1999; Hartman et al., 1999): "pulmonary maldevelopment that presents with cystic replacement of pulmonary parenchyma" (Hartman et al., 1999, p. 1013). There are two types: *Type I* ([lobar cystic adenomatoid malformation] large cysts replace one entire lobe of a lung; associated with ascites; more resectable and better prognosis than Type II); *Type II* ([diffuse cystic adenomatoid malformation] microscopic cysts are pervasive throughout entire lung; ascites is common; not resectable; neonatal death often ensues).

1. Clinical manifestations:
   a. May be asymptomatic if the cysts are small and occupy only a small portion of a lung.
   b. Respiratory distress is typically present if the cysts are microscopic but replace a large portion of a lung and lead to hydrops or macroscopic and involve a large portion of lung parenchyma.
   c. Hydrops fetalis
2. Interventions:
   a. *Respiratory support*; correct hypoxia and acid-base imbalances.
   b. Correct hypoperfusion and hypotension with volume replacement; consider inotropic agents to maintain systemic blood pressure; maintain appropriate fluid and electrolyte balance.
   c. *Surgical resection* of the affected lung

B. Congenital diaphragmatic hernia (CDH) (Casey, 1999): a diaphragmatic defect that allows herniation of the abdominal contents into the pleural cavity. Most defects (85% to 90%) are left sided. There is hypoplasia of the ipsilateral lung tissue and possible mediastinal shift compressing and causing hypoplasia of the contralateral lung. The defect can range in size from a small opening to complete absence of the diaphragm on the affected side.

1. Clinical manifestations:
   a. Barrel chest appearance; *scaphoid abdomen*
   b. *Respiratory distress* at birth or shortly thereafter; cyanosis and hypoxia; hypercapnia and respiratory acidosis
   c. *Decreased breath sounds on the side of the defect*; heart sounds can be shifted from their normal position.
   d. Hypoperfusion and hypotension; PPHN
2. Diagnosis: prenatal ultrasound; history of polyhydramnios; chest x-ray reveals bowel loops in chest.
3. Interventions:
   a. *Immediate endotracheal intubation* and positive pressure ventilation in the delivery room; mechanical ventilation **(bag/mask ventilation will increase gastric distention and further compromise ventilatory efforts)**
   b. Surfactant administration; correct hypoxia and acid-base imbalance; maintain appropriate fluid and electrolyte balance.
   c. *Insert nasogastric tube* to decompress the stomach.
   d. *Inotropic agents* to support systemic blood pressure
   e. Be prepared to insert chest tube in contralateral side in the event of a pneumothorax.
   f. Consider *ECMO* if the infant's pulmonary status cannot be stabilized with conventional ventilation.
   g. *Surgical correction of the defect*

VI. Apnea

A. Definition: absence of breathing for a period of 20 seconds or of shorter duration if the apnea is accompanied by cyanosis and/or bradycardia (heart rate < 100 bpm) (Papageorgiou & Bardin, 1999); present in most infants < 1,000 g

B. Types of apnea:

1. Primary: "initial cessation of respiratory movements after a period of rapid respiratory effort as a result of asphyxia during the delivery process" (Goodwin, 1999, p. 152)

2. Secondary: "apnea occurring after a period of deep, gasping respirations and fall in blood pressure and heart rate, brought about by prolonged asphyxia during the delivery process. The gasping becomes slower and weaker and then ceases" (Goodwin, 1999, p. 152). *(At delivery it is impossible to distinguish between primary and secondary apnea.)*

3. Central: complete absence of breathing movements and airflow that may be attributed to the following: immature respiratory center (incomplete CNS myelinization, fewer synapses, and decreased dendritic arborization); chest wall instability; and diaphragmatic fatigue.

4. Obstructive: breathing movements are present but there is no airflow. Obstructive apnea is attributed to blockage of the upper, and in some instances, lower airway (eg, hyperextension or flexion of the neck, mechanical blockage secondary to anatomic abnormalities, and aspiration) (Goodwin, 1999; Papageorgiou & Bardin, 1999).

5. Mixed: both central and obstructive components are present.

6. Apnea of prematurity: recurring episodes of apnea present in the premature infant who does not have any other abnormalities; usually presents itself within the first week of life and resolves (95% of cases) by the time the infant is term.

C. Etiology of apnea:

1. *Prematurity*

2. RDS and pulmonary disorders; *hypoxia; asphyxia*

3. CNS disorders (eg, *intracranial hemorrhages* [ICH] and masses, congenital malformations, and *seizures*)

4. Cardiovascular disorders (eg, hypoperfusion, hypotension)

5. *Sepsis*

6. GI disorders (eg, *NEC, bowel perforation, gastroesophageal [GE] reflux*)

7. Metabolic (eg, *hypothermia*, hypocalcemia, *hypoglycemia*, *hypermagnesemia*, hyperammonemia, and hyponatremia)

8. Maternal drugs (eg, *narcotics, magnesium sulfate*, and general anesthesia)

9. Neonatal drugs (eg, morphine and *fentanyl* [observe for chest wall rigidity], versed, ativan, and PGE_1)

10. Other (eg, polycythemia, *anemia*, warm environmental temperature, *stooling, feeding*, and *pain*)

D. Interventions: evaluate the infant and eliminate obvious causes; respiratory support; methylxanthines (eg, caffeine, aminophylline, and theophylline) stimulate the respiratory center, with resultant increased respiratory rate, increased tidal volume and minute ventilation, and decreased diaphragmatic fatigue.

Part B: Diagnostic Procedures and Calculations

I. Radiographic interpretation: examine radiographic studies systematically:

A. Exposure: overexposure (entire film is too dark, thereby obscuring pertinent details); underexposure (entire film is too light)

B. Densities: different tissue and fluid densities will appear in varying shades of white and gray; air will appear black (Dettenmeier, 1995): Metal (bright white) → bone → fluid and water → fat (least white).

C. Rotation (AP view): *the posterior ribs appear longer on the side towards which the infant is rotated.* Rotation can distort the proper size and location or internal organs, thereby leading to inaccurate radiographic interpretation.

D. Identify structures: skeleton (eg, 12 paired ribs, vertebral anomalies, or fractures); internal organs (eg, left-sided stomach bubble and right-sided liver, left cardiac border in left hemithorax, or air leaks); soft tissue (eg, anasarca); invasive catheters and tubes (eg, endotracheal tube [ETT], umbilical venous catheter [UVL] and umbilical arterial catheter [UAL] placement, nasogastric tube [NGT] placement)

II. Calculations

A. Measurements of respiratory function (Table 13.2)

1. Alveolar-arterial gradient (A-aDO$_2$) (Harris & Wood, 1996): A-aDO$_2$ is the difference between O$_2$ tension in the alveolus (A) and in the arterial blood (a) and reflects the level of gas exchange through the lungs. Etiology includes:

a. V/Q (ventilation/perfusion) mismatch (eg, atelectasis, BPD, MAS, pulmonary embolism, and pneumonia)

b. Hypoventilation

c. Noncardiac, intrapulmonary shunt (right-to-left shunt) (eg, PPHN)

d. Decreased cardiac output (eg, hypovolemia)

e. Diffusion block (eg, methemoglobinemia, severe pneumonia)

f. Normal A-a gradient = **10 to 15 TORR**

2. Arterial/alveolar O$_2$ tension ratio (PaO$_2$/PAO$_2$ or a/A ratio): "a measurement of the difference in the partial pressures of O$_2$ in the arterial blood and alveolar gas, and as such is a comparison of the actual amount of O$_2$ entering the blood with the absolute amount delivered to the alveoli for O$_2$ uptake" (Harris & Wood, 1996, p. 156). **PaO$_2$/PAO$_2$ values: < 0.75 is abnormal**; < 0.30 indicates severe respiratory compromise.

3. Oxygen index (OI): a measurement of disease severity in which "the OI factors in the pressure cost of achieving a certain level of postductal oxygenation" (Harris & Wood, 1996, p. 59). **OI values: > 15 indicates severe respiratory compromise**; OI 30 to 35 indicates failure to respond to mode of ventilation; several consecutive OI > 40 increases the risk of mortality to approximately 80% and justifies the use of ECMO.

TABLE 13.2 A-aDO$_2$, A-aRatio, and Oxygen Index (OI) Calculations

A-aDO$_2$	A-aDO$_2$ = [(FiO$_2$ × 713*) − (PaCO$_2$ ÷ 0.8)] − PaO$_2$
	or
	(PaCO$_2$ × 1.25)]
	Example: [(1.00 × 713) − (65 ÷ 0.8)] − 60 = 571.75 TORR
	or
	(65 × 1.25)]

*713 = barometric pressure (760 mmHg at sea level)—partial pressure of H$_2$O (47 mmHg)

a/A ratio	A-a ratio = PaO$_2$ ÷ PAO$_2$*
	Example: 80 ÷ ([713 × 1.00] − 50) = 0.12
	*PAO$_2$ = (713 × FiO$_2$) − PaCO$_2$
OI	OI = (Paw* × FiO$_2$ × 100) ÷ PaO$_2$ (postductal)
	Example: (21 × 1.00 × 100) ÷ 60 = 35

*Paw = mean airway pressure.

TORR = the pressure of 1/760 of standard atmospheric pressure; equivalent to the pressure of 1 mm of mercury (1 mmHg)

B. Blood gas calculations:
    1. Blood gas analysis directly measures pH, PaCO$_2$, and PaO$_2$ and calculates base deficit/excess, bicarbonate (HCO$_3^-$), and O$_2$ saturation.
    2. Blood gas values: normal acid-base values vary slightly according to different reference labs, textbooks, the gestational age of the infant, and whether the blood specimen is arterial, venous, or capillary.
    3. Venous blood gases generally have a lower pH, higher PvCO$_2$, and lower PvO$_2$ than ABGs (Hamm, 1999); capillary blood gas samples, properly arterialized by warming the extremity, correspond roughly with arterial pH, PaCO$_2$, and HCO$_3^-$ (Table 13.3) (Czervinske, 1993).
    4. Calculating pH from arterial blood gas (Box 13.1)
    5. Calculating base deficit (see Box 13.1)
    6. Calculating acid-base balance on an ABG (Box 13.2)

Part C: Respiratory Support

I. Assisted mechanical ventilation (Goldsmith & Karotkin, 1996)
    A. Reasons to initiate assisted ventilation in the neonate (Harris & Wood, 1996): maintain normal PaO$_2$, thereby minimizing hypoxia; maintain normal PaCO$_2$, thereby optimizing alveolar ventilation; reduce the work of breathing and decrease respiratory muscle fatigue; and recruit atelectatic lung segments.
    B. Types of mechanical ventilation: intermittent negative-pressure ventilation (rarely used); intermittent positive-pressure ventilation (6 basic types):

TABLE 13.3 Blood Gas Values

	pH	PCO₂	HCO₃	Base Excess and Base Deficit
Normal values*	7.34–7.45	35–40 mmHg	18–26 mEq/L	± 4
Respiratory acidosis	↓	↑	Normal	———
Metabolic acidosis	↓	Normal	↓	Base deficit
Respiratory alkalosis	↑	↓	Normal	———
Metabolic alkalosis	↑	Normal	↑	Base excess
Compensated respiratory acidosis	Normal or ↓	↑	↑	
Compensated metabolic acidosis	Normal or ↓	↓	↓	Variable deficit
Compensated respiratory alkalosis	Normal or ↑	↓	↓	
Compensated metabolic alkalosis	Normal or ↑	↑	↑	Variable excess

*Values adapted from Kirby, E. (1999). Assisted ventilation. In J. Deacon & P. O'Neill (Eds.), *Core curriculum for neonatal intensive care nursing* (2nd ed., pp. 164–191). Philadelphia: WB Saunders; Hamm, C. R. (1999). Respiratory management. In T. L. Gomella, M. D. Cunningham, F. G. Eyal, & K. E. Zenk (Eds.), *Neonatology: management, procedures, on-call problems, diseases, drugs* (4th ed., pp. 43–67). Stamford, CT: Appleton & Lange; and Christiana Care Health Systems laboratory reference, 2001.

1. Volume cycled (inspiration is terminated when a preset volume is reached)
2. Pressure cycled (inspiration is terminated when a preset pressure is reached)
3. Time cycled (inspiration is terminated when a preset time is reached)

▼ BOX 13.1   Calculating pH and Base Deficit/Excess

Calculating pH from arterial blood gas (ABG)
- For every ± 10 from PaCO₂ of 40 → pH ↑ or ↓ by .08 from 7.40.
- Assume a normal PaCO₂ = 40 and a normal pH = 7.40.
- Example: If the PaCO₂ = 50, then the pH decreases by .08 from 7.40 [7.40 − .08 = 7.32 *calculated pH*]

Calculating base deficit (three steps)
- *Calculate* the pH (see Calculating pH formula above).
- Determine the difference between *calculated* pH and *measured* pH (on ABG). 7.32 (*Calculated* pH) − 7.18 (*measured* pH) = 0.14
- For every .15 difference between *calculated* pH and *measured* pH there is ± of 10 in the base (deficit/excess)
- Example: 0.15 : 10 :: 0.14 : x = 9.3 base deficit

▼ **BOX 13.2** | **Calculating Acid–Base Balance**

Normal values
- Assume normal pH = 7.35–7.45
  (< 7.35 = acidosis and > 7.45 = alkalosis)
- Assume normal PCO_2 = 35–45 mmHg **(ventilation status)**
  > 45 = hypoventilation and respiratory acidosis
  < 35 = hyperventilation and respiratory alkalosis
- Assume normal HCO_3 = 22–26 mEq/L **(metabolic status)**
  < 22 (or base **deficit** of −2 mEq/L or more) = metabolic acidosis
  > 26 (or base **excess** of +2 mEq/L or more) = metabolic alkalosis

Primary and compensating disorder
- When both PCO_2 and HCO_3 are abnormal, one is the **primary acid–base disorder** and the other is the **compensating disorder**. "To decide which is which, check the pH. Only a process of acidosis can make the pH acidic; only a process of alkalosis can make the pH alkaline" (Anderson, 1990).
- **Determine the primary disorder** (with complete compensation) when the pH is 7.35–7.45
  Primary acidosis (pH 7.35–7.40)
  Primary alkalosis (pH 7.40–7.45)
- **Determine type of compensation**
  Noncompensated: only PCO_2 or HCO_3 is abnormal; pH is abnormal
  Partial compensation: PCO_2 and HCO_3 and pH are abnormal
  Complete compensation: PCO_2 and HCO_3 are abnormal; pH is normal

Adapted from Anderson, S. (1990). Six easy steps to interpreting blood gases. *American Journal of Nursing* (1990, August), pp. 42–45.

---

    4. Flow cycled (inspiration is terminated when flow reaches a critical low level)

    5. *Mixed cycle* (two or more of the independent cycled mechanisms are present in the same ventilator) (eg, time cycled/pressure limited ventilation—commonly used with neonates)

    6. *High-frequency jet and oscillatory ventilation* (ventilators that cycle at > 150 breaths per minute)

C. Conventional ventilation:

    1. *$PaCO_2$ is affected by PIP, RR,* and changes in minute ventilation:

      a. Minute ventilation = tidal volume* × RR (*TV = 4–8 mL/kg)

      b. To decrease $PaCO_2$ → increase minute ventilation by ↑ *PIP and/or* ↑ RR, or ↓ PEEP.

      c. To increase $PaCO_2$ → decrease minute ventilation by ↓ *PIP and/or* ↓ RR, or ↑ PEEP.

    2. *PaO_2 is affected by FiO_2, PEEP, mean airway pressure (MAP),* and flow:

      a. To increase PaO_2 → ↑ *FiO_2* ↑ *PEEP,* ↑ *MAP,* or ↑ flow

      b. To increase MAP → ↑ PEEP

D. High-frequency oscillatory ventilation (HFOV):

    1. Indications for HFOV (Kirby, 1999): severe respiratory failure unresponsive to conventional ventilation; treatment for air leak syndromes; and PPHN

2. Settings:

a. MAP (*affects oxygenation*): ranges from 3 to 45 cm H_2O; to increase $PaO_2 \rightarrow \uparrow$ MAP; excessive MAP will hyperexpand the lungs and impede cardiac output.

b. Oscillatory power (or ΔP or *amplitude*) (*affects ventilation*): ranges from 0 to 100 cm H_2O; to decrease $PaCO_2 \rightarrow \uparrow \Delta P$; *chest wall vibration ("wiggle") is essential.*

c. Percent I time: ranges from 33% to 50% (33% is typical beginning parameter); to decrease $PaCO_2 \rightarrow \uparrow$ I time will $\uparrow$ tidal volume

d. Frequency: ranges from 3 to 15 Hz (1 Hz = 60 breaths per minute); 8 to 10 Hz is a usual beginning parameter; to decrease $PaCO_2 \rightarrow \downarrow$ Hz will $\uparrow$ tidal volume

e. FiO_2: follow ABGs and pulse oximetry and adjust the FiO_2 accordingly.

f. HFOV requires background sighs via conventional ventilator to recruit atelectatic alveoli.

E. High-frequency jet ventilation (HFJV) (Kirby, 1999): effective machine for eliminating CO_2

1. Settings:

a. Conventional ventilator, used concurrently with HFJV, provides PEEP, background sigh rate, and medical gases.

b. *PIP is usually set the same as that which is needed with conventional ventilation.* A background PIP (2 to 5 cm H_2O lower than HFJV) is set on the conventional ventilator. PIP adjustments will affect $PaCO_2$ (*ventilation*).

c. Respiratory rate: 400 to 500 breaths per minute (Bunnell Life PulseJet ventilator default is *420/min*); background sigh rate on the conventional ventilator is 5 to 20 breaths per minute.

d. Jet valve on time *(I-time)* is typically *0.02 seconds.*

e. *FiO_2* is set on the jet and conventional ventilators and affects *oxygenation*.

f. *"Vibration of the chest wall* is an indicator of lung compliance, airway patency, and effectiveness of ventilator settings" (Kirby, 1999, p. 180).

F. Lung compliance:

1. The greater the lung compliance (eg, term infants without lung disease), the less pressure needed to move a fixed amount of gas.

2. The less the lung compliance (eg, premature infants with surfactant deficiency), the more pressure required to move a fixed amount of gas.

3. Premature infants have less lung compliance (stiff lungs) and more chest wall compliance (pliable chest walls), thereby making them difficult to ventilate.

II. Oxygen delivery systems

A. Free-flow oxygen: delivered via O_2 tubing, oxygen mask, or flow inflating (anesthesia) resuscitation bag to an infant with spontaneous respirations. This method of oxygen administration is fast, convenient, and easy. This method should be used only for emergency and/or short-term situations (eg, in the delivery room, during care-giving activities).

B. Oxy-Hood: "warm, humidified oxygen is provided at a measured concentration via a plastic hood placed over the infant's head" (Kirby, 1999, p. 169). This method requires proper hood size for the infant, pulse oximetry monitoring, proper monitoring of O_2 concentration by means of a calibrated oxygen analyzer, and adequate gas flow through the hood to eliminate a buildup of CO_2.

C. Nasal cannula: "humidified O_2 is delivered at a set flow rate via a cannula, with the flow directed into the nares" (Kirby, 1999, p. 169). The amount of oxygen delivered to the infant varies, depending upon the flow rate (L/min) and the concentration of blended oxygen (eg, 100% and 1 L/min ≈ 66%, 100% and 1/4 L/min ≈ 34%; 40% and 1 L/min ≈ 27%, 40% and 1/4 L/min ≈ 22%).

D. CPAP: continuous distending airway pressure is applied to a spontaneously breathing infant via mask (short-term situations, such as respiratory support before intubation), nasal prongs, nasally inserted endotracheal tube whose tip is located in the nasopharynx, or endotracheally intubated infants. Distending pressures do not usually exceed 8 cm H_2O. CPAP may be used for the following: mild respiratory distress to improve PaO_2 and eliminate CO_2 (institutional practices vary regarding the implementation and maintenance of CPAP and the level of permissive hypercapnia); postextubation to stabilize airway; and recruitment of atelectatic alveoli.

E. Extracorporeal membrane oxygenation: "ECMO is the process of prolonged cardiopulmonary bypass that provides cardiorespiratory support for infants in reversible, profound respiratory and/or cardiac failure" (Lund, 1999, p. 192).

  1. Indications: respiratory failure unresponsive to conventional modes of ventilatory support (eg, RDS and meconium aspiration); persistent pulmonary HTN; sepsis and/or pneumonia; congenital diaphragmatic hernia; and postcardiac surgery

  2. Entry criteria (Gleason, 1999; Lund, 1999; Short, 1999): gestation > 34 weeks and weight > 2 kg; reversible pulmonary disease; ventilatory support for less than 10 to 14 days; no bleeding diathesis; no major intracranial hemorrhage; no major cardiac lesion; no major congenital anomalies; and one or more of the following:

    a. A-a gradient > 605 to 620 for 4 to 12 hours

    b. PaO_2 35–50 mmHg for 2 to 12 hours

    c. OI > 35 for 30 minutes to 6 hours

    d. Acute deterioration

    e. Barotrauma

  3. Methods:

    a. Venoarterial perfusion: deoxygenated blood drained from a catheter threaded into the right atrium (via the jugular vein) and oxygenated blood returned to the systemic circulation via a catheter placed into the ascending aorta (via right common carotid artery)

    b. Venovenous perfusion: a double lumen catheter is threaded into the right atrium where deoxygenated blood is removed via the inflow port and oxygenated blood is returned to the right atrium via the outflow port with the side holes pointed toward the tricuspid valve

4. Complications (Gomez, Hansen, & Corbet, 1998; Lund, 1999):
  a. Emboli (air or particulate matter)
  b. Carotid artery ligation (for arteriovenous perfusion)
  c. Hemorrhagic complications secondary to heparin therapy
  d. "Cardiac stun syndrome": the infant's cardiac output decreases as the ECMO flow is reduced, thereby possibly prolonging time on the ECMO circuit.
  e. Increased pulmonary edema with further decrease in lung compliance secondary to compliment activation and increased leukotriene production. Often responds to high PEEP pressures and exogenous surfactant administration.
  f. Decreased urine output is experienced as the pulmonary and generalized edema increases and hypotension ensues. It may be necessary to administer colloids and vasopressors to maintain blood pressure, loop diuretics to facilitate diuresis, and/or hemofiltration if pulmonary edema does not resolve.
  g. Systemic hypertension secondary to circulation overload. Often responds to diuretics and hemofiltration.

F. iNO: potent, selective, gaseous, pulmonary vasodilator delivered to the lungs via the ventilator circuit (Hamm, 1999). iNO is indistinguishable from endogenously produced endothelial-derived relaxing factor (EDRF). "NO is rapidly bound by hemoglobin, limiting its action to the site of production or administration (Hamm, 1999, p. 55)", thereby reducing pulmonary HTN and improving oxygenation without causing systemic hypotension. It is used to treat PPHN.
  1. Dosage: 5–80 ppm (parts per million) delivered via conventional or high-frequency ventilator circuit. > 40 ppm is not particularly beneficial and rarely used.
  2. Complications (Spitzer, Greenspan, Antunes, & Shaffer, 1996): NO_2 (oxidized product of NO) can potentially cause pulmonary toxicity when NO is administered at high concentrations; methemoglobinemia, resulting in decreased oxygen carrying capacity and hypoxia, may occur with high NO exposure.

III. Noninvasive monitoring

A. Oxygenation (Koff, Eitzman, & Neu, 1993): most oxygen is attached to Hb molecules within the red blood cell while a small portion is dissolved in the plasma. Adult (Hb A) and fetal (Hb F) hemoglobin Hb present in the infant's system affect oxygenation. *Hb A* comprises two α and two β chains and has a decreased affinity for oxygen. This affinity varies directly with pH and inversely with temperature and 2,3-DPG (2,3-diphosphoglycerate, a byproduct of glucose metabolism). *Hb F* comprises two α and two γ chains and has an increased affinity for oxygen. Hb F decreases appreciably by 6 months of age and is replaced by Hb A.
  1. PaO_2 is the direct measurement of oxygen present in the plasma whereas other parameters (eg, SaO_2) are calculated or measured and relate to oxygen delivery at the tissue level.
    a. Hypoxemia is a decreased level of oxygen in arterial blood; hypoxia is a decreased level of oxygen at the tissue level.
    b. Cyanosis becomes apparent when ≥ 5 g of Hb are not bound to oxygen per 100 cc of blood, ie, when the PaO_2 is 75% to 85% (Bell, 1999).
  2. Pulse oximetry (Hodson & Truog, 1999; Koff, et al., 1993; Martin,

Sosenko & Bancalari, 2001): noninvasive assessment of tissue oxygenation by use of infrared spectrometry. The pulse oximetry probe contains two electrodes that emit and absorb light at two different wavelengths. The ratio of the light absorbed at these two wavelengths is used to calculate the SaO_2 value and is dependent on (1) the light absorption characteristics and (2) the amount of Hb-oxygen (HbO_2) and deoxyhemoglobin present in arterial blood (Figure 13.1). SaO_2, expressed as a percentage, is related to PaO_2 by the oxyhemoglobin dissociation curve (OHDC).

   a. OHDC is the mathematical relationship between the partial pressure of oxygen and the percentage of saturation of hemoglobin with oxygen.

      (1) OHDC shifts to the *right* with acidosis, presence of Hb A, increased CO_2, increased metabolic state, increased 2,3-DPG, and increased temperature, thereby decreasing Hb's affinity for oxygen. This aids with O_2 off-loading to the tissues (Czervinske, 1993; Hamm, 1999).

      (2) OHDC shifts to the *left* with alkalosis, decreased CO_2, decreased 2,3-DPG, presence of Hb F, high altitude, decreased metabolism, and decreased temperature, thereby increasing Hb's affinity for oxygen. Oxygen is not delivered as readily to the tissues, but on-loading of oxygen in the lungs is facilitated (Czervinske, 1993; Hamm, 1999).

      (3) 30-60-60-90 rule (Czervinske, 1993): assuming a normal pH, PCO_2, and temperature, Hb at a PaO_2 of 30 mmHg will be 60% saturated; Hb at a PaO_2 of 60 mmHg will be 90% saturated.

   b. Clinical implications: noninvasive, rapid response time, and no manual calibration required; inaccurate in the presence of tissue ischemia, movement of the extremity, improper placement of the probe, and ambient light (eg, phototherapy)

  3. Transcutaneous oxygen ($tcPO_2$): measurement of partial pressure of oxygen at the skin surface by means of an electrochemical sensor equipped with an O_2-permeable membrane. An electrode heats the skin to a temperature of approximately 43°C to 44°C and measures the partial pressure of oxygen that has diffused from the arterialized capillary bed to the surface of the skin.

   a. Clinical implications: noninvasive and be may be used as an adjunct to other methods of assessing oxygenation (eg, blood gas analysis); requires daily calibration; requires probe site relocation several times a day to prevent skin irritation and injury; inaccurate readings in the face of hypoperfusion and tissue ischemia, tissue edema, hypothermia, and acidosis

B. Ventilation:

  1. End tidal CO_2 ($ETCO_2$) (Hamm, 1999): end tidal CO_2 measurements are taken by in-line infrared monitoring equipment. At the end of each breath the amount of CO_2 at the mouth and nose reaches a plateau, is measurable, and reflects alveolar CO_2.

   a. Clinical indications: noninvasive and responds rapidly to changes in CO_2; sensor attached to the ETT may significantly increase dead space; inaccurate readings may occur when respiratory rates exceed 60 breaths per minute, there is excessive humidity in the inspired gases, or the a/A ratio is < 0.3.

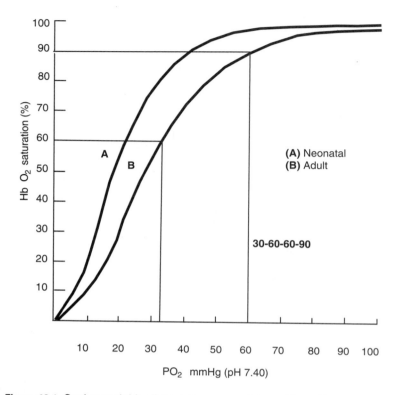

Figure 13.1. Oxyhemoglobin dissociation curve. Adapted from Hamm, C. R. (1999). Respiratory Management. In T. L. Gomella, M. D. Cunningham, F. G. Eyal, & K. E. Zenk (Eds.), *Neonatology: Management, procedures, on-call problems, diseases, drugs* (4th ed., pp. 43–67). Stamford, CT: Appleton & Lange.

2. Transcutaneous PCO_2 ($tcPco_2$) (Hamm, 1999): "the $tcPco_2$ electrode operates by tissue CO_2 equilibration across the skin and generation of an electrical charge proportional to the change in pH of the contact electrolyte solution" (Hamm, 1999, p. 47).
   a. Clinical implications: noninvasive; requires daily recalibration and frequent probe site changes; readings can be fairly accurate and, thus, decrease the need for frequent blood gas analysis; skin injury may result from frequent site changes and probe temperature.

▼ References

Alpan, G. (1999). Persistent pulmonary hypertension of the newborn. In T. L. Gomella, M. D. Cunningham, F. G. Eyal, & K. E. Zenk (Eds.), *Neonatology: Management, procedures, on-call problems, diseases, drugs* (4th ed., pp. 345–350). Stamford, CT: Appleton & Lange.

Anderson, S. (1990). Six easy steps to interpreting blood gases. *American Journal of Nursing*, August 1990. 42–45.

Bell, S. G. (1999). An introduction to hemoglobin physiology. *Neonatal Network*, *18*(2), 9–15.

Casey, P. M. (1999). Respiratory distress. In J. Deacon & P. O'Neill (Eds.), *Core curriculum for neonatal intensive care nursing* (2nd ed., pp. 118–150). Philadelphia: WB Saunders.

Czervinske, M. P. (1993). Arterial blood gas analysis and other cardiopulmonary monitoring. In P. B. Koff, D. Eitzman, & J. Neu (Eds.), *Neonatal & pediatric respiratory care* (2nd ed., pp. 302–323). St. Louis: Mosby.

Desai, T. R., Statter, M. B., & Arensman, R. M. (1996). Surgical management of the airway. In J. P. Goldsmith & E. H. Karotkin (Eds.), *Assisted ventilation of the neonate* (3rd ed., pp. 353–354). Philadelphia: WB Saunders.

Dettenmeier, P. A. (1995). *Radiographic assessment for nurses*. St. Louis: Mosby.

Eichenwald, E. C. (1998). Meconium aspiration. In J. P. Cloherty & A. R. Stark (Eds.), *Manual of neonatal care* (4th ed., pp. 388–391). Philadelphia: Lippincott-Raven.

Gleason, C. A. (1999). Extracorporeal membrane oxygenation. In T. L. Gomella, M. D. Cunningham, F. G. Eyal, & K. E. Zenk (Eds.), *Neonatology: Management, procedures, on-call problems, diseases, drugs* (4th ed., pp. 125–128). Stamford, CT: Appleton & Lange.

Goldsmith, J. P., & Karotkin, E. H. (1996). Introduction to assisted ventilation. In J. P. Goldsmith & E. H. Karotkin (Eds.), *Assisted ventilation of the neonate* (3rd ed., pp. 1–20). Philadelphia: WB Saunders.

Gomella, T. L. (1999a). Chest tube placement. In T. L. Gomella, M. D. Cunningham, F. G. Eyal, & K. E. Zenk (Eds.), *Neonatology: Management, procedures, on-call problems, diseases, drugs* (4th ed., pp. 160–161). Stamford, CT: Appleton & Lange.

Gomella, T. L. (1999b). Transient tachypnea of the newborn. In T. L. Gomella, M. D. Cunningham, F. G. Eyal, & K. E. Zenk (Eds.), *Neonatology: Management, procedures, on-call problems, diseases, drugs* (4th ed., pp. 510–512). Stamford, CT: Appleton & Lange.

Gomez, M., Hansen, T., & Corbet, A. (1998). Therapies for intractable respiratory failure. In H. W. Taeusch & R. A. Ballard (Eds.), *Avery's diseases of the newborn* (7th ed., pp. 595–601). Philadelphia: WB Saunders.

Goodwin, M. (1999). Apnea of the newborn infant. In J. Deacon & P. O'Neill (Eds.), *Core curriculum for neonatal intensive care nursing* (2nd ed., pp. 151–163). Philadelphia: WB Saunders.

Hamm, C. R. (1999). Respiratory management. In T. L. Gomella, M. D. Cunningham, F. G. Eyal, & K. E. Zenk (Eds.), *Neonatology: Management, procedures, on-call problems, diseases, drugs* (4th ed., pp. 43–67). Stamford, CT: Appleton & Lange.

Hansen, T., & Corbet, A. (1998a). Chronic lung disease. In H. W. Taeusch & R. A. Ballard (Eds.), *Avery's diseases of the newborn* (7th ed., pp. 634–647). Philadelphia: WB Saunders.

Hansen, T., & Corbet, A. (1998b). Diseases of the airway. In H. W. Taeusch & R. A. Ballard (Eds.), *Avery's diseases of the newborn* (7th ed., pp. 661–667). Philadelphia: WB Saunders.

Hansen, T., & Corbet, A. (1998c). Disorders of the transition. In H. W. Taeusch & R. A. Ballard (Eds.), *Avery's diseases of the newborn* (7th ed., pp. 602–629). Philadelphia: WB Saunders.

Harris, T. R., & Wood, B. R. (1996). Physiologic principles. In J. P. Goldsmith & E. H. Karotkin (Eds.), *Assisted ventilation of the neonate* (3rd ed., pp. 21–68). Philadelphia: WB Saunders.

Hartman, G. E., Boyajian, M. J., Choi, S. S., Eichelberger, M. R., Newman, K. D., Powell, D. M. (1999). General surgery. In G. B. Avery, M. A. Flecher, & M. G. MacDonald (Eds.), *Neonatology: Pathophysiology and management of the newborn* (5th ed., pp. 1005–1044). Philadelphia: Lippincott Williams & Wilkins.

Hodson, W. A., & Truog, W. E. (1999). Principles of management of respiratory problems. In G. B. Avery, M. A. Fletcher, & M. G. MacDonald (Eds.), *Neonatology: Pathophysiology and management of the newborn* (5th ed., pp. 533–556). Philadelphia: Lippincott Williams & Wilkins.

Kirby, E. (1999). Assisted ventilation. In J. Deacon & P. O'Neill (Eds.), *Core curriculum for neonatal intensive care nursing* (2nd ed., pp. 164–191). Philadelphia: WB Saunders.

Koff, P. B., Eitzman, D., & Neu, J. (Eds.). (1993). *Neonatal & pediatric respiratory care* (2nd ed.). St. Louis: Mosby.

Korones, S. B., & Bada-Ellzey, H. S. (1993). *Neonatal decision making*. St. Louis: Mosby-Year Book, Inc.

Lund, C. H. (1999). Extracorporeal membrane oxygenation in the neonate. In J. Deacon & P. O'Neill (Eds.), *Core curriculum for neonatal intensive care nursing* (2nd ed., pp. 192–204). Philadelphia: WB Saunders.

Martin, R. J., Sosenko, I. & Bancalari, E. (2001). Respiratory problems. In M. H. Klaus & A. A. Fanaroff (Eds.), *Care of the high-risk neonate* (5th ed., pp. 243–276). Philadelphia: WB Saunders.

Papageorgiou, A., & Bardin, C. L. (1999). The extremely-low-birth-weight infant. In G. B. Avery, M. A. Fletcher, & M. G. MacDonald (Eds.), *Neonatology: Pathophysiology and management of the newborn* (5th ed., pp. 445–472). Philadelphia: Lippincott Williams & Wilkins.

Pauly, T. H. (1999). Pulmonary diseases. In T. L. Gomella, M. D. Cunningham, F. G. Eyal, & K. E. Zenk (Eds.), *Neonatology: Management, procedures, on-call problems, diseases, drugs* (4th ed., pp. 490–514). Stamford, CT: Appleton & Lange.

Short, B. L. (1999). Extracorporeal membrane oxygenation. In G. B. Avery, M. A. Fletcher, & M. G. MacDonald (Eds.), *Neonatology: Pathophysiology and management of the newborn* (5th ed., pp. 557–568). Philadelphia: Lippincott Williams & Wilkins.

Silverman, G. A. (1998). Air leak: Pneumothorax, pulmonary interstitial emphysema, pneumomediastinum, pneumopericardium. In J. P. Cloherty & A. R. Stark (Eds.), *Manual of neonatal care* (4th ed., pp. 358–364). Philadelphia: Lippincott-Raven.

Spitzer, A. R., Greenspan, J. S., Antunes, M. J., & Shaffer, T. H. (1996). Special ventilatory techniques ii: Liquid ventilation, nitric oxide therapy, and negative-pressure ventilation. In J. P. Goldsmith, & E. H. Karotkin (Eds.). *Assisted ventilation of the neonate* (3rd ed., pp. 229–240). Philadelphia: WB Saunders.

Van Marter, L J. (1998). Persistent pulmonary hypertension of the newborn. In J. P. Cloherty & A. R. Stark (Eds.), *Manual of neonatal care* (4th ed., pp. 364–369). Philadelphia: Lippincott-Raven.

Whitsett, J. A., Pryhuber, G. S., Rice, W. R., Warner, B. B., & Wert, S. E. (1999). Acute pulmonary disorders. In G. B. Avery, M. A. Fletcher, & M. G. MacDonald (Eds.), *Neonatology: Pathophysiology & management of the newborn* (5th ed., pp. 485–508). Philadelphia: Lippincott Williams & Wilkins.

Zayek, M. (1999). Bronchopulmonary dysplasia. In T. L. Gomella, M. D. Cunningham, F. G. Eyal, & K. E. Zenk (Eds.), *Neonatology: Management, procedures, on-call problems, diseases, drugs* (4th ed., pp. 498–502). Stamford, CT: Appleton & Lange.

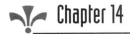 **Chapter 14**

Cardiovascular Disorders

Theresa M. McGreevy, MSN, RNC, NNP

I. Assessment of the neonate with suspected or confirmed congenital heart disease

  A. History

    1. Family history: congenital heart disease (CHD) is the most common congenital malformation, with an incidence of 0.8% of live births. A family history of heart disease increases the risk for first-degree relatives. The recurrence risk for all forms of structural heart disease in a family in which one child has heart disease is 3% to 5% in general, and higher for some lesions, such as left-sided obstructive lesions (Huhta, 1996). The probability of recurrence is substantially higher when the mother is the affected parent (Park, 1997).

    2. Maternal history: maternal conditions that increase the infant's chances for developing CHD include maternal viral infections, medications, diabetes, autoimmune disease, and congenital disorders (Flanagan, Yeager, & Weindling, 1999; Park, 1997).

  B. Physical assessment:

    1. Color (acyanosis versus cyanosis):

      a. Cyanosis: produced by a significant amount of deoxygenated hemoglobin (Hb) (usually > 5 g Hgb/dL) in the peripheral circulation; dependent on the total blood Hb concentration (Santulli, 1993). An anemic infant may have a severe desaturated arterial oxygen level without cyanosis.

      b. Cyanosis without lung disease is usually indicative of structural heart disease. It is difficult to differentiate between primary lung disease and heart disease that causes pulmonary edema.

    2. Hyperoxia test (determines whether hypoxemia is due to intrapulmonary shunting or intracardiac shunting): place the infant in 100% oxygen and then measure the rise in the arterial PO_2 (Hsu & Gersony, 1996).

      a. Intrapulmonary shunting or hypoventilation: alveolar PO_2 rises and raises the arterial PO_2.

      b. Intracardiac shunting: increase in alveolar PO_2 does not significantly affect the arterial PO_2 because the deoxygenated blood does not pass through the lungs. The exception is persistent pulmonary hypertension of the newborn (PPHN) (assume heart disease until there is echocardiogram confirmation).

    3. Respiratory rate: persistent tachypnea without respiratory distress can be associated with heart disease. Tachypnea with heart disease is the result of increased pulmonary blood flow leading to pulmonary edema.

4. Heart sounds (Fletcher, 1998):
   a. First heart sound (S1): represents closure of the atrioventricular valves at the beginning of systole. S1 is best heard over the apex of the heart.
   b. Second heart sound (S2): represents closure of the aortic and pulmonary valves at the end of systole. S2 is loudest at the left upper sternal border (LUSB).
   c. Third heart sound (S3): occurs early in diastole and represents the transition from rapid to slow-filling phases. S3 is heard best at the apex or left lower sternal border (LLSB).
   d. Fourth heart sound (S4): dull low-frequency indistinct soft thuds that precedes S1; it is abnormal.
   e. Gallop: implies pathology and results from the combination of a loud S3 or S4, and tachycardia; common in congestive heart failure (CHF)
   f. Thrill: coarse low-frequency vibrations occurring with loud murmurs
   g. Murmur: generated by turbulent blood flow. Murmurs can be analyzed in terms of timing, intensity, location, transmission, and quality.
      (1) Timing: systolic murmurs (holosystolic or systolic ejection murmur [SEM]) occur between S1 and S2; diastolic murmurs (early, mid, or late); and continuous murmurs (indicate turbulence beginning in systole and extending into diastole).
      (2) Intensity: Grade I (barely audible); Grade II (soft but easily audible); Grade III (moderately loud but without a thrill); Grade IV (louder with a thrill); Grade V (audible with the stethoscope barely on the chest); and Grade VI (audible with the stethoscope off the chest)
      (3) Location: maximum intensity of the murmur on the thorax (listen over both sides of the back in infants and children); aortic area (along the mid-left sternal border to beneath the right clavicle); pulmonary area (along the LUSB and beneath the left clavicle); tricuspid area (along the lower left and right sternal border); and mitral area (cardiac apex)
      (4) Transmission: reflects the direction of turbulent flow.
      (5) Quality: describes the pitch of the murmur as high, medium, or low.
5. Heart rate (HR):
   a. Bradycardia: **consider heart block when there is a fixed rate**.
   b. Tachycardia: may be a compensatory mechanism used to increase cardiac output because the infant has reduced capacity to increase stroke volume. Distinguish between sinus tachycardia versus tachydysrhythmia.
   c. Point of maximal impulse (PMI) in infants should be located in the fourth intercostal space at the midclavicular line.
6. Perfusion: evaluate by palpating peripheral pulses, timing capillary refill, and measuring blood pressure. Decreased peripheral

pulses and prolonged capillary refill result from decreased cardiac output. Measure blood pressure in all four extremities. A significant difference between the upper and lower extremities warrants further evaluation.

7. CHF:

    a. Etiology: develops secondary to left ventricular dysfunction, ventricular overload, cardiomyopathy, or rhythm disturbances.

    b. Clinical manifestations: pallor, mottled skin, cool extremities, and prolonged capillary refill; tachypnea, increased work of breathing, rales, and pulmonary edema; tachycardia, weak peripheral pulses, possible murmur, gallop rhythm, and hepatomegaly; poor feeding and failure to thrive

    c. Diagnosis: chest x-ray reveals cardiomegaly and increased pulmonary vascular markings.

    d. Interventions: treat underlying physiologic abnormality; provide respiratory/ventilatory support; improve cardiac output by increasing contractility; alter the preload and/or afterload on the heart; treat metabolic acidosis.

C. Diagnostic tools:

    1. Chest x-ray findings: although rarely diagnostic for specific cardiac defects, it provides valuable information regarding the absence/presence of lung disease; increased/decreased pulmonary vascular markings; absence/presence of cardiomegaly; presence of a right aortic arch; associated noncardiac anomalies.

    2. Electrocardiography: identifies cardiac dysrhythmias and aids in the diagnosis of cardiac disease.

    3. Echocardiography: identifies heart structures, anomalies, shunts, and blood flow velocities.

II. Congenital heart lesions most commonly diagnosed in the neonatal period

A. Acyanotic lesions with increased pulmonary blood flow:

    1. Patent ductus arteriosus (PDA): the ductus arteriosus forms a connection between the pulmonary artery and the distal aorta. At birth, multiple factors (eg, increased oxygen tension, levels of circulating prostaglandins, and available ductal mass) cause ductal constriction (Flanagan, et al., 1999). At term, it is a muscular contractile structure that undergoes functional closure in the first few hours to days after birth. PDA is frequently seen in premature infants, especially those with respiratory distress syndrome (RDS). The incidence of PDA is inversely related to the gestational age.

    a. Hemodynamics: with decreased pulmonary vascular resistance and increased systemic vascular resistance, blood **shunts left to right** from the aorta to the pulmonary artery via the ductus arteriosus. If the ductus arteriosus is small, the shunt remains small; if there is a moderate to large PDA, it is usually associated with a significant shunt and resultant increased pulmonary blood flow and volume overload of the left ventricle (Wood, 1997).

b. Clinical manifestations:

(1) Term infant (clinical presentation depends upon the decreasing pulmonary vascular resistance): murmur (usually a systolic murmur; infrequently a continuous murmur); bounding peripheral pulses; widened pulse pressure; CHF (usually seen later); poor weight gain; and recurrent pulmonary infections

(2) Preterm infant (clinical presentation usually occurs 2 to 4 days after birth, especially after surfactant therapy): murmur (usually a systolic murmur but some infants have the classic continuous murmur; a murmur is not always audible with a large PDA); bounding peripheral pulses; widened pulse pressure with low diastolic pressures; hypotension; worsening respiratory status; decreased urinary output; and chest x-ray (increased heart size and increased pulmonary vascular markings)

c. Interventions:

(1) Term infant: PDA is abnormal and does not usually respond to pharmacologic closure (ie, indomethacin). If there is no cardiovascular compromise, perform catheter closure or surgical ligation between 6 months and 1 year of age. Term infants with CHF often benefit from treatment with diuretics and digoxin.

(2) Preterm infant (management depends on the infant's symptoms): increase ventilatory support as needed; *fluid restriction* and possible use of diuretics; treat hypotension (dopamine or dobutamine); packed red blood cell (PRBC) transfusion for an anemic infant; and *indomethacin* administration

(3) Indomethacin (prostaglandin synthetase inhibitor) decreases cerebral, renal, and gastrointestinal (GI) blood flow. Contraindications to therapy include severe renal dysfunction, evidence of necrotizing enterocolitis (NEC), significant thrombocytopenia, or active bleeding (Young & Magnum, 2001). Side effects include transient renal dysfunction (decreased urine output, sodium and water retention, weight gain, dilutional hyponatremia). Treat indomethacin-induced oliguria in preterm infants with furosemide given simultaneously, or with low-dose dopamine (1–3 µg/kg/min) (Drummond, 1996).

(4) Surgical interruption of the ductus arteriosus is indicated for infants with a persistent hemodynamically significant PDA when indomethacin has failed or is contraindicated.

2. Ventricular septal defect (VSD) (Wood, 1997) defect in the ventricular septum that is variable in size. Often associated with other cardiac anomalies. It is the most common form of CHD.

a. Hemodynamics: determined by the size of the defect and the difference between systemic and pulmonary vascular resistance; not usually symptomatic in the neonatal period unless there is a significant left-to-right shunt

b. Clinical manifestations: murmur (classic holosystolic murmur at LLSB); tachypnea; poor feeder; chest x-ray (may be normal or show cardiomegaly with increased pulmonary vascular markings with a significant left-to-right shunt); and electrocardiogram [ECG] (left ventricular hypertrophy [LVH] or right ventricular hypertrophy [RVH])

   c. Interventions: diuretics and digoxin; surgical closure

3. Endocardial cushion defect (atrioventricular [AV] canal): malformation of the endocardial cushion (partial or complete defect) often associated with Down syndrome. *Partial* defect consists of an atrial septal defect [ASD] located low in the atrial septum, a cleft in the mitral valve with mitral regurgitation; *complete* defect consists of an ASD located low in the atrial septum that is continuous with a large VSD and a common atrioventricular valve.

   a. Hemodynamics:

     (1) Partial defect: left-to-right shunt across the ASD or regurgitation from the left ventricle to the right atrium through the cleft mitral valve (Flanagan, et al., 1999)

     (2) Complete defect: left-to-right shunt across the left atrium to the right atrium, left ventricle to the right ventricle, and left ventricle to the right atrium with resultant volume overload on the right atrium and right ventricle as well as increased pulmonary blood flow. These infants develop pulmonary hypertension (HTN).

   b. Clinical manifestations:

     (1) Partial defect: usually not symptomatic in the newborn period unless there is severe mitral regurgitation. These infants have recurrent pulmonary infections and later may show signs of CHF.

     (2) Complete defect: mild cyanosis; murmur ([holosystolic murmur at LLSB]; pulmonary systolic ejection murmur [SEM]; middiastolic murmur at apex); gallop rhythm in severe CHF; loud S2; CHF; chest x-ray (cardiomegaly and increased pulmonary vascular markings); and ECG (RVH, LVH)

   c. Interventions:

     (1) Partial defect: treat CHF.

     (2) Complete defect: treat CHF; most of these infants have surgery in the newborn period due to refractory CHF or pulmonary HTN.

B. Right ventricular outflow obstruction:

   1. Tetralogy of Fallot (TOF) (Spilman & Furdon, 1998): consists of four defects (large VSD, pulmonary stenosis or atresia, overriding aorta, and right ventricular hypertrophy).

   a. Hemodynamics: the degree of cyanosis is dependent on the severity of the right ventricular outflow obstruction. Pressures equalize between the ventricles through the large VSD. Severe right ventricular outflow obstructions have a right-to-left intracardiac shunt and infants are usually *cyanotic*; mild to moderate right ventricular outflow obstructions have a left-to-right intracardiac shunt and infants are initially *acyanotic*.

   b. Clinical manifestations: varying degrees of cyanosis; mild tachypnea; murmur (pulmonary stenosis [SEM at left sternal border] and pulmonary atresia [continuous murmur]); single

S2; chest x-ray (**normal size "boot-shaped" heart**; normal or decreased pulmonary vascular markings); and ECG (RVH)

  c. Interventions: severe cyanosis (Prostaglandin E₁ [PGE₁] administration to maintain ductal patency and increase pulmonary blood flow); mild cyanosis (closely observe infants for worsening cyanosis after ductal closure; these infants will need surgical correction during the neonatal period)

2. Critical pulmonary stenosis (PS) (Spilman & Furdon, 1998): a narrowing at the entrance of the pulmonary artery. The obstruction may occur below the valve in the infundibular area (subvalvular), above the valve (supravalvular), or at the valve (valvular).

  a. Hemodynamics: the flow to the pulmonary artery from the right ventricle is obstructed if the ventricular septum is intact. Severe valvular obstruction produces cyanosis due to right-to-left shunting via the patent foramen ovale (PFO). In the most severe form of stenosis, ductal patency is required for adequate pulmonary blood flow and systemic arterial oxygenation.

  b. Clinical manifestations: cyanosis; murmur (SEM at LUSB radiating to the back); single S2; chest x-ray (normal size heart; decreased pulmonary vascular markings); and ECG (RVH)

  c. Interventions: PGE₁ infusion to maintain ductal patency; infant will require percutaneous balloon valvuloplasty or surgical valvotomy.

3. Pulmonary atresia with intact ventricular septum: no outflow from the right ventricle due to the total fusion of the valve leaflets. Because blood cannot pass from the right ventricle, there is a small hypoplastic right ventricle.

  a. Hemodynamics: there is an obligatory right-to-left shunt across the PFO to the left atrium; pulmonary blood flow is supplied through a PDA. As the ductus arteriosus closes, pulmonary perfusion is greatly reduced, causing severe cyanosis. Right ventricular and tricuspid valve hypoplasia are found in 90% of cases (Hsu & Gersony, 1996).

  b. Clinical manifestations: severe cyanosis; severe respiratory distress, bradycardia, hypotension, and severe metabolic acidosis; murmur (holosystolic murmur along LLSB and right lower sternal board [RLSB]); single S2; chest x-ray (heart size mildly enlarged; decreased pulmonary vascular markings); and ECG (right atrial hypertrophy [RAH], LVH)

  c. Interventions: PGE₁ infusion; treat underlying conditions; and surgical intervention as soon as possible

4. Tricuspid atresia: complete failure in the development of the tricuspid valve. There is no connection between the right atrium and the right ventricle. The right ventricle is hypoplastic, and there is pulmonary stenosis. Almost all of these infants have a VSD.

  a. Hemodynamics: systemic venous return flows from the right atrium across the foramen ovale or ASD to the left atrium.

The systemic and pulmonary venous blood mixes in the left atrium and flows into the left ventricle and out to the aorta. Some of this blood passes through the VSD into the hypoplastic right ventricle. The degree of pulmonary blood flow is dependent on the size of the VSD and the severity of the pulmonary stenosis (Spilman & Furdon, 1998).

b. Clinical manifestations: varying degrees of cyanosis; murmur (SEM of PS and/or holosystolic murmur of VSD); single S2; CHF if large VSD with minimal PS; chest x-ray (heart size normal or slightly enlarged; decreased pulmonary vascular markings); ECG (right atrial enlargement [RAE], LVH)

c. Interventions: PGE_1 infusion; surgical intervention required

5. Ebstein's anomaly: the leaflets of the tricuspid valve are displaced into the right ventricular cavity so that a portion of the right ventricle is incorporated into the right atrium with resultant small right ventricle and dysfunctional tricuspid valve.

a. Hemodynamics: in the newborn period when pulmonary vascular resistance is high, tricuspid regurgitation is more pronounced, resulting in increased right-to-left shunting at the atrial level through the foramen ovale. This decreases the amount of pulmonary blood flow from the right ventricle, causing cyanosis. As pulmonary vascular resistance decreases and right ventricular pressure falls, tricuspid insufficiency decreases and cyanosis improves or resolves. Infants with severe regurgitation and pulmonary hypoplasia have a high mortality rate (Flanagan, et al., 1999).

b. Clinical manifestations: varying degrees of cyanosis; murmur (holosystolic); presence of one or more extra heart sounds during systole; CHF; chest x-ray (cardiomegaly; decreased pulmonary vascular markings); ECG (Wolf-Parkinson-White [WPW] and sinoventricular tachycardia [SVT] are common)

c. Interventions: severe cyanosis (PGE_1 infusion to maintain PDA); treat CHF; may need antiarrhythmic therapy for WPW or SVT; may need surgical intervention if cyanosis persists.

C. Cyanotic mixing lesions:

1. D-transposition of the great arteries (TGA) (Flanagan, et al., 1999): the aorta arises from the right ventricle, and the pulmonary artery arises from the left ventricle. The systemic and pulmonary circulations are separate and parallel. A communication (PFO, ASD, VSD, or PDA) must exist between the right and left sides of the heart to allow for mixing.

a. Hemodynamics: systemic venous blood returns to the right atrium, enters the right ventricle, and exits via the aorta. Pulmonary venous blood coming from the lungs enters the left atrium, goes to the left ventricle, and then returns to the pulmonary arteries back to the lungs. Unless there is a mechanism for mixing between the two circulations, oxygenated blood cannot be delivered to the systemic circulation and systemic venous blood cannot pick up oxygen in the lungs. Infants with intact ventricular septum become extremely cyanotic after birth due to the closure of the foramen ovale and the ductus arteriosus.

   b. Clinical manifestations: varying degrees of cyanosis; tachypnea without increased work of breathing; murmur (holosystolic murmur of VSD); single S2; CHF for infants with a large VSD; chest x-ray (cardiomegaly; cardiac silhouette has a characteristic **"egg-shaped"** appearance; increased pulmonary vascular markings); ECG (RVH)

   c. Interventions: PGE$_1$ infusion; oxygen administration has little benefit; treat CHF; surgical intervention required

2. Total anomalous pulmonary venous return (TAPVR): an abnormal connection of the pulmonary veins to the right atrium either directly or indirectly. The pulmonary veins connect with a systemic venous channel that delivers pulmonary venous blood to the right atrium. This abnormal drainage may be **supracardiac** (into the right or left SVC), **intracardiac** (into the coronary sinus and right atrium), **infracardiac** *or* **subdiaphragmatic** (through the portal system, IVC), or **mixed sites** of drainage. A PFO or ASD is usually present to allow venous return to the left side of the heart. Infants with TAPVR can be divided into two major categories: nonobstructive veins and obstructive veins (Flanagan, et al., 1999).

   a. Hemodynamics: pulmonary venous return drains into the right atrium. There is mixing of systemic and pulmonary venous blood. Oxygen saturations in the systemic and pulmonary circulations are the same. Blood then flows through the ASD or PFO to the left side of the heart in the left atrium.

      (1) TAPVR with nonobstructed veins: results in a large right-to-left shunt at the atrial level. Systemic output is maintained by the right-to-left shunt through the ASD or PFO. This mixing of the blood in the right atrium usually produces only cyanosis.

      (2) TAPVR with obstructed veins: an obstruction can be present in the channel returning pulmonary venous blood to the right atrium. This obstruction and inadequate pulmonary venous drainage causes a backflow of blood into the pulmonary system, resulting in increased pulmonary vascular resistance (PVR) with resultant pulmonary edema and potential pulmonary HTN. These infants become severely cyanotic.

   b. Diagnosis: often misdiagnosed as pulmonary disease; ECG may be misleading; therefore, cardiac catheterization and angiography may be necessary to distinguish pulmonary disease from this form of cardiac disease (Johnson & Moller, 2001).

   c. Clinical manifestations:

      (1) TAPVR with nonobstructed veins (infants usually become symptomatic after the neonatal period when PVR is decreased and have a large right-to-left shunt): mildly cyanotic; murmur (SEM); wide fixed splitting of S2; CHF; chest x-ray (cardiomegaly; **"snowman" sign** is seen in older infants with the supracardiac type of TAPVR); and ECG (RAE, RVH)

(2) TAPVR with obstructed veins (infant is usually critically ill): severe cyanosis; respiratory distress; no murmur; loud single S2 with gallop rhythm; chest x-ray (size is normal; pulmonary edema); ECG (RAE, RVH)

d. Interventions:

(1) TAPVR with nonobstructed veins: temporary medical management before surgical intervention

(2) TAPVR with obstructed veins: treat respiratory distress; consider PGE₁ infusion; treat other underlying conditions; emergent surgical intervention

3. Truncus arteriosus: a single arterial trunk (with a truncal valve) arises from the ventricle and gives rise to the pulmonary, systemic, and coronary circulations. A large VSD is always present. Classifications of truncus arteriosus are based on the level at which the pulmonary vessels arise off the trunk. More than 75% of infants show deletion of a portion of chromosome 22 and other laboratory findings of DiGeorge syndrome, such as hypocalcemia and reduced T lymphocytes (Johnson & Moller, 2001).

a. Hemodynamics: due to the large VSD and the common arterial trunk, there is mixing of the systemic and pulmonary venous blood and the infant is cyanotic. The degree of cyanosis is dependent on the amount of pulmonary blood flow that can be altered if there is an obstruction in the pulmonary arteries. If there is no obstruction, there is increased pulmonary blood flow resulting in CHF.

b. Clinical manifestations: varying degrees of cyanosis; CHF; murmur (loud holosystolic murmur of VSD; diastolic murmur); single S2; chest x-ray (cardiomegaly; increased pulmonary vascular markings; right aortic arch is seen in approximately 30% to 35% of infants); and ECG (bilateral ventricular hypertrophy [BVH])

c. Interventions: medical management of CHF; close monitoring of calcium levels; and surgical intervention

4. Hypoplastic left heart syndrome (HLHS): characterized by a combination of anomalies that includes hypoplasia of the left ventricle, aortic atresia, and severe mitral valve stenosis or atresia. HLHS is the most common cause of death from CHD during the first months of life (Park, 1997).

a. Hemodynamics: a severe obstruction to both left ventricular inflow and outflow. Pulmonary venous return to the left atrium is unable to enter the left ventricle due to obstruction at the mitral valve; therefore, blood flows from the left atrium to the right atrium via the PFO. The right ventricle supplies both the pulmonary and systemic circulation. The systemic circulation is supplied by right-to-left flow through the ductus arteriosus. Coronary blood flow is retrograde from the hypoplastic ascending aorta via the PDA (Hsu & Gersony, 1996). Decompensation occurs as the ductus arteriosus constricts, causing increased pulmonary circulation with decreased systemic blood flow and poor coronary perfusion.

b. Clinical manifestations (symptoms not usually seen until constriction of the ductus arteriosus): CHF; hypotension and shock; single S2; chest x-ray (mild to moderate cardiomegaly with pulmonary edema); ECG (RVH)

c. Interventions: PGE_1 infusion; supplemental oxygen and hyperventilation are usually discouraged because they decrease PVR; treat CHF/shock; and surgical repair or heart transplantation

D. Left ventricular outflow obstruction:

1. Aortic stenosis (AS): left ventricular outflow obstruction can occur at any level along the transition from the left ventricle to the ascending aorta. The most common cause of AS is valvular and occurs when the aortic valve is bicuspid instead of tricuspid (Wood, 1998). AS is commonly associated with a significant murmur at birth and occurs three times more frequently in males (Johnson & Moller, 2001). AS that presents in the neonatal period is called critical AS.

    a. Hemodynamics: owing to the aortic valve stenosis, the left ventricular pressure rises to maintain a normal cardiac output. The result is LVH. Blood flow to the systemic circulation is from the right ventricle via a PDA. Infants with critical AS present with acute and severe left ventricular failure.

    b. Clinical manifestations: CHF; murmur (SEM at right upper sternal border [RUSB] or left middle sternal border [LMSB]); single S2; chest x-ray (cardiomegaly; increased pulmonary vascular markings); ECG (LVH)

    c. Interventions: PGE_1 infusion; treat CHF; immediate surgical intervention (balloon valvuloplasty or surgical valvotomy)

2. Coarctation of the aorta: a narrowing of the descending aorta that usually occurs in the vicinity of the ductus arteriosus. Coarctation of the aorta can be described as either preductal, postductal, or juxtaductal.

    a. Hemodynamics: the location of the narrowing in relation to the ductus arteriosus determines the blood supply to the descending aorta. LVH develops secondary to the elevated systolic pressure proximal to the coarctation. The pressure proximal to the coarctation is higher than the pressure distal to the coarctation.

    b. Clinical manifestations: CHF; blood pressure difference (upper extremity BP > lower extremity BP); murmur (SEM at LUSB radiating to the back; continuous murmur of a PDA); chest x-ray (cardiomegaly; increased pulmonary vascular markings); ECG (RVH)

    c. Interventions: consider PGE_1 infusion (depends upon location of coarctation in relation to the ductus arteriosus); treat CHF; ductal-dependent lesion (surgical intervention); nonductal-dependent lesion (close monitoring of upper and lower BP readings; when BP gradient increases then surgical intervention is necessary)

3. Interrupted aortic arch (IAA): absence of a segment of the aortic arch. A VSD is associated with this lesion. This lesion is also associated with DiGeorge syndrome.
   a. Hemodynamics: the left ventricle supplies the blood flow to the ascending aorta proximal to the interruption. The ductus arteriosus supplies the blood flow to the aorta distal to the interruption. When the ductus arteriosus constricts there is decreased systemic perfusion.
   b. Clinical manifestations: CHF; shock; absent lower extremity pulses; chest x-ray (cardiomegaly; increased pulmonary vascular markings); ECG (RVH)
   c. Interventions: PGE_1 infusion; treat CHF/shock; close monitoring of calcium levels; surgical intervention

III. **ECG fundamentals** (Vargo, 1998)
   A. ECG paper: measures time and voltage.
      1. Recording speed of the paper is 25 mm per second.
      2. Time is measured on the horizontal axis: each small square = 0.04 seconds; each large square = 0.2 seconds.
      3. Voltage or amplitude is measured on the vertical axis: measures the upward and downward deflection of a cardiac impulse; each small square = 1 mm of amplitude; two large squares (10 mm) = 1 millivolt (mV).
   B. Evaluating the heart rate: determine the heart rate by counting the number of R-to-R cycles in six large squares and multiplying by 50.
   C. Cardiac cycle:
      1. P wave: represents atrial depolarization; should be upright (positive) in Lead II; maximum duration of the P wave in infants < 12 months of age is 0.08 seconds (2 small boxes).
      2. QRS complex: represents ventricular depolarization; QRS duration will increase with age.
      3. T wave: represents ventricular repolarization.
   D. Cardiac rhythm:
      1. Refers to the regularity of the ECG pattern; sinus rhythm is the normal cardiac rhythm.
      2. Only one P wave should occur consistently before each QRS complex; the QRS complex is consistently followed by a T wave; the pattern should repeat itself at regular intervals.

IV. **Common neonatal dysrhythmias**
   A. Premature atrial contractions (PACs): results from premature atrial depolarization.
      1. ECG: each conducted PAC is represented by a premature P wave followed by a correspondingly premature QRS complex; a nonconducted PAC is represented by a premature P wave that is not followed by a corresponding QRS complex.
      2. Outcome: essentially benign; frequent, blocked, or nonconducted PACs can result in ventricular bradycardia; often resolve by 3 months of age without treatment.
   B. Premature ventricular contractions (PVCs):
      1. ECG: PVCs are early QRS complexes with a different morphology from the sinus QRS and are not preceded by P waves.
      2. Outcome: usually benign but warrant further evaluation for pos-

sible electrolyte imbalances, structural heart disease, or long-QT syndrome; usually resolve by 2 to 3 months of age without treatment in the healthy neonate.

C. Tachydysrhythmias: all infants with documented tachydysrhythmias should have a complete cardiac evaluation. With persistent tachydysrhythmias, the infant can develop heart failure.
   1. ECG: determine whether the QRS complex is wide or narrow during the tachycardia: ventricular tachycardia (the QRS complex remains wide); supraventricular tachycardia ([SVT] narrow normal QRS complex; up to 25% of infants with SVT have structural heart disease) (Flanagan, et al., 1999). Determine whether the heart rate is fixed or variable; determine whether there is a visible P wave and the P wave axis.
   2. SVT: the most common tachydysrhythmia in the fetus, neonate, and young child (Anisman, Eshaghpour, & Robinson, 1996). SVT involves a reentry circuit using an accessory atrioventricular conduction pathway (always retrograde). Interventions include: attempt to convert to sinus rhythm by implementing vagal maneuvers; adenosine administration when vagal maneuvers are ineffective (start with 50 µg/kg via rapid intravenous [IV] push); synchronized direct current (DC) cardioversion (begin with 0.5 Joules/kg); and prophylactic therapy (digoxin is usually prescribed secondary to an approximate 20% recurrence risk) (Flanagan, et al., 1999).
   3. WPW syndrome: a tachydysrhythmia in which some pathways conduct impulses in antegrade and retrograde directions. During sinus rhythm there is a characteristic delta wave, short PR interval, and wide QRS complex. Propanolol is the usual drug of choice.
D. Complete heart block: the inability of an electrical impulse to be conducted to the ventricles; the ventricular rate is slower (~ 50 to 100 bpm) and independent of the atrial rate. P waves usually occur at the normal neonatal rate; QRS complexes occur more slowly and occur completely dissociated from the atrial rhythm; and there is little variability in the HR.
E. Complete congenital heart block (CCHB): heart block present in a newborn infant who had a prenatal onset
   1. Etiology:
      a. Structural heart disease: approximately 50% of the infants with CCHB have associated structural cardiovascular anomalies (Flanagan, et al., 1999).
      b. Transplacental passage of maternal autoantibodies that interact with the developing fetus' conduction systems (eg, maternal lupus erythromatosis)
   2. Outcome:
      a. CCHB without structural heart disease: usually do well in the newborn period because the stroke volume increases to compensate for the low ventricular rate and maintain adequate cardiac output.
      b. CCHB with associated cardiovascular anomalies: most die in the neonatal period despite pacemaker management and surgical attempts to repair the cardiovascular anomalies (Anisman, et al., 1996).

▼ References

Anisman, P., Eshaghpour, E., & Robinson, B. (1996). Cardiac dysrhythmias. In A. R. Spitzer (Ed.), *Intensive care of the fetus and neonate* (pp. 797–822). St. Louis: Mosby.

Bell, S. G. (1998). Neonatal cardiovascular pharmacology. *Neonatal Network*, *17*(2), 7.

Drummond, W. H. (1996). Ductus arteriosus. In A. R. Spitzer (Ed.), *Intensive care of the fetus and neonate* (pp. 760–771). St. Louis: Mosby.

Flanagan, M. F., Yeager, S. B., & Weindling, S. N. (1999). Cardiac disease. In G. B. Avery, M. A. Fletcher, & M. G. MacDonald (Eds.), *Neonatology: Pathophysiology and management of the newborn* (5th ed., pp. 577–646). Philadelphia: Lippincott Williams & Wilkins.

Fletcher, M. A. (1998). *Physical diagnosis in neonatology.* Philadelphia: Lippincott-Raven.

Furdon, S. A. (1997). Recognizing congestive heart failure in the neonatal period. *Neonatal Network*, *16*(7), 5.

Hsu, D. T., & Gersony, W. M. (1996). Medical management of the neonate with congenital heart disease. In A. R. Spitzer (Ed.), *Intensive care of the fetus and neonate* (pp. 787–796). St. Louis: Mosby.

Huhta, J. C. (1996). Fetal echocardiography in the detection and management of fetal heart disease. In A. R. Spitzer (Ed.), *Intensive care of the fetus and neonate* (pp. 772–786). St. Louis: Mosby.

Johnson, Jr., W. H., & Moller, J. H. (2001). *The pediatric cardiology handbook.* Philadelphia: Lippincott Williams & Wilkins.

Klassen, L. R. (1999). Complete congenital heart block: A review and case study. *Neonatal Network*, *18*(3), 33.

Park, M. K. (1997). *The pediatric cardiology handbook* (2nd ed.). St. Louis: Mosby.

Ruth-Sanchez, V. (1998). Cardiac anomalies restricting blood flow to the left atrium. *Neonatal Network*, *17*(6), 7.

Santulli, T. V. (1993). An approach to the newborn with heart disease. In J. J. Pomerance & C. J. Richardson (Eds.), *Neonatology for the clinician* (pp. 339–362). Norwalk, CT: Appleton & Lange.

Spilman, L. J., & Furdon, S. A. (1998). Recognition, understanding, and current management of cardiac lesions with decreased pulmonary blood flow. *Neonatal Network*, *17*(4), 7.

Vargo, L. (1998). The basics of neonatal ECG interpretation. *Neonatal Network*, *17*(8), 7.

Wood, M. K. (1997). Acyanotic lesions with increased pulmonary blood flow. *Neonatal Network*, *16*(3), 17.

Wood, M. K. (1998). Acyanotic cardiac lesions with normal pulmonary blood flow. *Neonatal Network*, *17*(3), 5.

Young, T. E. & Mangum, B. (Eds.). *Neofax 2001.* (14th ed.). Raleigh, NC: Acorn Publishing, INC.

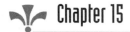 **Chapter 15**

Neurologic and Musculoskeletal Disorders

Paulette S. Haws, MSN, RNC, NNP

Part A: Gestational Age, Cranium, Spine, Cranial and Peripheral Nerves, and Global Neurologic Insults

I. Gestational age (GA) assessment (Gomella, 1999; Wolcott & Conry, 2000):

   A. Date of last menses: estimated date of conception (EDC) = last menstrual period (LMP) − 3 months + 7 days (Nägele's rule).

   B. Early fetal ultrasound: crown-rump measurements made between 6 to 11 weeks' gestation are accurate to within 3 days.

   C. Date of first fetal heart sounds: heard by a Doppler instrument between 10 and 12 weeks' gestation and by a fetoscope between 18 and 20 weeks' gestation

   D. Date of first fetal movement: *quickening* (fluttering movements in the abdomen perceived by the mother) normally occurs between 16 and 20 weeks' gestation.

   E. Uterine size: the distance (in centimeters) between the symphysis pubis and the uterine fundus is approximately the GA (in weeks), if measured before the middle of the third trimester.

   F. Newborn physical maturity and neuromuscular maturity examination (Figure 15.1)

   G. Lens vascularity (Figure 15.2)

II. The cranium

   A. Fontanels (Gomella, 1999; Tappero & Honeyfield, 1993): the unossified membranes lying between the cranial bones of the fetus and infant. The fontanels of the infant's skull are the *anterior* (diamond-shaped area formed by the junction of the coronal, frontal, and sagittal sutures; closes by 18 to 24 months of age), *posterior* (triangular-shaped area formed by the junction of the lambdoid and sagittal sutures; closes by 12 months of age), *sphenoid* (irregularly shaped area located anterior to the ear and bordered by the frontal, parietal, and temporal bones), and *mastoid* (irregularly shaped area bordered by the parietal, temporal, and occipital bones). Alterations from normal appearance may indicate the following:

      1. Enlarged anterior fontanel: hypothyroidism, hypophosphatasia (perinatal and congenital autosomal-recessive disorder with signs of rickets secondary to alkaline phosphatase deficiency), chromosomal abnormalities, skeletal disorders (eg, osteogenesis imperfecta), and small-for-gestational-age (SGA) infants

      2. Small anterior fontanel: hyperthyroidism, microcephaly, and craniosynostosis

      3. Bulging fontanels: increased intracranial pressure (ICP), hydrocephalus, and meningitis

      4. Depressed fontanels: dehydration

Neuromuscular Maturity

	-1	0	1	2	3	4	5
Posture							
Square Window (wrist)	>90°	90°	60°	45°	30°	0°	
Arm Recoil		180°	140°-180°	110°-140°	90-110°	<90°	
Popliteal Angle	180°	160°	140°	120°	100°	90°	<90°
Scarf Sign							
Heel to Ear							

Physical Maturity

Skin	sticky friable transparent	gelatinous red, translucent	smooth pink, visible veins	superficial peeling &/or rash, few veins	cracking pale areas rare veins	parchment deep cracking no vessels	leathery cracked wrinkled
Lanugo	none	sparse	abundant	thinning	bald areas	mostly bald	
Plantar Surface	heel-toe 40-50 mm: -1 <40 mm: -2	>50mm no crease	faint red marks	anterior transverse crease only	creases ant. 2/3	creases over entire sole	
Breast	imperceptible	barely perceptible	flat areola no bud	stippled areola 1-2mm bud	raised areola 3-4mm bud	full areola 5-10mm bud	
Eye/Ear	lids fused loosely:-1 tightly:-2	lids open pinna flat stays folded	sl. curved pinna; soft; slow recoil	well-curved pinna; soft but ready recoil	formed &firm instant recoil	thick cartilage ear stiff	
Genitals male	scrotum flat, smooth	scrotum empty faint rugae	testes in upper canal rare rugae	testes descending few rugae	testes down good rugae	testes pendulous deep rugae	
Genitals female	clitoris prominent labia flat	prominent clitoris small labia minora	prominent clitoris enlarging minora	majora & minora equally prominent	majora large minora small	majora cover clitoris & minora	

Figure 15-1. Ballard exam form. Used with permission from Ballard, J. L., Khoury, J. C., Wedig, K., Wang, L., Eilers-Walsman, B.L., & Lipp, R. (1991). New Ballard Score, expanded to include extremely premature infants. *The Journal of Pediatrics*, 119, 417–423.

B. Cranial sutures (Tappero & Honeyfield, 1993): the lines of articulation between the skull bones; *sagittal* suture extends from the anterior fontanel to the posterior fontanel and separates the parietal bones; *metopic* suture extends down the forehead from the anterior fontanel and separates the frontal bones; *coronal* sutures extend laterally from the anterior fontanel to the sphenoid fontanel (midway

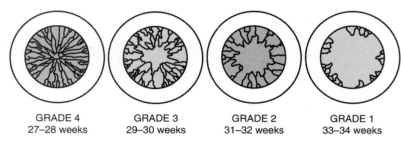

| GRADE 4 | GRADE 3 | GRADE 2 | GRADE 1 |
| 27–28 weeks | 29–30 weeks | 31–32 weeks | 33–34 weeks |

Figure 15-2. Lens Vascularity Diagram. Adapted from Hittner, H. M., Hirsch, N. J., & Rudolph, A. J. (1977). Assessment of gestational age by examination of the anterior vascular capsule of the lens. *The Journal of Pediatrics, 91,* 455–458.

between the eye and the ear) and separate the parietal bones from the frontal bones; *squamosal* sutures extend from the sphenoid fontanel (anterior to the ear) to the mastoid fontanel (posterior to the ear) and separate the parietal bones from the temporal bones; *lambdoidal* sutures extend from the lateral aspect of the posterior fontanel to the mastoid fontanels (posterior to the ear) and separate the parietal bones from the occipital bone.

  C. Bone and soft tissue abnormalities:

    1. Cutis aplasia (Witt, 1993): lesions occurring, most often on the scalp, in which there is a congenital absence of some or all layers of the skin. It may be associated with midline defects or chromosomal syndromes, or occur in isolation. Interventions: keep area clean and dry; topical antibiotic therapy may be required; and surgical intervention may be necessitated.

    2. Cleft lip and palate:

      a. Associated malformations (skeletal spinal and limb anomalies, congenital heart disease [atrial septal defect (ASD), ventricular septal defect [VSD], patent ductus arteriosus [PDA], transposition], gastrointestinal [GI] tract [stenoses, atresias, hernias, fistulas]) are more often seen with cleft lip and palate than with isolated cleft lip or isolated cleft palate (Milerad, Larson, Hagberg, & Ideberg, 1997).

      b. Etiology: associated with genetic and chromosomal abnormalities (eg, trisomy 13, Apert syndrome, and Velocardiofacial syndrome); teratogens (eg, maternal phenytoin ingestion during pregnancy); and multifactorial

      c. Clinical manifestations:

        (1) Cleft lip may be unilateral (majority are on the left) or bilateral (often associated with cleft palate); the gum may be involved, ranging from a small notch to a complete division into separate parts; distorted nares

(2) Cleft palate (soft *or* soft and hard palate) may be an isolated finding. Palate should be examined with the initial physical examination.

d. Interventions: breast or bottle feeding may be possible with cleft lip; special nipples, cleft palate nipples, or squeeze bottles may be necessary for infants with cleft palates; and surgical intervention

e. Outcome (Schiefelbein, 1999): favorable outcome with surgical intervention; aspiration; dentition problems; feeding difficulties; hearing loss secondary to frequent bouts of otitis media and upper respiratory tract infections; and speech delays

3. Craniosynostosis (McCulloch, 1999; Volpe, 2001): premature fusion of one or more of the cranial sutures that may result in restricted brain growth. Asymmetric skull shape may be present at birth or may not be detectable until later in infancy. Etiology may be idiopathic or part of a genetic syndrome (eg, Apert or Crouzon syndrome) or metabolic disorder (eg, hyperthyroidism and idiopathic hypercalcemia).

   a. Clinical manifestations: asymptomatic, abnormal head shape

   b. Diagnosis: physical examination (differentiate between overriding sutures and sutures that are ridged and fixed); radiographic skull films; and computed tomography (CT) scan

   c. Interventions: depending upon the extent of the premature fusion, surgical intervention may be necessitated.

4. Cephalohematoma: bleeding beneath the periosteum of a skull bone. The hemorrhage is *confined within the suture line*.

   a. Diagnosis: radiographic skull films or CT scan if an underlying fractured skull is suspected

   b. Interventions: follow hematocrit (Hct) and serum bilirubin levels.

   c. Outcome: complete resolution within weeks to months

5. Caput succedaneum: diffuse scalp edema found over the presenting part of the fetal head and often *extending across suture lines* caused by venous constriction. No intervention is required, and resolution occurs within a few days.

6. Craniotabes (Buschbach, 1999): abnormally soft demineralized areas of skull bones, usually along the lambdoidal suture in the occipital and parietal regions

   a. Clinical manifestations: slight pressure over the affected area will indent the bone and then it will return to its normal position.

   b. Interventions: when there is a small affected area, no intervention is required and the condition resolves with time. If most of the skull is involved, then it may be associated with disorders that affect ossification, such as syphilis and osteogenesis imperfecta.

7. Skull fracture (Harris, 1999; McCulloch, 1999; Volpe, 2001):

a. Etiology: traumatic operative delivery (eg, forceps delivery) or excessive pressure against the maternal pelvic structures during labor

b. Clinical manifestations: the defect may be linear (relatively common and usually asymptomatic) or depressed (indented skull surface, does not cross suture lines, and possible separation of adjacent sutures).

c. Diagnosis: radiographic skull films and CT scan to identify bone fragments or the presence of extradural or subdural clot

d. Interventions:

    (1) Close observation to detect abnormal neurologic symptoms

    (2) Elevate a depressed fracture with a breast pump shield attached to a vacuum extractor, or fingertip pressure around the edges of the fracture.

    (3) Neurosurgical intervention may be needed in the following situations: fractures that are depressed > 0.5 cm; bone fragments within the cerebrum; increased ICP; cerebrospinal fluid (CSF) leakage from nose or ear or beneath the galea

    (4) Antibiotic administration with documented or suspected CSF leakage

e. Outcome:

    (1) Linear fractures usually heal within 3 months.

    (2) Depressed fractures: outcome is dependent upon extent of the injury.

D. Vascular injuries and malformations:

  1. Intraventricular hemorrhage (IVH) and periventricular hemorrhage: intraventricular bleeding that usually "originates (in the preterm infant) in the subependymal germinal matrix region with extension into the ventricular system and possibly into the aqueduct, cisterns, and subarachnoid spaces" (Goddard-Finegold, Mizrahi, & Lee, 1998, pp. 861–862). Extension of the hemorrhage into the periventricular white matter does not usually occur unless there has been previous white matter damage. This damage is probably secondary to substantial IVH-resultant periventricular venous occlusion.

    a. Risk factors (McCulloch, 1999) include: premature infants < 34 weeks' gestation and < 1,500 g; acidosis; asphyxia; blood pressure (BP) instability; coagulation disorders; acute blood loss; arteriovenous malformation; hypovolemia; maternal chorioamnionitis; neonatal transport; rapid fluid resuscitation; hyperosmolar fluid infusion (eg, sodium bicarbonate); respiratory distress with mechanical ventilation; air leak syndromes

    b. Diagnosis: cranial ultrasound (majority of IVHs occur within 72 hours after birth); CT scan

      (1) Grading is done according to extent and location of hemorrhage: *Grade I* (subependymal hemorrhage in periventricular germinal matrix); *Grade II* (bleeding into the lateral ventricle without ventricular dilation); *Grade III* (bleeding into the lateral ventricles with ventricular dila-

tion); *Grade IV* (intraventricular bleeding extending into the parenchymal tissue)

c. Clinical manifestations range from asymptomatic to acute deterioration: anemia; apnea and bradycardia; changes in level of consciousness and activity (hypotonia, lethargy, and seizures); hyperglycemia; metabolic acidosis; oxygen desaturation; respiratory distress

d. Interventions:
(1) Prevent preterm labor and delivery; encourage maternal transport to a tertiary care facility.
(2) Correct acidosis; correct clotting disorders; prevent situations that promote BP instability (eg, air leaks, excessive agitation and motor activity, and crying); and prevent hyperosmolar and/or rapid fluid administration.
(3) Observe for signs of worsening hemorrhage: bulging fontanel; increased ventilatory support; seizures; apnea; and change in level of consciousness or activity

e. Outcome depends upon the extent of the hemorrhage: there may be no neurologic sequelae; neurodevelopmental delays; posthemorrhagic hydrocephalus; periventricular leukomalacia; and death

2. Periventricular leukomalacia (PVL) (Bernbaum, 1999): PVL is "caused by ischemic infarction of the white matter adjacent to the lateral ventricles. A weakening in the integrity of the white matter in this area occurs, followed by either repair or the development of cysts" (Bernbaum, 1999, p. 1469).

a. Risk factors: prematurity; ischemia; hypoxia; IVH; events that alter cerebral blood flow (eg, sepsis, meningitis, seizures, cardiorespiratory arrest)

b. Diagnosis is confirmed by documenting the presence of fluid-filled periventricular cysts: cranial ultrasound; CT scan; and magnetic resonance imaging (MRI)

c. Clinical manifestations: no specific symptoms are noted in the neonatal period.

d. Outcome:
(1) Cerebral palsy (moderate or severe quadriplegia or diplegia) may be present when cyst formation is > 3 mm in areas of vital neural tissue; motor, visual, and auditory deficits; and mental retardation
(2) Little or no neurologic sequelae when cysts resolve

3. Subarachnoid hemorrhage (Volpe, 2001): intracranial bleeding (venous source) within the subarachnoid space commonly located over cerebral convexities (usually posteriorly) and in the posterior fossa. The bleeding is not an extension of subdural, intraventricular, or intracerebellar hemorrhages. It is more common in term than preterm infants. Etiology is usually trauma (in term infants) or hypoxia (in preterm infants).

a. Clinical manifestations (three major syndromes):
(1) Minor hemorrhage: infant exhibits few or no symptoms.

(2) Significant hemorrhage: may lead to seizures, beginning on the second day of life, in an apparently well infant. A preterm infant may have recurrent apnea.

(3) Massive hemorrhage (rare occurrence): severe deterioration and rapid demise

b. Diagnosis: CT scan detects acute blood accumulation; increased red blood cells (RBCs) and protein in CSF will raise suspicion of hemorrhage.

c. Outcome: complications are usually rare unless the hemorrhage is associated with severe traumatic or hypoxic insult.

4. Subdural hemorrhage (Hill & Volpe, 1999; Volpe, 2001): lacerations of the major veins or venous sinuses overlying the cerebral hemispheres or cerebellum, often associated with accompanying tear in the dura.

a. There are four major varieties of subdural hemorrhage: *tentorial laceration* (rupture of straight sinus, transverse sinus, vein of Galen, or infratentorial veins); *occipital osteodiastasis* (rupture of occipital sinus); *falx laceration* (rupture of the inferior sagittal sinus); and *rupture of superficial cerebral veins*

b. Etiology: traumatic delivery (eg, vacuum or forceps); vaginal delivery with malpresentation (eg, breech, brow, face, footling); cephalopelvic disproportion

c. Clinical manifestations (McCulloch, 1999; Volpe, 2001):

(1) Symptoms associated with a subdural hemorrhage range from "no clinical signs" to "coma and death." The severity of the clinical manifestations often depends upon the location and size of the hemorrhage; infants may present at birth, or soon thereafter (eg, tentorial laceration), after several days, or after several months of life (eg, chronic subdural effusion).

(2) Rapid lethal hemorrhages (symptoms appear soon after birth): stupor advancing to coma; lateral deviation of the eyes that is not affected by the doll's eyes maneuver; unequal pupils that become fixed and dilated; nuchal rigidity; opisthotonus; bradycardia; respiratory arrest

(3) Less severe hemorrhages (symptoms may appear several hours to several days after birth): signs of increased ICP (eg, bulging fontanels, lethargy, and irritability); signs of brain stem involvement (eg, eye deviation, oculomotor abnormalities, and respiratory abnormalities), hemiparesis, and focal seizures

d. Diagnosis: CT scan is better for the detection of supratentorial lesions; MRI is better for the detection of infratentorial lesions.

e. Interventions: close observation may be the only required intervention when there is neither brain stem involvement nor deterioration in neurologic status; surgical evacuation of the blood clot

f. Outcome: major hemorrhages are often lethal; hydrocephalus is possible; many infants have a favorable outcome.

5. Subgaleal hemorrhage (Harris, 1999): bleeding from emissary veins running between the periosteum and the galea aponeurot-

ica (fibrous membrane connecting the occipital and frontal muscles). The hemorrhage may extend from the infant's brow and root of the nose, laterally to the root of the ear, and to the nape of the neck. The hemorrhage is usually associated with forceps or vacuum-assisted deliveries.

a. Clinical manifestations: hemorrhage is a fluctuant mass that crosses suture lines and fontanels; hypovolemic shock

b. Interventions: volume replacement; tight turban-type head dressing (eg, Kling dressing and adhesive tape) applied within 2 to 4 hours of onset

c. Outcome: 25% to 50% of affected infants may die secondary to hypovolemia or complications such as disseminated intravascular coagulopathy (DIC).

6. Vascular malformations (Madsen & Frim, 1999; Volpe, 2001): two major intracranial vascular malformations are congenital arterial aneurysm and arteriovenous (AV) malformations (fistulous connection between an artery and vein, bypassing the capillary bed). In the neonate, the most common site (AV) involves the vein of Galen system (Madsen & Frim, 1999).

a. Clinical manifestations:

(1) Arterial aneurysm: abrupt neurologic deterioration; increased ICP (bulging anterior fontanel); focal seizures; and neurologic deficits relate to the location and extent of the lesion.

(2) AV malformation (Volpe, 2001): normally presents within the first 3 months of life as intracerebral and/or intraventricular hemorrhage; seizures; congestive heart failure (CHF) (due to high cardiac output); hydrocephalus; opisthotonus; and congenital or abrupt onset paraplegia

b. Diagnosis: head ultrasonography and angiography

c. Interventions: surgical excision of the lesion or embolic therapy for large or inoperative lesions

d. Outcome: varies according to the site and extent of the lesion and the brain injury incurred from the hemorrhage.

E. Neuronal developmental defects:

1. Holoprosencephaly (Goddard-Finegold, 1998; McCulloch, 1999; Volpe, 2001): abnormal formation of the telencephalon (cerebral hemispheres) and diencephalon (thalamus and hypothalamus). The extent of the defect varies.

a. Clinical manifestations:

(1) Microcephaly; hydrocephalus with macrocephaly

(2) Facial defects: hypotelorism; cebocephaly (single flattened nostril located between the eyes); cyclopia; cleft lip and palate (median with absent philtrum or bilateral)

(3) Neurologic and metabolic disturbances: apnea; seizures; hypothalamic dysfunction (diabetes insipidus [DI], syndrome of inappropriate antidiuretic hormone [SIADH])

b. Outcome:

(1) Mildly affected infants (subtle or no obvious facial anomalies) may escape detection until later in infancy. These infants may have a normal cognitive and motor outcome.

(2) Affected infants with severe facial anomalies have major cognitive and motor delays

(3) Spontaneous abortion; death

2. Dandy-Walker malformation (Goddard-Finegold, 1998; Volpe, 2001): a malformation consisting of partial or complete agenesis of the cerebellar vermis, cystic dilation of the fourth ventricle, and posterior fossa enlargement with resultant superior displacement of the lateral sinuses, tentorium, and torcular.

a. Clinical manifestations: hydrocephalus may be present at birth or develop during the first prenatal year; cranial nerve palsies; apnea; nystagmus; and truncal ataxia

b. Diagnosis: prenatal ultrasound and postnatal CT scan or MRI

c. Interventions: ventricular and posterior fossa shunting if diagnosis is made during the neonatal period

d. Outcome: varies depending upon the severity of the lesion and presence of other associated malformations; increased chance of cognitive delays

3. Lissencephaly (or agyria) and Pachygyria (Goddard-Finegold, 1998; Volpe, 2001):

a. Lissencephaly is a developmental disorder in which the brain has few or no gyri ("smooth brain" [Type I] or "cobblestone" appearance [Type II]). Pachygyria describes a brain with few and abnormally broad gyri.

b. Etiology: unknown; genetic association; vascular insult during the third and fourth months of gestation; fetal cytomegalovirus (CMV) infection

c. Clinical manifestations: normal head size and facial features are usually present at birth; hypotonia and decreased movement in the neonatal period; seizures in the neonatal period are possible; and feeding difficulties

d. Diagnosis: CT scan and MRI (better definition of parenchymal lesion)

e. Outcome: lissencephaly (seizures, spastic quadriplegia, and mental retardation) and pachygyria (motor and cognitive deficits, however, usually less than those with lissencephaly)

4. Porencephaly, hydranencephaly, and multicystic encephalomalacia (Volpe, 2001): these terms are used to describe focal or multifocal areas of brain necrosis during the prenatal and early postnatal period with resultant tissue dissolution and cavity formation. *Porencephaly* is "a single unilateral lesion in the cerebral hemisphere that may or may not communicate with the lateral ventricle" (Volpe, 2001, p. 316). *Hydranencephaly* has CSF-filled cavities located bilaterally in the cerebral hemispheres. *Multicystic encephalomalacia* has multiple areas of cavitation located, usually bilaterally, throughout the cerebral hemispheres.

a. Etiology:

(1) Maternal factors: hypotension; illicit drug use (eg, cocaine); and trauma

(2) Intrauterine and intrapartum factors: cord accidents; placental abruption; and twin-to-twin transfusion

(3) Neonatal: asphyxia; cerebral vascular malformation; congenital heart disease (CHD) with heart failure; fluid and electrolyte disturbances; hemorrhage; hypotension; persistent pulmonary hypertension of the newborn (PPHN); sepsis; and thromboembolic disorders/accidents

b. Clinical manifestations: vary according to the size and location of the destroyed neural tissue.

c. Outcome: cognitive and motor deficits

5. Schizencephaly (Volpe, 2001): neuronal migrational disorder in which there is complete agenesis of a portion of the germinative zones and cerebral wall with resultant clefts (deep in folding) of the cerebral cortex

a. Etiology: unknown; defect in the homeobox gene, EMX2; destructive lesions may be present during the third and fourth months of gestation.

b. Diagnosis: CT scan and MRI

c. Outcome: neurologic sequelae depend upon the extent of the lesion; seizures are possible (may begin in adulthood); mental retardation with bilateral clefts; less likely with unilateral lesions; motor deficits with frontal and open-lipped lesions

III. The spinal cord

A. Cranial nerves (Table 15.1)

B. Spinal cord and central nervous system (CNS) defects:

1. Spinal cord injuries (Volpe, 2001): injury to the spinal cord secondary to traction or rotation during the birthing process; injury to the lower cervical and upper thoracic regions principally occurs during breech delivery; and injury to upper and midcervical regions principally occurs with cephalic presentation and delivery.

a. Clinical manifestations:

(1) There are three basic syndromes: *stillbirth or rapid neonatal demise* when adequate respiratory function is not established (upper cervical cord and/or brain stem involvement); development of *respiratory failure* during the first few days of life leading to death; *survival with neurologic sequelae*

(2) Flaccid weakness and areflexia of lower limbs; variable involvement of upper limbs

(3) Diaphragmatic breathing; "paradoxical" respirations

(4) Abdominal muscle paralysis; atonic anal sphincter; neurogenic bladder

b. Interventions:

(1) "Appropriate management of breech presentations and any other obstetrical situation that might lead to dysfunctional labor" (Volpe, 2001, p. 823)

(2) Rule out surgically correctable lesions with spinal x-rays, ultrasonography, MRI, or CT scan.

(3) Supportive care: ventilatory support; thermoregulation; and prevention of urinary tract infections (UTIs) and contractures

c. Outcome: vary according to the location and severity of the injury.

2. Neural tube defects (Theda, 1999): malformations of the develop-

TABLE 15.1 Cranial Nerves

Cranial Nerve	Nerve Category	Sensory, Motor, or Both	Examination
I	Olfactory	Sensory	Smell
II	Optic	Sensory	Visual acuity; tracking
III	Oculomotor (eye muscles)	Motor	Pupils equal and reactive to light; opening eye; up inward and outward, lateral inward, and down outward eye movements; "doll's eye"
IV	Trochlear (superior oblique eye muscle)	Both	Motor: down inward eye movement; "doll's eye" Sensory: not tested
V	Trigeminal (3 divisions: mandibular, maxillary, ophthalmic) (sensory to face; motor to jaw)	Both	Motor: strength of biting portion of suck Sensory: "rooting reflex"; "corneal reflex"
VI	Abducens	Both	Motor: lateral outward eye movement; "doll's eye" Sensory: not tested
VII	Facial	Both	Motor: facial expressions and movements; close eyes and mouth Sensory: not tested
VIII	Auditory, acoustic, or vestibulocochlear	Sensory	Auditory: startle response to loud noise Vestibular: "doll's eye"
IX	Glossopharyngeal (tongue movement)	Both	Motor: swallow, gag Sensory: taste
X	Vagus (soft palate, larynx, pharynx)	Both	Motor: gag; hoarse cry; stridor Sensory: not tested
XI	Accessory (trapezius and sternocleidomastoid muscles)	Both	Evaluation of shoulder height; turn head against resistance; infant attempts to bring head midline when lying supine
XII	Hypoglossal (tongue movement)	Both	Motor: atrophy; abnormal tongue movement; gag; suck; swallow Sensory: not tested

Adapted in part from Carey, B. E. (1993). In E.P. Tappero & M. E. Honeyfield (Eds.), *Physical assessment of the newborn* (pp. 121–138). Petaluma, CA: NICU Ink; and Tortora, G. J. (1983). The brain and the cranial nerves. In G. J. Tortora (Ed.), *Principles of human anatomy* (3rd ed, pp. 414–452). New York: Harper & Row.

ing brain and spinal cord due to failure of the neural tube to close. Spina bifida occulta, anencephaly, and myelomeningocele are the most common neural tube defects.

   a. Etiology: maternal dietary deficiencies (folic acid, vitamin B_{12}, and zinc); chromosomal abnormalities (trisomy 13 and 18, and triploidy); single gene defects; and teratogens (nitrates, antifolates, thalidomide, and hyperglycemia in infants of diabetic mothers [IDMs])

   b. Diagnosis: maternal serum α-fetoprotein (AFP) levels at 14 to 16 weeks' gestation; level II prenatal ultrasound; and amniotic fluid AFP and acetylcholinesterase levels

3. Anencephaly (Goddard-Finegold, 1998; McCulloch, 1999): an early neurulation (formation of the embryonic neural plate and development and closure of the neural tube) defect, ie, failure of the anterior neuropore to close. There is no brain tissue above the brain stem. There may be partial absence of skull bones, cerebellum, brain stem, and spinal cord.

   a. Clinical manifestations: abnormally shaped skull with exposed hemorrhagic and degenerated neural tissue; infant's face and head have a frog-like appearance.

   b. Interventions: supportive measures; parental genetic counseling; and family support

   c. Outcome: most are stillborn; live-born infants usually die during the neonatal period.

4. Encephalocele (Goddard-Finegold, 1998; McCulloch, 1999): a postneurulation defect. There is neural tissue herniation that may or may not contain meninges or brain parenchyma. Most defects occur in the occipital region.

   a. Clinical manifestations: midline skin-covered out-pouching from the head or nape of the neck (usually a closed lesion); often associated with other malformations (cleft lip/palate, myelomeningocele, CHDs, agenesis of the corpus callosum, porencephaly, and hydrocephalus)

   b. Interventions: cranial ultrasound, CT scan, and MRI aid in determining the extent of the lesion; neurosurgical excision of the lesion may be indicated; ventriculoperitoneal shunt may be required to treat secondary hydrocephalus.

   c. Outcome: deficits vary according to the extent of the brain tissue involved; approximately one third of cases are fatal, posterior defects more so than anterior defects; hydrocephalus is a possible complication.

5. Arnold-Chiari malformation: "congenital anomaly in which the cerebellum and medulla oblongata, which is elongated and flattened, protrude down into the spinal canal through the foramen magnum" (On-line Medical Dictionary, 1998). The defect may present with or without aqueductal stenosis. Malformation is usually present with a myelomeningocele. Hydrocephalus is a common complication.

   a. Clinical manifestations (McCulloch, 1999): reflux and aspiration; laryngeal stridor; central hypoventilation; and apnea

    b. Diagnosis: CT scan or MRI

    c. Interventions: ventriculoperitoneal (VP) shunt may be required.

    d. Outcome: varies in severity.

  6. Hydrocephalus (McCulloch, 1999; Theda, 1999):

    a. Definition: "condition marked by dilation of the cerebral ventricles, most often occurring secondarily to obstruction of the cerebrospinal fluid pathways and accompanied by an accumulation of cerebrospinal fluid within the skull, the fluid is usually under increased pressure, but occasionally may be normal or nearly so" (On-line Medical Dictionary, 1998). Excessive CSF is secondary to decreased reabsorption or overproduction (rare).

    b. Etiology may be congenital (aqueductal stenosis, Dandy-Walker malformation, Arnold-Chiari malformation, congenital mass, congenital infection, or neural tube defects and neuronal developmental defects) or acquired (posthemorrhagic, infection and meningitis).

    c. Clinical manifestations: rapidly increasing head circumference; bulging anterior fontanel; widened cranial sutures; "sun-setting" eyes; prominent scalp veins; apnea; lethargy; and poor feeding

    d. Interventions: VP shunt

IV. Peripheral nerve injuries

A. Facial nerve palsy (Goddard-Finegold, Mizrahi, & Lee, 1998; Volpe, 2001): injury to the facial nerve secondary to probable hemorrhage or edema into the nerve sheath with resultant weakness or paralysis of the affected side of the face. Most are left-sided paralysis.

  1. Etiology includes: forceps delivery; excessive pressure in utero of the infant's face against the maternal sacral promontory or ischial spines; and congenital hypoplasia or absence of the facial nerve (usually unilateral).

  2. Clinical manifestations: weakness of upper and lower facial muscles; when the infant is at rest, the affected side has a widened palpebral fissure and flattened nasolabial fold; with activity the infant cannot wrinkle the brow, close the eye completely, move the corner of the mouth or the lower face during crying or grimacing, and dribbles feeding from the corner of the mouth on the affected side.

  3. Interventions:

    a. No intervention is usually required.

    b. Artificial tears for the infant who cannot close the lid completely; taping the lid closed to prevent corneal injury

B. Brachial plexus injury (Goddard-Finegold, Mizrahi & Lee, 1998; Gomella, 1999; McCulloch, 1999): excessive stretching of the brachial plexus during the birthing process with resultant injury to cervical and thoracic nerve roots (ranging from C5 through T1)

  1. Risk factors: abnormal presentations; macrosomia; multiparity; prolonged or augmented labor; and shoulder dystocia

2. Clinical manifestations vary depending upon the location of the nerve injury:
   a. Weakness or paralysis of the upper and/or lower arm; flaccid arm; asymmetric Moro and/or grasp reflexes
   b. Erb palsy (upper arm paralysis involving C5 and C6): shoulder is abducted and internally rotated, elbow is extended, forearm is in pronation, and wrist and fingers are flexed (waiter's tip position); abnormal Moro but intact grasp
   c. Klumpke palsy (lower arm paralysis involving C7 through T1): arm is flexed, forearm supinated, shoulder is normally positioned, wrist and fingers are flaccid; rare occurrence
   d. Erb-Klumpke palsy (entire arm is affected involving C5 through T1): occurs more often than an isolated Klumpke palsy.
3. Interventions:
   a. Gentle immobilization of the arm across the chest for the first week, followed by passive range of motion (after the inflammation subsides); physical therapy; possible splinting; and serial electromyography to note progress
   b. Surgical intervention for injuries that do not resolve spontaneously by 4 months of age
4. Outcome: most recover spontaneously within 3 weeks of life (Volpe, 2001).

C. Phrenic nerve palsy (Goddard-Finegold, Mizrahi, & Lee, 1998; McCulloch, 1999): diaphragmatic paralysis as a result of stretch injury and tearing of the nerve sheaths of C3 through C5
   1. Risk factors: often associated with brachial plexus injury; macrosomia; prolonged labor; and shoulder dystocia
   2. Clinical manifestations vary depending upon the severity of the nerve injury: tachypnea; respiratory distress; possible cyanosis; irregular labored breathing; decreased breath sounds on the affected side
   3. Diagnosis: fluoroscopy demonstrates paradoxical diaphragmatic movement.
   4. Interventions: ventilatory support; surgical placation of the affected diaphragm
   5. Outcome: most occurrences spontaneously resolve.

V. Global neurologic insults

A. Hypoxic-ischemic encephalopathy (HIE) (Volpe, 2001; Yang, 1999): HIE is a disturbance of the neural tissue secondary to a deficit in oxygen supply. Oxygen deprivation to the perinatal brain occurs as a result of (1) *hypoxemia*, ie, decreased amount of oxygen in the blood supply, or (2) *ischemia*, ie, deceased blood supply to the brain. Both hypoxemia and/or ischemia are the result of *asphyxia*, ie, impaired oxygen and carbon dioxide gas exchange. Ischemia is believed to be the more serious cause of oxygen deprivation; the period of reperfusion, when the most adverse consequences of ischemia occur, affects brain metabolism and neural structure (Volpe, 2001).
   1. Perinatal asphyxia as defined by the American Academy of Pediatrics (AAP)/American College of Obstetricians and Gynecologists

(ACOG) (Uebel & Lott, 1999): APGAR score of 0 to 3 for > 5 minutes; umbilical cord arterial blood pH < 7.00; neurologic sequelae (hypotonia, seizures, coma, or HIE); and multiple organ dysfunction in the immediate neonatal period

2. Etiology is multifactorial:
   a. Antenatal: uteroplacental insufficiency; maternal hypotension; fetal malformation or congenital disorder (eg, hydrops fetalis); and prematurity
   b. Intrapartum: traumatic delivery; acute blood loss (eg, abruption, cord accident); prolapsed cord; and infection
   c. Postpartum: severe respiratory disease; CHD; and shock (eg, hypovolemic or septic)

3. Clinical manifestations:
   a. Metabolic or mixed acidosis
   b. Neurologic symptoms depend upon the severity and duration of the hypoxic-ischemic insult: seizures (within 12 to 24 hours usually indicative of intrapartum injury; may be the result of hypoglycemia); hypotonia; decreased spontaneous movements; stupor or coma; decreased reflexes; ischemic injury to the anterior horn cells within the spinal cord gray matter
   c. Multiple organ damage: liver (elevated liver enzymes, indirect hyperbilirubinemia, and decreased clotting factors); heart (tricuspid insufficiency, ventricular dysfunction, and CHF); kidneys (decreased urine output, acute tubular necrosis, and renal shutdown); lungs (respiratory distress syndrome [RDS] secondary to surfactant deficiency or dysfunction, and PPHN); and GI system (necrotizing enterocolitis [NEC])
   d. Interventions: immediate and aggressive resuscitation; correct acidosis; correct perfusion problems; control seizures with anticonvulsants; and prevent cerebral edema with fluid restriction and by avoiding hyperosmolar fluid infusion (eg, sodium bicarbonate).
   e. Outcome:
      (1) Many survivors do not have adverse neurologic sequelae.
      (2) Neurologic deficits depend upon the severity and duration of the hypoxic-ischemic insult. Risk factors for deficits include:
         (a) APGAR score # 3 at 20 minutes of age; multiple organ involvement, especially oliguria persisting past 24 hours of age.
         (b) Seizures difficult to control or occur within the first 12 hours of life; abnormal brain stem function; abnormal visual, auditory, or somatosensory evoked potential occurring after 7 days of life
         (c) Abnormal MRI obtained within the first 24 to 72 hours of life; electroencephalograph (EEG) abnormalities (moderate to severe findings), especially burst-suppression and/or isoelectric pattern at any time, or EEG depression after the 12th day of life
      (3) Death

B. Neonatal abstinence syndrome (NAS) (Botham, 1999; Volpe, 2001; Wong et al., 1999): symptoms of withdrawal exhibited by (1) an infant born to an opiate-dependent mother or (2) a critically ill infant who has had prolonged opiate administration for analgesia and/or sedation

1. Clinical manifestations: onset of symptoms ranges from shortly after birth to 2 weeks of age but usually occurs within 72 hours after birth. Duration of symptoms may be weeks to months. Onset of symptoms depends upon (1) the amount of the maternal dose, (2) the time of mother's last dose, (3) the length of mother's addiction, and (4) the infant's GA.

   a. CNS symptoms: jitteriness; hypertonicity and hyperreflexia; irritability; sleep disturbances; high-pitched cry; and seizures (rare)

   b. GI symptoms: poor feeding; regurgitation; diarrhea; and frantic sucking but poor swallowing

   c. Autonomic nervous system symptoms: fever; sweating; yawning; nasal stuffiness and sneezing; and mottled skin

2. Interventions:

   a. Recognition of opiate withdrawal: implementation of the NAS scoring (aids in documenting the onset and progression of withdrawal symptoms, and the infant's response to pharmacotherapy); three consecutive scores ≥ 8 warrants consideration for pharmacotherapy; withdrawal symptoms mimic metabolic disturbances and/or infection; therefore, screen infant's electrolytes, blood glucose, serum calcium, and complete blood count (CBC).

   b. Supportive care: maintain fluid and electrolyte balance; provide adequate nutrition; provide a dark quit environment; and bundle the infant snugly.

   c. Pharmacotherapy (eg, oral morphine, tincture of opium, phenobarbital, chlorpromazine, and diazepam)

3. Outcome: subacute withdrawal symptoms may persist for months, placing a great deal of stress upon the primary caregivers; increased risk for sudden infant death syndrome (SIDS); usually have normal cognitive and neurologic developmental.

Part B: Neurological Assessment, Neuromuscular Disorders, and Skeletal Abnormalities

I. Neurologic physical examination

A. Elements of an abnormal neurologic examination include: alterations in consciousness (eg, lethargy, stupor, or coma); asymmetric bilateral movements; absent or weak reflexes (eg, absent anal wink, absent suck or gag); alterations in tone (eg, hypertonicity or hypotonicity); and abnormal gross or fine motor movement (eg, jittery, bicycling movements, lip smacking, tonic-clonic jerking).

B. Neonatal seizures (McCulloch, 1999; Wong et al., 1999):

1. Etiology: seizures are clinical signs of a serious underlying disorder.

   a. Metabolic: decreased adenosine triphosphate production (eg, ischemia, hypoxemia, hypoglycemia, HIE); electrolyte imbalance; hypocalcemia; hypomagnesemia; inborn errors of metabolism; hyperammonemia; pyridoxine deficiency; and kernicterus

b. Chromosomal and genetic disorders (eg, trisomy 13, Zellweger syndrome, autosomal-dominant inheritance)

c. Structural defects: neural tube and neuronal tissue malformation; intracranial hemorrhage; and hydrocephalus

d. Infection: meningitis and congenital TORCH infection

e. Maternal drug addiction (rare cause of neonatal seizures)

2. Clinical manifestations: signs of seizures range from overt to very subtle and/or unrecognized.

   a. Subtle: apnea; bicycling movements (lower extremities) and rowing movements (upper extremities); lateral eye deviation; blinking; staring; lip smacking; nonnutritive sucking; drooling; and twitching

   b. Tonic: more common in premature infants with IVH; *extension of all extremities or upper extremity flexion with lower extremity extension*; appears to be decorticate positioning.

   c. Clonic: multifocal (no specific pattern *as rhythmic jerking movements* move from one part of the body to another; typical pattern seen with HIE) and focal (*localized jerking movements*)

   d. Myoclonic: one or more *flexion jerk(s) of an extremity*

3. Diagnosis:

   a. Obtain maternal and family history; close observation of abnormal movements

   b. Obtain electrolyte values, serum glucose, calcium, and magnesium levels.

   c. Obtain spinal fluid for culture, cell count, glucose, and protein.

   d. EEG; CT scan or MRI may be required to identify intracranial abnormality.

4. Interventions: correct electrolyte or metabolic imbalance; treat infection with antibiotics; anticonvulsants

C. Primary (or primitive) reflexes (Carey, 1993; Volpe, 2001):

1. Babinski: extension or flexion of the toes when the sole of the foot is stimulated; absence of this reflex is abnormal during the neonatal period.

2. Doll's eye: while rotating the infant's head from side to side the eyes should deviate away from the direction of the rotation. Fixed-eye position indicates possible brain stem dysfunction; eyes that move in the same direction as head rotation indicate possible oculomotor nerve or brain stem dysfunction.

3. Grasp (palmar): infant's fingers will grasp the examiner's finger when the palmar surface of the hand is stimulated. Reflex disappears at approximately 2 months of age.

4. Moro: while holding the infant in a supine position, remove support from the infant's head and allow it to fall into the examiner's hand. The infant should respond with (1) abduction and extension of upper extremities with outstretched hands, followed by

(2) bilateral upper extremity flexion (ie, "embracing" motion, and an audible cry). Reflex usually disappears by 6 months of age.

5. Rooting: when the corner of the mouth or cheek is stroked the infant will turn his or her head toward the stimulus. Reflex usually disappears by 3 to 4 months of age.

6. Suck: in response to gently stroking the infant's lips her/his mouth will open and sucking movements will begin. Reflex disappears at approximately 1 year of age.

7. Stepping: stepping movements occur as a response to stimulating the dorsum of the foot by the edge of a table. Reflex usually disappears by 3 to 4 months of age. Significance of this response is unclear (Volpe, 2001).

8. Tonic neck (or fencing position): with the infant lying supine and head turned to one side, the upper extremity on the side to which the head is facing should extend and the opposite upper extremity should flex; the lower extremity on the side to which the head is facing should extend and the opposite lower extremity should flex. Reflex usually disappears by 6 to 7 months of age.

9. Truncal incurvation: while the infant is held aloft in a prone position, firm pressure is applied parallel to the thoracic spinal area. The infant's pelvis should flex toward the side of the stimulus. Reflex usually disappears by 3 to 4 months of age.

II. Neuromuscular disorders

A. Arthrogryposis multiplex congenita (Sterk, 1999): nonprogressive congenital joint contractures involving upper and/or lower extremities. There are decreased numbers of anterior horn cells within the spinal cord.

1. Etiology: exact cause is unknown; may be secondary to fetal CNS abnormality, decreased fetal movement, uterine environment, or infection.

2. Clinical manifestations:

   a. Multiple joint contractures: shoulder adduction and internal rotation, elbow extension, and wrist and finger flexion; hip and knee flexion, feet deformities

   b. Wax-like appearance of skin and no creases at the joints

3. Interventions: radiographic studies to determine the presence of fractures, congenital hip dysplasia, and spinal deformities; range of motion exercises; and orthopedic intervention

4. Outcome: normal intelligence is likely; favorable functional prognosis is possible.

B. Fetal alcohol syndrome (see Chapter 19: Dysmorphism)

C. Myasthenia gravis (Volpe, 2001): a transient or congenital disorder that affects neurotransmission at the level of the neuromuscular junction.

1. Etiology: *transient* myasthenia gravis occurs in 10% to 15% of infants born to mothers with myasthenia gravis and is related to the maternal autoimmune process. The infant has elevated levels of circulating antibody to acetylcholine receptor protein. *Congenital* myasthenia gravis is the result of a genetic defect at the neuromuscular junction.

2. Clinical manifestations: generally characterized by muscle weakness brought on by activity and relieved by rest

    a. Transient disease: onset is between birth and 3 days of life, but usually within the first 24 hours of life; feeding difficulties, at times, requiring tube feedings; generalized muscle weakness and hypotonia; respiratory depression; weak cry; weak suck and swallow; ptosis and oculomotor dysfunction (less common symptoms)

    b. Congenital disease: onset is usually within the first few weeks of life; ptosis and ophthalmoplegia; facial weakness, feeble suck and cry; and muscle weakness and hypotonia present after activity.

  3. Diagnosis: marked decrease in muscle fatigue following administration of an anticholinesterase agent (eg, edrophonium chloride [Tensilon] or neostigmine methylsulfate)

  4. Interventions: administration of an anticholinesterase agent; exchange transfusion (with transient disease); supportive care with feedings; and good pulmonary toilet

D. Spinal muscular atrophy (SMA) (or anterior horn cell disease) (Goddard-Finegold, Mizrahi & Lee, 1998; Volpe, 2001): SMA is a degenerative disease involving the anterior horn cells of the spinal cord and motor nuclei of the cranial nerves.

  1. Etiology: autosomal-recessive inheritance with the locus mapped to chromosome 5q11.2-13.3. There are three types: SMA I (*Werdnig-Hoffman Disease*) usually manifests itself at birth or in early infancy. Life expectancy is usually 2 to 4 years. SMA II and SMA III have a later onset and longer life expectancy.

  2. Clinical manifestations:

    a. Decreased fetal movement during the later part of gestation

    b. Severe generalized hypotonia; muscle weakness is more pronounced in (1) lower extremities rather than upper extremities and (2) proximal rather than distal muscle groups; areflexia and muscle atrophy; poor head control in prone and supine positions; alert expression and normal eye movements

    c. Weak respiratory effort secondary to affected intercostal muscles; diaphragm is less affected; therefore, increased abdominal breathing movements; weak cry

    d. Poor suck and swallow; drooling; aspiration of secretions; tongue fasciculations and atrophy

  3. Diagnosis: abnormal electromyography (EMG); muscle biopsy identifies atrophied Type 1 and Type 2 muscle fibers; and elevated serum creatine kinase

  4. Interventions: supportive care; tube feedings; aggressive pulmonary toilet; range of motion to prevent contractures; and parent education and genetic counseling

III. Skeletal abnormalities

A. Achondroplasia (see Chapter 19: Dysmorphism)

B. Congenital developmental dysplasia of the hip (DDH) (Butler, 1998; Griffin & Robertson, 1999): embryologically normal hip that presents at birth or shortly thereafter with instability that ranges from subluxation to dislocation. DDH occurs in utero probably secondary to (1) maternal hormones that relax fetal tissues and (2) mechanical forces during the perinatal period.

1. Risk factors for DDH: female:male ratio is 6:1; first-born children; breech presentation; and positive history for DDH
2. Clinical manifestations: may not appear until 6 weeks of age; approximately 60% are on the left, 20% are on the right, and 20% are bilateral; asymmetric gluteal folds; limited abduction; and discrepancy in bilateral leg length
3. Diagnosis:
   a. Ortolani maneuver (may be positive for 6 to 8 weeks): place fingers on the trochanter, thumb on inner aspect of the thigh, and flex the hip; while applying inward and upward pressure with the fingers over the greater trochanter, lift the femur forward and abduct the thigh. The femoral head will move back into the acetabulum if the hip is dislocated. There will be a *distinctive "clunk."* "Clicks" are normal, high-pitched sounds that refer to snapping of ligaments or tendons.
   b. Barlow maneuver: with the hands in the same position as described, adduct the thigh when applying outward and downward pressure to the inner thigh with the thumb. Hip dislocation will be seen and heard (clunk) as the femoral head moves over the acetabulum.
   c. Hip ultrasound
4. Interventions: use of a splint (eg, Pavlik harness) to maintain reduction of the affected hip
C. Fractures (Sterk, 1999): occur most often secondary to difficult deliveries (eg, macrosomia and cephalopelvic disproportion, and malpresentation).
   1. Clinical manifestations: common fractures are the clavicle (snap heard during delivery, lump palpated over the clavicle, upper chest and shoulder crepitus, decreased arm movement, and asymmetric Moro), humerus (loss of spontaneous arm movement, edema, and pain elicited with passive range of motion), and femur (decreased or absent movement, edema, pain elicited with passive range of motion).
   2. Diagnosis: radiographic evaluation
   3. Interventions: clavicle (no special treatment; arm abduction and shoulder immobilization if the infant exhibits signs of pain); humerus (immobilize arm at the infant's side with elbow flexed 90° for 10 to 14 days; pain control); femur (splinting for 2 to 4 weeks; pain control)
D. Isolated deformities of the extremities:
   1. Amniotic band syndrome (Butler, 1998): uncommon, asymmetric, congenital deformity that ranges from limb amputations, constriction bands, and clubfoot, to syndactyly, and craniofacial defects. Clinical manifestations depend upon which type of defect is present: simple ring constriction; ring constrictions with bony fusion distally; ring constriction with fusion of soft tissue parts; or intrauterine amputations.
      a. Etiology: "localized rupture of the amniotic sac results in entanglement of the body parts in amniotic threads" (Sterk, 1999, p. 571).

      b. Interventions: depends upon the type of defect and body part that is involved; close monitoring of circulation distal to the defect; surgical intervention to release constrictions and improve venous and lymphatic drainage

  2. Polydactyly of the hand (Butler, 1998): more than five digits. There are three types: Type 1 (soft tissue connected by a pedicle); Type 2 (partial duplication of the phalanges); and Type 3 (complete duplication of phalanges and metacarpals).

      a. Interventions: Type 1—simple excision; Types 2 and 3—surgical correction to enhance function and appearance

  3. Syndactyly (Butler, 1998): fusion or webbing of two or more digits. The fusion may be: simple (connection with skin or soft tissue); complex (osseous connection); complete (fusion from base to tip of digit); or incomplete (fusion does not extend to tip of digit).

      a. Etiology: spontaneous mutations and familial tendency

      b. Interventions: surgical correction to promote function and normal appearance. Digits of unequal length should be separated within 6 to 12 months of age.

  4. Talipes equinovarus (or clubfoot) (Butler, 1998): congenital deformity of the foot involving taut hyperextension and in-curving of the foot

      a. Etiology: multifactorial (genetic predisposition and environmental factors)

      b. Clinical manifestations: apparent at birth; taut skin laterally; increased skin folds medially; affected foot may be smaller that opposite foot; decreased range of motion; resists dorsiflexion

      c. Interventions: serial casting; corrective surgery; parent education

  5. Talipes calcaneovalgus: usually benign flexible-foot deformity that presents with marked dorsiflexion and eversion (outward positioning) of the foot and the heel in valgus (away from midline) position. Passive range of motion can move the foot back into proper alignment.

      a. Etiology: abnormal in utero positioning

      b. Interventions: range of motion to bring foot back into plantarflexed varus (toward midline) position; casting for more serious defects

 E. Osteogenesis imperfecta (see Chapter 19: Dysmorphism)

▼ References

Ballard, J. L., Khoury, J. C., Wedig, K., Wang, L., Eilers-Walsman, B. L., & Lipp, R. (1991). New Ballard Score, expanded to include extremely premature infants. *The Journal of Pediatrics, 119,* 417–423.

Bernbaum, J. C. (1999). Medical care after discharge. In G. B. Avery, M. A. Fletcher, & M. G. MacDonald (Eds.), *Neonatology: Pathophysiology and management of the newborn* (5th ed., pp. 1463–1478). Philadelphia: Lippincott Williams & Wilkins.

Botham, S. (1999). Perinatal substance abuse. In J. Deacon & P. O'Neill (Eds.), *Core curriculum for neonatal intensive care nursing* (2nd ed., pp. 618–634). Philadelphia: WB Saunders.

Buschbach, D. (1999). Physical assessment of the newborn infant. In J. Deacon & P. O'Neill (Eds.), *Core curriculum for neonatal intensive care nursing* (2nd ed., pp. 74–100). Philadelphia: WB Saunders.

Butler, J. (1998). Assessment and management of musculoskeletal dysfunction. In C. Kenner, J. W. Lott, & A. A. Flandermeyer (Eds.), *Comprehensive neonatal nursing: A physiologic perspective* (2nd ed., pp. 608–619). Philadelphia: WB Saunders.

Carey, B. E. (1993). Neurologic assessment. In E. P. Tappero & M. E. Honeyfield (Eds.), *Physical assessment of the newborn* (pp. 121–138). Petaluma, CA: NICU Ink.

Goddard-Finegold, J. (1998). The intrauterine nervous system. In H. W. Taeusch & R. A. Ballard (Eds.), *Avery's diseases of the newborn* (7th ed., pp. 802–831). Philadelphia: WB Saunders.

Goddard-Finegold, J., Mizrahi, E. M., & Lee, R. T. (1998). The newborn nervous system. In H. W. Taeusch & R. A. Ballard (Eds.), *Avery's diseases of the newborn* (7th ed., pp. 839–892). Philadelphia: WB Saunders.

Gomella, T. L. (1999). Assessment for gestational age. In T. L. Gomella, M. D. Cunningham, F. G. Eyal, & K. E. Zenk (Eds.), *Neonatology: Management, procedures, on-call problems, diseases, drugs* (4th ed., pp. 21–28). Stamford, CT: Appleton & Lange.

Gomella, T. L. (1999). Newborn physical examination. In T. L. Gomella, M. D. Cunningham, F. G. Eyal, & K. E. Zenk (Eds.), *Neonatology: Management, procedures, on-call problems, diseases, drugs* (4th ed., pp. 29–37). Stamford, CT: Appleton & Lange.

Griffin, P. P., & Robertson, W. W. (1999). Orthopedics. In G. B. Avery, M. A. Fletcher, & M. G. MacDonald (Eds.), *Neonatology: Pathophysiology & management of the newborn* (5th ed., pp. 1269–1284). Philadelphia: Lippincott Williams & Wilkins.

Harris, T. R. (1999). Birth trauma: Identification and management. *Perinatal update 1999: Parallels in maternal/neonatal outcomes.* 15th Annual Conference sponsored by the Department of Neonatology and Department of Perinatology, Memorial Medical Center, Savannah, Georgia.

Hill, A., & Volpe, J. J. (1999). Neurological and neuromuscular disorders. In G. B. Avery, M. A. Fletcher, & M. G. MacDonald (Eds.), *Neonatology: Pathophysiology & management of the newborn* (5th ed., pp. 1231–1252). Philadelphia: Lippincott Williams & Wilkins.

Madsen, J. R., & Frim, D. M. (1999). Neurosurgery of the newborn. In G. B. Avery, M. A. Fletcher, & M. G. MacDonald (Eds.), *Neonatology: Pathophysiology and management of the newborn* (5th ed., pp. 1253–1268). Philadelphia: Lippincott Williams & Wilkins.

McCulloch, M. (1999). Neurologic disorders. In J. Deacon & P. O'Neill (Eds.), *Core curriculum for neonatal intensive care nursing* (2nd ed., pp. 474–509). Philadelphia: WB Saunders.

Milerad, J., Larson, O., Hagberg, C., & Ideberg, M. (1997). Associated malformations in infants with cleft lip and palate: A prospective, population-based study. *Pediatrics, 100*(2), 180.

On-line Medical Dictionary (1998). Retrieved from http://www.graylab.ac.uk (2001, Nov.).

Schiefelbein, J. (1999). Genetics and fetal anomalies. In J. Deacon & P. O'Neill (Eds.), *Core curriculum for neonatal intensive care nursing* (2nd ed., pp. 540–559). Philadelphia: WB Saunders.

Sterk, L. (1999). Neonatal orthopedic conditions. In J. Deacon & P. O'Neill (Eds.), *Core curriculum for neonatal intensive care nursing* (2nd ed., pp. 560–577). Philadelphia: WB Saunders.

Tappero, E. P., & Honeyfield, M. E. (1993). *Physical assessment of the newborn: A comprehensive approach to the art of physical examination.* Petaluma, CA: NICU Ink.

Theda, C. (1999). Neural tube defects. In T. L. Gomella, M. D. Cunningham, F. G. Eyal, & K. E. Zenk (Eds.), *Neonatology: Management, procedures, on-call problems, diseases, drugs* (4th ed., pp. 470–479). Stamford, CT: Appleton & Lange.

Tortora, G. J. (Ed.). (1983). *Principles of human anatomy* (3rd ed.). New York: Harper & Row.

Uebel, P., & Lott, J.W. (1999). A case study of antenatal distress and consequent neonatal respiratory distress. *Neonatal Network, 18*(5): 68.

Volpe, J. J., (Ed.). (2001). *Neurology of the newborn* (4th ed.). Philadelphia: WB Saunders.

Witt, C. (1993). Skin. In E. P. Tappero & M. E. Honeyfield (Eds.), *Physical assessment of the newborn* (pp. 27–39). Petaluma, CA: NICU Ink.

Wolcott, H. D., & Conry, J. A. (2000). Normal labor. In A. T. Evan & K. R. Niswander (Eds.), *Manual of obstetrics* (6th ed., pp. 392-424). Philadelphia: Lippincott Williams & Wilkins.

Wong, D. L., Hockenberry-Eaton, M., Winkelstein, M. L., Wilson, D., Ahmann, E., & DiVito-Thomas, P. A. (Eds.). (1999). *Whaley & Wong's nursing care of infants and children* (6th ed.). St. Louis: Mosby.

Yang, L. (1999). Perinatal asphyxia. In T. L. Gomella, M. D. Cunningham, F. G. Eyal, & K. E. Zenk (Eds.), *Neonatology: Management, procedures, on-call problems, diseases, drugs* (4th ed., pp. 480–489). Stamford, CT: Appleton & Lange.

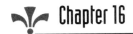 **Chapter 16**

Gastrointestinal Disorders
Donna DiSciascio Mann, MSN, RNC, NNP

I. Abdominal wall defects

   A. Omphalocele (Cooney, 1998; Dillon & Cilley, 1993; Nakayama, 1997k):

      1. Definitions: a midline defect covered with a translucent, avascular membrane onto which the umbilical cord attaches, ranges in size from 4–12 cm, and is central at the umbilical ring. The defect may include large and small intestine, stomach, and liver; all have nonrotation of the intestines; may be ruptured prenatally or at delivery. Hernia of the umbilical cord is usually < 4 cm in diameter; least severe type of omphalocele containing few or no loops of intestine

      2. Associated defects include craniofacial region, diaphragm, heart, and genitourinary system. Associated chromosomal abnormalities include trisomies 13, 15, 18, and 21 and other disorders (eg, Pentalogy of Cantrell and Beckwith-Wiedemann Syndrome).

      3. Etiology: results from any arrest or deviation of the central migration and fusion at the umbilical ring of the cephalic, two lateral, and caudal folds at approximately 18 weeks of gestation.

      4. Interventions (see Gastroschisis)

      5. Outcome: outcome is dependent on the degree of visceroabdominal disproportion and the severity of associated anomalies. Approximately half of the infants have gastroesophageal reflux (GER).

   B. Gastroschisis (Cooney, 1998; Davies & Stringer, 1997; Howell, 1998; Nakayama, 1997d):

      1. Definition: full-thickness abdominal wall defect that varies in size and usually presents to the right of the umbilical cord. The herniated abdominal contents (eg, intestines, stomach, bladder, liver) are fully exposed to amniotic fluid when in utero, causing them to appear thick and matted.

      2. Etiology: probably the result of rupture at the base of the umbilical cord in an area that has been weakened by the involution of the right umbilical vein, thereby allowing abdominal contents to herniate into the amniotic cavity

      3. Associated anomalies and problems: bowel atresias and stenoses; nonrotation of the intestines; possible preterm delivery and small for gestational age (SGA); not usually associated with chromosomal and structural anomalies

      4. Outcome: survival rate is approximately 90%; primary repair leads to a better survival rate, reduced risk of sepsis, and shorter hospital stay than a staged repair; GER occurs in 40% to 50% of infants.

      5. Interventions for omphalocele and gastroschisis (Howell, 1998; Strodtbeck, 1998):

    a. Initial delivery room management:

        (1) Delivery mode (vaginal versus cesarean section) is still controversial (Cooney, 1998; How et al., 2000).

        (2) Follow Neonatal Resuscitation Program (NRP) guidelines for initial resuscitation.

        (3) For respiratory distress, intubate immediately to avoid bowel distention resulting from positive pressure bag-mask ventilation.

        (4) Sterile gloves and sterile blankets or towels should be used to handle and dry the infant.

        (5) Cover the defect with a saline-soaked gauze and plastic wrap (intact defects) *or* a clear sterile bowel bag (intact or ruptured defects).

    b. Observe the bowel for evidence of vascular compromise.

    c. Decompress stomach with nasogastric tube (NGT)/orogastric tube (OGT) attached to suction drainage.

    d. Intravenous (IV) access in an upper extremity; initiate antibiotic therapy; maintain fluid and electrolyte balance; and strict intake and output measurements

    e. Nonoperative treatment:

        (1) Delaying surgery may be necessary (eg, coexisting life-threatening anomalies, awaiting results of chromosome analysis [particularly with omphalocele], or premature infant with respiratory distress syndrome [RDS]).

        (2) Pharmacotherapy: application of silver sulfadiazine (silvadene), 0.5% silver nitrate solution, 70% alcohol (if used sparingly), or biologic dressings to the exposed viscera

    f. Operative treatment:

        (1) Bowel resection may be necessary secondary to poor perfusion or ischemia.

        (2) Primary closure versus staged repair depends on the size of the defect and the abdominal cavity and whether bowel perfusion and respiratory status will be compromised.

        (3) Large defects may be covered with a silo, a covered pouch created outside the abdomen that encloses the intestines. The silo is sequentially reduced until the intestines are within the abdominal cavity, then the abdominal wall is surgically closed.

    g. Postoperative management:

        (1) Monitor respiratory status.

        (2) Maintain fluid and electrolyte balance; antibiotic administration

        (3) Pain management

        (4) NGT/OGT attached to suction drainage; monitor gastrointestinal (GI) output and replace fluids appropriately.

        (5) Monitor color and temperature of lower extremities to assess for vascular compromise.

C. Prune belly syndrome (or Eagle-Barrett syndrome) (Docimo, Jeffs, & Gearhart, 1997; Druschel, 1995; Georges, 1997; Jones, 1997):

    1. Definition: a triad of anomalies consisting of deficient abdominal wall musculature, bilateral cryptorchidism, and dilation of the urogenital tract of varying degree (95% of cases are males) (Noh, Cooper, Winkler, Zderic, Snyder, & Canning, 1999)

2. Etiology (several theories):
   a. A disorder of embryogenesis in the lateral mesenchyme affects the development of the abdominal musculature and the smooth muscle of the urinary tract.
   b. Lower urinary tract obstruction (eg, posterior urethral valves) causes a progressive backup of urine flow leading to possible bladder or ureter rupture.
   c. Ascites, not associated with urinary obstruction, has been associated with the abdominal wall findings of prune belly.
3. Associated findings: oligohydramnios; impaired renal function; respiratory distress in newborn period; chronic respiratory infections secondary to poor abdominal musculature and inability to cough and effectively clear secretions; ascites; intestinal duplication; volvulus; pulmonary stenosis; cystic adenomatoid malformation; deafness; and mental retardation
4. Diagnosis: frequently diagnosed on prenatal ultrasound
5. Interventions (Hendren, Carr, & Adams, 1998): respiratory support; antibiotics for urosepsis prophylaxis; monitor serial creatinine values, renal function studies, and urine cultures; and possible surgical urinary diversion or reconstructive surgery of the urinary tract
6. Outcome: depends upon renal and pulmonary function; moderate renal involvement may require dialysis or transplantation.

II. Hernias
   A. Umbilical hernia (Cilley & Krummel, 1998; Gomella, 1999; O'Donnell, Glick, & Caty 1998; Scherer & Grosfeld, 1993):
      1. Definition: a skin-covered defect (rarely > 2 cm in diameter) of the fascia at the umbilical ring that allows protrusion of the abdominal contents
      2. Etiology: results from incomplete development, imperfect attachment, or weakness within the structures of the umbilical ring.
      3. Diagnosis: palpation of abdominal contents through the umbilical ring. The diameter of the defect, not the length of the protrusion, is of prognostic significance. Hernias < 1 cm are more likely to close spontaneously than those of larger diameters (> 1.5 cm).
      4. Interventions: most hernias close spontaneously by 3 years of age; incarcerated "nonreducible" hernia is a surgical emergency.
      5. Outcome: infection and recurrence of the hernia are both rare.
   B. Inguinal hernia (Kapur, Caty, & Glick, 1998; Lloyd & Rintala, 1998; Nakayama, 1997g; Scherer & Grosfeld, 1993):
      1. Definition: a protrusion of intestine, bowel, bladder, or ovary through a patent processus vaginalis that is seen as a groin bulge. In males the bulge may extend into the scrotum. The right side is more often affected than the left.
      2. Etiology: results from a prolonged patency of the processus vaginalis.
      3. Clinical manifestations:

   a. Appears as a bulge in the suprainguinal area that enlarges with increased abdominal pressure. When the infant is quiet, the hernia may reduce spontaneously or may be reduced manually with gentle pressure.
   b. Differentiate between a hydrocele (scrotal swelling), a descending testis, and hernia. An undescended testis may coexist with an inguinal hernia.
   c. Signs and symptoms of an incarcerated hernia include: irritability; groin and abdominal pain; vomiting (may become bilious or feculent); bloody stools secondary to bowel ischemia; and groin mass that is tense and will not reduce.
 4. Interventions:
   a. Sixty-nine percent of hernias that incarcerate will occur before 1 year of age; therefore, elective repair is recommended within the first 6 months of life.
   b. Incarcerated hernia: attempt reduction by gentle pressure; sedation and Trendelenburg position may help to reduce the hernia; and emergency surgery for nonreducible hernia *or* if there is a concern regarding the viability of the bowel
 5. Outcome: inguinal hernias do not resolve spontaneously; complications of incarcerated hernias include testis infarction, injury to the spermatic cord or vas deferens, infection, and hernia recurrence.

III. Atresias, stenoses, mechanical blockages, and masses
 A. Definitions:
  1. Atresia: an obstruction resulting in the complete occlusion of the intestinal lumen and possibly a lack of communication between two segments of the bowel
  2. Stenosis: partial obstruction of the intestinal lumen where a narrow opening separates the two involved segments
  3. Mechanical blockages: obstruction of the lumen of the intestine caused by either the bowel itself or some other entity, such as meconium
  4. Masses: palpable masses (smooth, cystic, and usually mobile) in the GI tract are rare and are caused by either a mesenteric cyst or an intestinal duplication. Other abdominal masses may be renal, ovarian, or hepatic in origin.
 B. Small bowel obstructions (Gomella, 1999; Grosfeld, 1998; Kays, 1996; Nakayama, 1997a, c; Pollack, 1996; Rescorla, 2001; Stauffer & Schwoebel, 1998; Touloukian & Smith, 1998):
  1. Etiology: pyloric web (varies in degree from a membranous web to a complete separation between the stomach and the duodenum); duodenal stenosis; duodenal atresia; annular pancreas (pancreatic tissue encircles and partially or completely obstructs the descending duodenum); malrotation (abnormal rotation of the intestinal tract that leads to a lack of fixation of the small bowel with resultant total or partial obstruction); midgut volvulus (occurs with a malrotation and is a twisting of the intestine that leads to total obstruction and bowel ischemia); jejunoileal atresia (there may be an isolated small atresia, multiple areas of atresia, or the "apple-peel" deformity that involves a large section

of the jejunum and ileum); meconium ileus (distal small bowel obstruction caused by thick meconium; it is the earliest sign of cystic fibrosis and occurs in 10% to 20% of infants with the disorder)

2. Clinical manifestations (vary with the defect):
   a. Many present with polyhydramnios.
   b. Feeding intolerance with increased residuals
   c. Vomiting (Kays, 1996): bilious vomiting if obstruction occurs beyond the ampulla of Vater; nonbilious if obstruction occurs proximal to the ampulla of Vater
   d. Gastric distention; firm abdomen
   e. Abnormal bowel gas pattern: no distal gas pattern with complete obstruction; distal bowel gas may present with partial obstruction.
   f. Bloody stool; delay in passage of meconium
   g. Hypovolemia and shock

3. Diagnosis:
   a. Anterior-posterior abdominal radiograph:
      (1) General findings: air-fluid levels and "thumb-sized" intestinal loops with no distal air with intestinal obstructions
      (2) "Double-bubble" sign of duodenal atresia: air distends the stomach (first bubble) and the first portion of the duodenum (second bubble) with no distal air.
      (3) Scattered amounts of distal air: duodenal stenosis, malrotation, and volvulus (Kays, 1996)
      (4) Colonic gas in the right upper abdomen: malrotation
      (5) Calcified extraluminal meconium: prenatally ruptured meconium ileus
   b. Upper GI series: identifies the duodenum and ligament of Treitz; intestines do not cross the midline in malrotation.
   c. Contrast enema: identifies small caliber of large colon in the presence of a small bowel obstruction or meconium ileus; may be therapeutic intervention for meconium ileus (Kays, 1996).

4. Interventions:
   a. NPO; NGT/OGT attached to suction drainage
   b. Fluid resuscitation; monitor fluid and electrolytes; broad-spectrum antibiotics
   c. Water-soluble contrast enema for nonsurgical management of meconium ileus without perforation
   d. Surgical management: surgery without radiographic imaging if the infant presents with signs of intestinal ischemia (Pollack, 1996); end-to-end anastomosis or the creation of an ostomy, depending upon the condition of the bowel
   e. Postoperative management (Kays, 1996):
      (1) Bowel decompression until bowel function returns and patency is assured
      (2) Antibiotics administration; maintain fluid and electrolyte balance.
      (3) Feedings are reintroduced slowly.

(4) Pancreatic enzymes with feedings when cystic fibrosis is suspected (Kays, 1996)

5. Outcome: depends upon the amount of functional bowel that remains (Kays, 1996).

C. Large bowel obstruction (Gomella, 1999; Kays, 1996; Kiely & Pena, 1998; Nakayama, 1997e, f, h, i; Pollack, 1996; Rescorla, 2001; Teitelbaum, Coran, Weitzman, Zeigler, & Kane, 1998; Young, 1998):

1. Etiology: meconium plug (obstruction of the distal colon by a large white meconium plug); colonic atresia; small left colon syndrome; Hirschsprung's disease ([aganglionic megacolon] absence of ganglion cells in the mesenteric and submucosal areas of the large colon ranging in severity from only a small distal portion to the entire colon); imperforate anus (severity, location, and involvement of other systems vary; there is often a fistula between the lower portion of the bowel and either the genitourinary system or a small opening along the perineum); and intussusception (terminal portion of the ileum prolapses through the ileocecal valve into the colon)

2. Clinical manifestations: vary depending upon the abnormality

  a. Abnormal physical examination (eg, abnormally placed *or* no anus, fistulous perineal opening, and meconium passage via urethral opening or vagina)

  b. Bilious emesis; abdominal distention; palpable loops of bowel; crampy abdominal pain

  c. Delayed passage of meconium; bloody or "currant jelly" stool (eg, intussusception) (Pollack, 1996)

  d. Lethargy; cardiovascular collapse

3. Diagnosis:

  a. Abdominal radiographs:

    (1) Multiple loops of dilated small bowel with air-fluid levels

    (2) Distended large colon to the level of the aganglionosis (eg, Hirschsprung's disease)

    (3) Paucity of rectal air (eg, imperforate anus)

    (4) Gasless area with concentric lines to the right of the spine (specific to intussusception) (Pollack, 1996)

  b. Ultrasound: useful for imperforate anus and intussusception

  c. Barium enema (BE) evaluation:

    (1) Microcolon to the level of an atresia (colonic atresia)

    (2) Transition zone in the left colon (small left colon syndrome)

    (3) Large meconium plug in the rectosigmoid portion of the colon (meconium plug syndrome)

    (4) BE may be normal with Hirschsprung's disease and there may be delayed emptying of the barium (24 to 48 hours).

    (5) BE may be used for evaluation of intussusception.

  d. Biopsy: suction biopsy (at bedside) to determine the presence/absence of ganglion cells; full thickness rectal biopsy (in operating room) when there is any question about the validity of the suction biopsy results

4. Interventions:

  a. NPO; NGT/OGT attached to suction drainage

b. IV fluids; antibiotic administration; maintain fluid and electrolyte balance.

c. Nonoperative management:
  (1) Small left colon syndrome usually resolves with supportive care.
  (2) BE enema is both diagnostic and therapeutic for meconium plug syndrome.
  (3) Intussusception: may be reduced by pneumatic reduction, or ultrasound-guided hydrostatic reduction. Surgical reduction is done when there is concern about perforation of the bowel, if the infant appears toxic, if there has been a prolonged course, or if the infant is in shock (Pollack, 1996).

d. Operative management:
  (1) Bowel resection with primary anastomosis *or* creation of an ostomy with delayed anastomosis
  (2) Hirschsprung's disease: creation of an ostomy proximal to the area of aganglionosis *or* a transanal pull-through procedure
  (3) High/intermediate imperforate anus: creation of a colostomy and full correction at 3 to 6 months of age. Low anomalies in males and low anomalies in females without a fistula: cut back anoplasty in the newborn period.

e. Postoperative management:
  (1) Monitor fluid and electrolyte balance; antibiotic administration; hyperalimentation
  (2) Observe for return of bowel function; reintroduce enteral feedings.
  (3) Voiding cystourethrography (VCUG) is recommended after imperforate anus repair to determine vesicoureteral reflux.

f. Outcome:
  (1) Meconium plug syndrome usually resolves within 24 hours after passage of the plug.
  (2) Hirschsprung's disease: 95% survival rate. Complications include anastomotic leak, enterocolitis, urinary and fecal incontinence, and constipation (Nakayama, 1997e).
  (3) Imperforate anus (Kiely & Pena, 1998): high defect (bowel continence); low anomaly (approximately 90% achieve bowel continence); complications include fistulas, retracting of the bowel, voiding dysfunction, and anal stenosis.
  (4) Intussusception: 10% recurrence rate for nonsurgical reduction and 1% to 4% recurrence for surgical reduction (Pollack, 1996)

IV. Esophageal and tracheal defects (Gomella, 1999; Harmon & Coran, 1998; Nakayama, 1997b):
  A. Definitions:
    1. Esophageal atresia (EA) ("A-type" tracheoesophageal anomaly): blind esophageal pouch proximally and a blind distal pouch that has no connection to the trachea or the proximal portion of the esophagus

    2. Esophageal atresia and tracheoesophageal fistula (TEF):
- **a.** "B-type" TEF: fistula between the proximal esophageal pouch and the trachea with a distal blind portion of the esophagus
- **b.** "C-type" TEF (most common): proximal esophageal blind pouch with a fistula between the lower trachea and the distal esophagus
- **c.** "D-type" TEF: EA with both the proximal and distal portions of the esophagus having a fistulous connection to the trachea

    3. TEF without an EA ("H-type"): the esophagus is fully connected and there is a fistula between the esophagus and the trachea.

B. Etiology: EA and TEF are believed to be the result of incomplete separation of the lung bud from the foregut during early fetal development.

C. Associated findings: VACTERL sequence, chromosomal abnormalities (eg, trisomies 13 and 18), DiGeorge sequence, polysplenia sequence, Holt-Oram syndrome, and Pierre Robin sequence

D. Clinical manifestations:
1. Prenatally: > 90% of fetuses with EA with/without TEF have polyhydramnios.
2. Isolated EA: copious oral secretions; vomiting of undigested formula; coughing and choking; and inability to pass a NGT into the stomach
3. TEF with EA: clinical manifestations of "isolated EA"; aspiration pneumonia; coughing, choking, and cyanosis; excess air entering the stomach can distend it and exert pressure on the diaphragm with resultant basilar atelectasis.
4. "H-type" TEF: recurrent aspiration; no manifestations of an EA

E. Diagnosis:
1. Chest and abdominal radiograph:
   - **a.** EA: NGT will be coiled in the upper mediastinum; no air in the stomach or bowel may indicate an EA without TEF.
   - **b.** Distal TEF: air in the stomach and distal portions of the bowel
2. A contrast study is recommended to determine the presence of an H-type fistula.
3. Bronchoscopy allows for direct visualization of a TEF.

F. Interventions:
1. Attach sump tube to continuous suction.
2. Head of the bed elevated 30° to 45°
3. NPO and parenteral IV fluids; broad-spectrum antibiotics; maintain fluid and electrolyte balance.
4. Respiratory support. Avoiding routine intubation will decrease the risk of gastric perforation and worsening respiratory distress that results from ventilating through a distal TEF.
5. G-tube insertion (at bedside) may be required to decompress the stomach in the case of a distal TEF.
6. Surgery:
   - **a.** Ligation of the fistula and esophageal repair
   - **b.** Primary repair: end-to-end anastomosis of the two portions of the esophagus

       c. Staged repair: necessary when the two portions of the esophagus are too far apart for primary anastomosis; gastrostomy tube placement for feedings; continuous suction of the proximal esophageal pouch or placement of an esophagostomy; reanastomosis within a couple months to 1 year of age

    7. Postoperative: extrapleural chest drain usually remains until a barium swallow confirms an intact anastomosis. Oral feedings are started after an intact anastomosis is confirmed.

    8. Complications and outcome: postoperative esophageal leak; esophageal strictures; recurrent aspiration from either a stricture or a fistula; tracheomalacia; and GER (approximately 40% of patients)

V. Infection (Freij & McCracken, 1994; Vanderhoof, Zach, & Adrian, 1994):

  A. Bacterial enterocolitis:

    1. Causative agents: salmonella; shigella; invasive *Escherichia coli*; campylobacter jejuni; *clostridium difficile*

    2. Clinical manifestations:

       a. General: diarrhea; heme-positive stools; the presence of leukocytes in the stool

       b. Shigella: may present with diarrhea or a "toxic or septic-appearing" infant.

       c. *E. coli*: frequent watery green stools within a 24-hour period that usually do not contain blood or mucus. Infants usually appear well.

       d. Campylobacter: may cause bloody diarrhea.

       e. *C. difficile*: possible pseudomembranous colitis, severe watery or bloody diarrhea, and colonic perforations in severe cases. Often occurs after a course of broad-spectrum antibiotics.

  B. Viral enterocolitis:

    1. Causative agents: rotavirus; enteric adenovirus; and enteroviruses

    2. Clinical manifestations: watery stool; carbohydrate malabsorption due to mucosal injury in the proximal jejunum

    3. Diagnosis: stool cultures are often unreliable due to the presence of rotavirus and *C. difficile* in cultures from asymptomatic infants. However, they may be helpful isolating other pathogens.

    4. Interventions:

       a. Contact isolation and strict infection control measures

       b. Monitor and maintain strict fluid and electrolyte balance.

       c. Invasive bacterial diarrhea (eg, Shigella): ampicillin or trimethoprim-sulfamethoxazole

       d. Noninvasive organisms that produce an enterotoxin (eg, *E. coli*): oral neomycin or colistin sulfate

       e. Antibiotics do not alter the clinical course of Salmonella, but may be indicated if there is prolonged illness or signs and symptoms of bloodstream invasion.

    5. Outcome: diarrhea in the newborn period is usually self-limited, but it can cause significant morbidity for some infants; rotavirus has caused fatal disease in a small number of infants and has been implicated as a cause of an outbreak of necrotizing enterocolitis (NEC).

C. NEC (Albanese & Rowe, 1998; Hebra & Ross III, 1996; Nakayama, 1997; Weiss, Williams, Ledbetter, & Neu, 2001):

1. Definition: predominantly a premature infant disease that is multifactorial in origin and ranges in severity from localized mucosal necrosis in a small segment of bowel to transmural necrosis of the entire small bowel and colon

2. Etiology: NEC results from a complex pathophysiologic process that involves the following four factors: hypoxia-ischemia reperfusion injury, enteral alimentation, bacteria, and inflammatory mediators.

3. Clinical manifestations:
   a. Often presents with nonspecific symptoms: lethargy, temperature instability, apnea, bradycardia, hypoglycemia, and shock
   b. More specific symptoms: abdominal distention, higher gastric residuals with feeding, vomiting, diarrhea, occult or gross blood in the stools
   c. Progression of the disease: worsening abdominal distention, abdominal wall tenderness, visible loops of bowel, and abdominal wall crepitus, edema, and erythema
   d. Laboratory findings include neutropenia, thrombocytopenia, and metabolic acidosis. Blood cultures are positive in 30% to 35% of patients with NEC.
   e. Radiologic findings include ileus pattern, pneumatosis intestinalis, portal vein gas, pneumoperitoneum, intraperitoneal fluid, and persistently dilated loops of bowel on plain anteroposterior and left lateral decubitus films.

4. Interventions:
   a. Supportive medical therapy: possible approach when there is no evidence of intestinal necrosis or perforation
      (1) NPO; bowel rest and decompression
      (2) Monitor laboratory studies (complete blood cell count [CBC], platelet count, blood gas analysis, serum electrolytes, disseminated intravascular coagulopathy [DIC] screen, and blood culture)
      (3) Aggressive fluid and electrolyte replacement; blood product transfusions as needed; broad-spectrum antibiotics
      (4) Frequent physical examinations; serial abdominal radiographs every 6 to 8 hours
   b. Surgical interventions for the following indications: pneumoperitoneum; clinical deterioration despite aggressive treatment; palpable abdominal mass; fixed dilated loop of intestine on radiograph; presence of portal vein air on radiograph (controversial); and paracentesis that is positive for more than 0.5 mL of yellow-brown fluid that contains bacteria on Gram stain
   c. Surgical intervention includes laparotomy with resection of necrotic bowel and possible creation of an ostomy. Attempts are made to resect only perforated or clearly necrotic bowel and to preserve the ileocecal valve.
   d. Peritoneal drainage for treatment of perforation: penrose drain placement in the lower abdomen (bedside procedure) to provide decompression of air, fluid, and stool material

e. Postoperative therapy:
   (1) Respiratory support
   (2) Fluid resuscitation may be required secondary to third space losses and sepsis; antibiotics administration
   (3) Observe abdominal wall and stoma for color changes and swelling. Monitor CBC, platelets, electrolytes, and acid-base status. Persistent acidosis may indicate presence of necrotic bowel.
f. Stoma closure: when an infant is tolerating feeds and gaining weight, reanastomosis may be delayed up to 4 months or more; excessive output from the stoma may necessitate earlier reanastomosis.
5. Complications include: strictures, malabsorption, gut hypermotility, hypersecretion of gastric acid, bacterial overgrowth, decreased intestinal transit time, and vitamin B_{12} and bile salt deficiency; short bowel syndrome.
6. Outcome: the mortality rate varies greatly depending on birth weight, coexisting disease, virulence of the disease process, and whether the patient was born locally or was referred.

VI. Other disorders
A. Short bowel syndrome (Georgeson, 1998; Taylor, 1997):
   1. Definition: a spectrum of malnutrition resulting from inadequate length or function of small bowel
   2. Etiology: in utero vascular accident leading to multiple atretic areas; in utero volvulus leaving the patient without a jejunum or ileum; complicated meconium ileus may result in necrotic ileum if the ileum twists on itself; aganglionosis of large and small bowel resulting in functional short bowel syndrome; NEC; abdominal wall defects; jejunal ileal atresia; midgut volvulus; and "functional" short bowel syndrome may occur when a stoma is created with inadequate bowel proximal to the stoma.
   3. Clinical manifestations:
      a. Diarrhea; steatorrhea
      b. Malabsorption (type and severity depends upon the segment of lost bowel):
         (1) Duodenum: absorption site for iron, calcium, folic acid, carbohydrate, fat, and protein; production site for cholecystokinin and secretin
         (2) Jejunum: absorption site for carbohydrate, fat, and protein
         (3) Ileum: absorption site for B_{12}, bile salts, and fat-soluble vitamins
         (4) Ileocecal valve is important for retarding intestinal transit and acting as barrier to colonic organisms
         (5) Colon: not as critical as the small bowel with regard to absorption; however, it is important for fluid and electrolyte balance.
   4. Interventions:
      a. Monitor and correct fluid, electrolyte, and metabolic balance; monitor stool volume and the amount of reducing substances in the stool.

    b. Provide adequate nutrition: hyperalimentation; enteral feeds (use an elemental formula [eg, Pregestimil, Alimentum, or Nutramigen])

    c. Medications:

       (1) Ranitidine: decreases acid hypersecretion.

       (2) Loperamide, codeine, paregoric, diphenoxylate: aid in slowing intestinal transit time.

       (3) Oral neomycin: decreases bacterial overgrowth.

       (4) Somatostatin and cholestyramine may decrease diarrhea.

    d. Surgery:

       (1) Stoma closure

       (2) Tapering a length of bowel that has become too dilated may aid with stasis and bacterial overgrowth.

       (3) Bowel lengthening procedures using dilated bowel are risky and considered only when a patient is total parenteral nutrition (TPN) dependent.

       (4) Small bowel transplantation can be performed when enteral feeds have failed, there is TPN-induced liver failure, and access for TPN is no longer possible.

  5. Outcome and complications: long-term survival is approximately 85%; sepsis from bacterial translocation from the bowel; central catheter sepsis or thrombosis; TPN-induced liver disease; and cholelithiasis

B. GER (Bernbaum, Gerdes, & Spitzer, 1996; Boix-Ochoa & Rowe, 1998; Faubion Jr, & Zein, 1998; Nakayama, 1997b):

  1. Definition: a condition in which the esophagus is exposed to gastric contents due to the retrograde movement of contents from the stomach to the esophagus and sometimes into the mouth

  2. Etiology is multifactorial: immaturity of the lower esophageal sphincter; transient relaxation of the sphincter; gastric distention stimulates transient relaxation of the sphincter; impaired clearance of gastric acid due to esophageal dysmotility or delayed gastric emptying; high osmolality feedings worsens reflux; previous esophageal surgery; and neurologic impairment

  3. Clinical manifestations range from subtle to severe:

    a. Regurgitation or vomiting; aspiration

    b. Growth failure; irritability

    c. Hematemesis due to esophagitis; food rejection due to esophagitis; Sandifer's syndrome (an abnormal posturing and neck craning associated with reflux)

    d. The association between apnea and reflux is not well defined; however, apnea associated with reflux remains a common indication for fundoplication.

  4. Diagnosis:

    a. Barium swallow demonstrates anatomic obstructions and visualizes the presence of reflux.

    b. Esophageal pH monitoring better indicates the severity and frequency of the reflux.

    c. Endoscopy detects the presence of esophagitis and strictures.

   d. Esophageal biopsy can detect the presence of eosinophils, which is sensitive for diagnosing reflux.
5. Interventions:
   a. Position the infant upright at a 30° angle after feeds and when asleep.
   b. Thicken feedings with rice or oatmeal cereal; smaller more frequent feedings
   c. Medications: prokinetic agents (eg, metaclopramide); acid blockade (eg, ranitidine or omeprazole)
   d. Surgery (Nissan fundoplication) may be indicated for growth failure, chronic aspiration, life-threatening apnea, or development of a peptic stricture from esophagitis. Complications of surgery include gas-bloat syndrome, dysphagia, and inability to burp or vomit.
6. Outcome: many infants have self-limited course of reflux resolved by 12 to 18 months of age.

▼
References

Albanese, C. T., & Rowe, M. I. (1998). Necrotizing enterocolitis. In J. A. O'Neill (Ed.), *Pediatric surgery* (5th ed., pp. 1297–1320). St. Louis: Mosby-Year Book.

Bernbaum, J. C., Gerdes, M., & Spitzer, A. R. (1996). Follow-up of the high-risk neonate. In A. R. Spitzer (Ed.), *Intensive care of the fetus and neonate* (pp. 729–741). St. Louis: Mosby-Year Book.

Boix-Ochoa, J., & Rowe, M. I. (1998). Gastroesophageal reflux. In J. A. O'Neill (Ed.), *Pediatric surgery* (5th ed., pp. 1029–1043). St. Louis: Mosby-Year Book.

Cilley, R. E., & Krummel, T. M., (1998) Disorders of the umbilicus. In J. A. O'Neill (Ed.), *Pediatric surgery* (5th ed., pp. 1029–1043). St. Louis: Mosby-Year Book.

Cooney, D. R. (1998). Defects of the abdominal wall. In J. A. O'Neill (Ed.), *Pediatric surgery* (5th ed., pp. 1045–1069). St. Louis: Mosby-Year Book.

Davies, B. W., & Stringer, M. D. (1997). The survivors of gastroschisis. *Archives of Disease in Childhood, 77*(2), 158–160.

Dillon, P. W., & Cilley, R. E. (1993). Newborn surgical emergencies: Gastrointestinal anomalies, abdominal wall defects. *Pediatric Clinics of North America, 40*(6), 1289–1313.

Docimo, S. G., Jeffs, R. D., & Gearhart, J. P. (1997). Bladder, cloacal exstrophy, and prune belly syndrome. In K. T. Oldham, P. M. Colombani, & R. P. Foglia (Eds.), *Surgery of infants and children: Scientific principles and practice* (pp. 1095–1122). Philadelphia: Lippincott-Raven.

Druschel, C. M. (1995). A descriptive study of prune belly in New York state, 1983 to 1989. *Archives of Pediatrics & Adolescent Medicine, 149*(1), 70–76.

Faubion, W. A., & Zein, N. N. (1998). Gastroesophageal reflux in infants and children. *Mayo Clinic Proceedings, 73*(2), 166-173.

Freij, B. J., & McCracken, G. H. (1994). Acute infections. In G. B. Avery, M. A. Fletcher, & M. G. MacDonald (Eds.), *Neonatology: Pathophysiology and management of the newborn* (4th ed., pp. 1082–1116). Philadelphia: JB Lippincott.

Georges, L. S. (1997). Anesthesia for genitourinary surgery in the newborn. In D. K. Nakayama, C. L. Bose, N. C. Chescheir, & R. D. Valley (Eds.), *Critical care of the surgical newborn* (pp. 555–558). Armonk, NY: Futura Publishing.

Georgeson, K. E. (1998). Short-bowel syndrome. In J. A. O'Neill (Ed.), *Pediatric surgery* (5th ed., pp. 1223–1231). St. Louis: Mosby-Year Book.

Gomella, T. L. (1999). Surgical diseases of the newborn. In T. L. Gomella, M. D. Cunningham, F. G. Eyal, & E. Zenk (Eds.), *Neonatology: Management, procedures, on-call problems, diseases, and drugs,* (4th ed., pp. 533–545). Stamford, CT: Appleton & Lange.

Grosfeld, J. L. (1998). Jejunoileal atresia and stenosis. In J. A. O'Neill (Ed.), *Pediatric surgery* (5th ed., pp. 1145–1158). St. Louis: Mosby-Year Book.

Harmon, C. M., & Coran, A. G. (1998). Congenital anomalies of the esophagus. In J. A. O'Neill, (Ed.), *Pediatric surgery* (5th ed., pp. 941–967). St. Louis: Mosby-Year Book.

Hebra, A., & Ross III, A. J. (1996). Necrotizing enterocolitis. In A. R. Spitzer (Ed.), *Intensive care of the fetus and neonate* (pp. 865–874). St. Louis: Mosby-Year Book.

Hendren, W. H., Carr, M. C., & Adams, M. C. (1998). Megaureter and prune-belly syndrome. In J. A. O'Neill (Ed.), *Pediatric surgery* (5th ed., pp. 1631–1651). St. Louis: Mosby-Year Book.

How, H. Y., Harris, B. J., Pietrantoni, M., Evans, J. C, Dutton, S., Khoury, J. & Siddiqi, T. A. (2000). Is vaginal delivery preferable to elective cesarean delivery in fetuses with a known ventral wall defect? *American Journal of Obstetrics and Gynecology, 182*(6), 1527–1534.

Howell, K. K. (1998). Understanding gastroschisis: An abdominal wall defect. *Neonatal Network, 17*(8), 17–25.

Jones, K. L. (1997). *Smith's recognizable patterns of malformation* (5th ed.). Philadelphia: WB Saunders.

Kapur, P., Caty, M. G., & Glick, P. L. (1998). Pediatric hernias and hydroceles. *Pediatric Clinics of North America, 45*(4), 773–789.

Kays, D. W. (1996). Surgical conditions of the neonatal intestinal tract. *Clinics in Perinatology, 23*(2), 353–375.

Kiely, E. M., & Pena, A. (1998). Anorectal malformations. In J. A. O'Neill (Ed.), *Pediatric surgery* (5th ed., pp.1425–1448). St. Louis: Mosby-Year Book.

Lloyd, D. A., & Rintala, R. J. (1998). Inguinal hernia and hydrocele. In J. A. O'Neill (Ed.), *Pediatric surgery* (5th ed., pp. 1071–1086). St. Louis: Mosby-Year Book.

Nakayama, D. K. (1997a). Duodenal atresia and stenosis. In D. K. Nakayama, C. L. Bose, N. C. Chescheir, & R. D. Valley (Eds.), *Critical care of the surgical newborn* (pp. 321–333). Armonk, NY: Futura Publishing.

Nakayama, D. K. (1997b). Esophageal atresia and tracheoesophageal fistula. In D. K. Nakayama, C. L. Bose, N. C. Chescheir, & R. D. Valley (Eds.), *Critical care of the surgical newborn* (pp. 227–249). Armonk, NY: Futura Publishing.

Nakayama, D. K. (1997c). Jejunoileal atresia. In D. K. Nakayama, C. L. Bose, N. C. Chescheir, & R. D. Valley (Eds.), *Critical care of the surgical newborn* (pp. 335–346). Armonk, NY: Futura Publishing.

Nakayama, D. K. (1997d). Gastroschisis. In D. K. Nakayama, C. L. Bose, N. C. Chescheir, & R. D. Valley (Eds.), *Critical care of the surgical newborn* (pp. 261–276). Armonk, NY: Futura Publishing.

Nakayama, D. K. (1997e). Hirschsprung's disease. In D. K. Nakayama, C. L. Bose, N. C. Chescheir, & R. D. Valley (Eds.), *Critical care of the surgical newborn* (pp. 419–447). Armonk, NY: Futura Publishing.

Nakayama, D. K. (1997f). Imperforate anus. In D. K. Nakayama, C. L. Bose, N. C. Chescheir, & R. D. Valley (Eds.), *Critical care of the surgical newborn* (pp. 449–473). Armonk, NY: Futura Publishing.

Nakayama, D.K. (1997g). Inguinal hernia and hydrocele. In D. K. Nakayama, C. L. Bose, N. C. Chescheir, & R. D. Valley (Eds.), *Critical care of the surgical newborn* (pp. 289–303). Armonk, NY: Futura Publishing.

Nakayama, D. K. (1997h). Malrotation of the intestine. In D. K. Nakayama, C. L. Bose, N. C. Chescheir, & R. D. Valley (Eds.), *Critical care of the surgical newborn* (pp. 367–382). Armonk, NY: Futura Publishing.

Nakayama, D. K. (1997i). Meconium ileus, meconium peritonitis, and meconium plug. In D. K. Nakayama, C. L. Bose, N. C. Chescheir, & R. D. Valley (Eds.), *Critical care of the surgical newborn* (pp. 347–365). Armonk, NY: Futura Publishing.

Nakayama, D. K. (1997j). Necrotizing enterocolitis. In D. K. Nakayama, C. L. Bose, N. C. Chescheir, & R. D. Valley (Eds.), *Critical care of the surgical newborn* (pp. 383–405). Armonk, NY: Futura Publishing.

Nakayama, D. K. (1997k). Omphalocele. In D. K. Nakayama, C. L. Bose, N. C. Chescheir, & R. D. Valley (Eds.), *Critical care of the surgical newborn* (pp. 277–288). Armonk, NY: Futura Publishing.

Noh, P. H., Cooper, C. S., Winkler, A. C., Zderic, S. A., Snyder, III, H. M., & Canning, D. A., (1999). Prognostic factors for long-term renal function in boys with the prune-belly syndrome. *The Journal of Urology, 162*(4), 1399–1401.

O'Donnell, K. A., Glick, P. L., & Caty, M. G. (1998). Pediatric umbilical problems. *Pediatric Clinics of North America, 45*(4), 791–799.

Pollack, E. S. (1996). Pediatric abdominal surgical emergencies. *Pediatric Annals,* 25(8), 448–457.

Rescorla, F. J. (1998). Meconium ileus. In J. A. O'Neill, (Ed.), *Pediatric surgery* (5th ed., pp. 1159–1172). St. Louis: Mosby-Year Book.

Rescorla, F. J. (2001). Surgical emergencies in the newborn. In R. A. Polin, M. C. Yoder, & F. D. Burg (Eds.), *Workbook in practical neonatology* (3rd ed. pp. 423–459). Philadelphia: WB Saunders.

Stauffer, U. G., & Schwoebel, M. (1998). Duodenal atresia and stenosis-annular pancreas. In J. A. O'Neill (Ed.), *Pediatric surgery* (5th ed., pp. 1133–1143). St. Louis: Mosby-Year Book.

Scherer, III, L. R., & Grosfeld, J. L. (1993). Inguinal hernia and umbilical anomalies. *Pediatric Clinics of North America, 40*(6), 1121–1131.

Strodtbeck, F. (1998). Abdominal wall defects. *Neonatal Network, 17*(8), 51–53.

Taylor, L. A. (1997). Short bowel syndrome. In D. K. Nakayama, C. L. Bose, N. C. Chescheir, & R. D. Valley (Eds.), *Critical care of the surgical newborn* (pp. 407–418). Armonk, NY: Futura Publishing.

Teitelbaum, D. H., Coran, A. G., Weitzman, J. J., Ziegler, M. M., & Kane, T. (1998). Hirschsprung's disease and related neuromuscular disorders of the intestine. In J. A. O'Neill (Ed.), *Pediatric surgery* (5th ed., pp. 1133–1143). St. Louis: Mosby-Year Book.

Touloukian, R. J., & Smith, E. I. (1998). Disorders of rotation and fixation. In J. A. O'Neill (Ed.), *Pediatric surgery* (5th ed., pp. 1199–1215). St. Louis: Mosby-Year Book.

Vanderhoof, J. A., Zach, T. L., & Adrian, T. E. (1994). Gastrointestinal disease. In G. B. Avery, M. A. Fletcher, & M. G. MacDonald (Eds.), *Neonatology: Pathophysiology and management of the newborn* (4th ed., pp. 605–629). Philadelphia: JB Lippincott.

Weiss, M. D., Williams, J. L., Ledbetter, D. J., & Neu, J. (2001). Necrotizing enterocolitis. In R. A. Polin, M. C. Yoder, & F. D. Burg (Eds.), *Workbook in practical neonatology* (3rd ed., pp. 460–477). Philadelphia: WB Saunders.

Young, D. G. (1998). Intussusception. In J. A. O'Neill (Ed.), *Pediatric surgery* (5th ed., pp. 1185–1196). St. Louis: Mosby-Year Book.

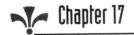 **Chapter 17**

Genitourinary and Renal Disorders

Kathy Keen, MSN, RNC, NNP, and Patricia A. Coates, MSN, RNC, NNP

Part A: **Genitourinary defects**

I. Lower abdominal wall defects

  A. Bladder exstrophy (Kaplan & McAleer, 1999; Murphy, 2000):

    1. Definition: eversion and extrusion of the urinary bladder through an abdominal wall defect, with the internal surface of the posterior wall of the bladder exposed. There are varying degrees of severity. Associated anomalies include epispadias, open urethra, widened pubic symphysis, and hypoplastic or bifid genital structures.

    2. Clinical presentation:

      a. Classic bladder exstrophy is an exposed bladder plate, open urethra, widened symphysis pubis, low umbilicus, and wide rectus. The exposed bladder mucosa is edematous and friable. The remainder of the urinary tract is usually normal.

      b. The penis is wide and short, the testes are usually descended, and the vas deferens and ejaculatory ducts are normal.

      c. The clitoris is bifid and the labia are separated; the vagina is shortened and displaced anteriorly; the uterus, ovaries, and tubes are generally normal, but duplication may occur.

    3. Interventions (see Cloacal exstrophy)

    4. Outcomes: 40% to 80% of patients achieve long-term continence; adequate sexual function is possible, but fertility in male patients is diminished.

  B. Cloacal exstrophy (Warner & Ziegler, 2000):

    1. Definition: severe complex of anomalies that includes bladder exstrophy with associated defects plus omphalocele, exposed bowel, and imperforate anus

    2. Clinical manifestations:

      a. Classically, there is an omphalocele superiorly and exposed bladder and bowel inferiorly. Small and large bowels are often short and may be malrotated.

      b. The genitals are always abnormal: males (the penis and scrotum may be absent or bifid and widely separated and testes are undescended); females (the clitoris and labia may be absent or bifid and widely separated and there is usually a duplex vagina and a bicornuate uterus)

      c. Anomalies of other organ systems (eg, upper urinary tract, vertebral anomalies, spinal cord defects, and lower extremity defects, such as club feet) occur in up to 85% of cases.

    3. Interventions for bladder and cloacal exstrophy:

      a. Physical examination for bladder plate size, genital structures, and sexual identity

b. Protect the bladder/intestines with a bowel bag, cellophane wrap, or Vaseline gauze immediately after birth to prevent mucosal drying. Avoid adherent dressings and protect the exposed mucosa from trauma.

c. Renal ultrasound to evaluate upper urinary tract. Evaluate all possible defects (eg, upper urinary tract, central nervous system [CNS], musculoskeletal deformities, and gender status).

d. Surgical intervention: bladder exstrophy (primary closure of the bladder within the first 48 to 72 hours); cloacal exstrophy (staged surgical correction with initial reconstruction occurring within the first few days of life; subsequent operative stages usually occur when the infant has reached 20 to 25 pounds)

4. Outcomes for cloacal exstrophy (Kaplan & McAleer, 1999):

    a. Most patients require a permanent colostomy and a urinary stoma or intermittent bladder catheterization.

    b. In males, a functional penis can rarely be constructed; in females, the genitalia can usually be reconstructed with a fairly normal external appearance.

    c. Pelvic, extremity, and spinal deformities may require prosthetics and various other orthopedic procedures. All patients require ongoing psychologic and emotional support secondary to multiple hospitalizations and reconstructive procedures.

II. Gonadal defects

  A. Undescended testes (UDT) (or cryptorchidism) (Tappero & Honeyfield, 1996; Wallen & Shortliffe, 2000):

    1. Definition: cryptorchidism is present when one or both testes have not descended completely into the scrotum. Most UDT will descend by 3 months of age. Spontaneous descent rarely occurs after 9 months of age.

    2. Diagnosis is made when the testes are not palpable within the scrotum.

    3. Intervention: orchiopexy (ie, freeing the UDT and implanting it into the scrotum) is recommended at approximately 1 year of age. Repair may be done earlier if a symptomatic inguinal hernia is present.

  B. Ambiguous genitalia (Moore, Persaud, & Shiota, 1994; Page, 1994; Repetto, 1999):

    1. Definition: the sex of the infant is not readily apparent after examination of the external genitalia. Appearance of the genitals reveals neither male, with normal penis, scrotum, and palpable testes, nor female, with a vaginal orifice or normal labia and clitoris.

    2. Etiology:

      a. Virilization of female infants (female pseudohermaphroditism) occurs in genetic females (46,XX) exposed to excessive fetal or maternal androgens in utero. Conditions include congenital adrenal hyperplasia (CAH) and less common causes such as virilizing maternal or fetal tumors, and maternal androgen ingestion or topical use.

b. Inadequate virilization of male infants (male pseudohermaphroditism): occurs in genetic males (46,XY), and results from inadequate androgen production or deficiency in end-organ response to androgen. *These abnormalities are uncommon* and require an extensive workup.

(1) Enzyme defects (autosomal-recessive disorders)

(2) Deficiency of mullerian-inhibiting substance (commonly presents in a male infant with inguinal hernias that contain the uterus or fallopian tubes)

(3) Testicular unresponsiveness to human chorionic gonadotropin and luteinizing hormone

(4) Anorchia

(5) Pituitary deficiency (associated with microphallus and hypoglycemia) with absence of gonadotropins, adrenocorticotropic hormone (ACTH), or growth hormone

(6) Defect in the androgen receptor (or testicular feminization): total (labial testes and otherwise normal-appearing female genitalia) or partial (incomplete virilization of a male)

(7) 5α-reductase deficiency: failure of the external genitalia to undergo male differentiation, with resultant ambiguous or external female genitalia; 46,XY karyotype; normally developed testes, and male internal ducts

c. Disorders of gonadal differentiation (Repetto, 1999):

(1) True hermaphroditism **(rare)**: presence of testis and ovary, ie, ovotestes, in the same individual; appearance of the genitalia is variable. Most infants are 46,XX karyotype, but 45,X and multiple X/multiple Y karyotype are possible.

(2) Gonadal dysgenesis: gonads exist in an undifferentiated form termed "streak gonads" that may be bilateral or unilateral. This condition has an X-chromosome and a Y-chromosome form. Streak gonads in the Y-chromosome form are at risk for tumor development and should be removed. Most common are infants with 45,X karyotype and signs of Turner's syndrome.

(3) Chromosome abnormalities, syndromes, and associations with possible, although not usual, ambiguous genitalia include: Turner's syndrome (45,XO) and Klinefelter's syndrome (47,XXY); Smith-Lemli-Opitz syndrome; Rieger's syndrome; camptomelic dysplasia; CHARGE association; and VACTERL association.

3. Diagnosis:

a. Be aware of family history of early neonatal deaths (may be secondary to CAH); paternal consanguinity; female relatives with amenorrhea and infertility; maternal history of virilization or CAH, and ingestion or topical application of androgens.

b. Physical examination:

(1) Palpate number, size, symmetry, and position of gonads; note appearance of external genitalia.

(**2**) *Palpable gonads below the inguinal canal are almost certainly testes. Ovaries are not found in scrotal folds or in the inguinal region.* Testes may be intra-abdominal.

(**3**) Measure the length of the phallus (at least 2 cm term infant).

(**4**) Labioscrotal folds range from unfused labia majora, varying degrees of posterior fusion and bifid scrotum, to fully fused normal-appearing scrotum.

4. Radiographic studies: ultrasound to evaluate presence/position of gonads, vagina, and uterus; contrast studies to outline the internal anatomy

5. Laboratory studies:
   a. Chromosome analysis:
      (**1**) Normal 46,XX: virilization of genetic female
      (**2**) Normal 46,XY: incompletely virilized genetic male
      (**3**) Abnormal karyotype: may indicate mixed gonadal dysgenesis with a dysplastic gonad.
   b. 17-Hydroxyprogesterone (17-OHP): precursor to the enzyme defect in 21-hydroxylase enzyme deficiency, and one step prior to that in 11-hydroxylase enzyme deficiency. 17-OHP plasma level will be 100 to 1,000 times the normal level.
   c. Daily electrolytes: 21-hydroxylase enzyme deficiency will have hyponatremia and hyperkalemia within the first 3 to 5 days of life.
   d. Testosterone: if 17-OHP is normal and there is no maternal virilization, elevated testosterone suggests hermaphroditism (most are 46,XX) or fetal testosterone-producing tumor.

6. Interventions:
   a. Delivery room management: *do not assign a gender*. Inform parents of the infant's "incompletely developed" genitalia. Use neutral terms (eg, infant/baby, gonad, or phallus) when describing the physical findings. *This is a medical emergency.*
   b. Medical management:
      (**1**) Urology, genetics, and endocrinology consults
      (**2**) Congenital adrenal hyperplasia: onset of adrenal insufficiency occurs 3 to 14 days of life in 50% of patients. Early diagnosis and replacement therapy with hydrocortisone (glucocorticoid) and Florinef (mineralocorticoid) is imperative to prevent vascular collapse.
      (**3**) Incompletely virilized genetic male: treatment with Depo-Testosterone is used to evaluate whether adequate growth of the phallus occurs.
      (**4**) Gender assignment and the sex of rearing should be determined only when the final diagnosis is secure. Goals guiding the selection of sex of rearing include: genitalia should be correctable to provide a normal body image and gender identity; genitalia should be of normal size and function to permit sexual function in adulthood; and retaining fertility.

    c. Outcomes: many patients are fertile as adults, some due to reproductive technology. Optimal social and psychologic outcomes depend on appropriate gender assignment and ongoing psychological support.

C. Hydrocele (Pulito, 1999; Tappero & Honeyfield, 1996; Weber, Thomas, & Tracy, 2000):

    1. Definition: circumscribed collection of clear fluid in the scrotum; may communicate with the inguinal canal and may be associated with a hernia; noncommunicating hydrocele is common in newborns.

    2. Etiology: persistence of a narrow patent processus vaginalis, too narrow to permit entrance of small intestine, but wide enough to allow peritoneal fluid to drip down and accumulate in the scrotum

    3. Diagnosis: appearance of unilateral/bilateral scrotal swelling; the soft, fluid-filled sac transilluminates brightly.

    4. Outcome: usually resolves without treatment within 6 to 12 months.

D. Hypospadias (Kaplan & McAleer, 1999; Murphy, 2000; Pulito, 1999):

    1. Definition: developmental anomaly characterized by abnormal location of the urethral meatus on the ventral surface of the penis, the scrotum or perineum; frequently associated with chordee (ventral curvature of the penis) and foreskin abnormality

    2. Diagnosis: there are different anatomic classifications, depending upon the location of the meatal opening (glanular, penal shaft, penoscrotal, scrotal, and perineal) and the degree of chordee. Severe cases may be confused with ambiguous genitalia. Associated anomalies include undescended testes and inguinal hernia.

    3. Interventions:

        a. Avoid circumcision (foreskin tissue may be needed for later surgical correction).

        b. Radiologic evaluation of the urinary system

        c. Surgical repair usually done between 6 and 12 months of age

        d. Objectives of hypospadias correction: complete straightening of the penis; placing the meatus at the tip of the glans; forming a symmetric cone-shaped glans; constructing a urethra of uniform caliber; and completing a satisfactory cosmetic skin coverage

E. Testicular torsion (Kaplan & McAleer, 1999; Noseworthy, 2000; & Tappero & Honeyfield, 1996):

    1. Definition: condition in which the testis and its tunica vaginalis rotate in the scrotal sac, inguinal canal, or abdomen and compromise blood flow to the testis, with resultant ischemic infarction

    2. Etiology: uncertain; may occur in utero.

    3. Diagnosis: usually presents as a firm nontender slightly enlarged testis; scrotal skin may appear normal, discolored, ecchymotic, or edematous; often detected on initial examination after delivery

    4. Intervention: urgent operation may be necessary to distinguish torsion from incarcerated inguinal hernia; surgical exploration is performed as soon as possible (< 6 hours) when there is a change in testicular examination; obvious infarcted testis (non-emergent surgery is indicated to remove the affected testis and provide fixation for the remaining testis)

5. Outcome: usually there is complete infarction with loss of the affected testis.

III. Bladder defects and malfunctions

A. Posterior urethral valves (Kaplan & McAleer, 1999; Lantz, 2000; Pulito, 1999):

1. Definition: abnormal tissue folds along the male membranous urethra, causing bladder outflow obstruction and subsequent dilation of the upper urinary tract

2. Clinical manifestations: depends upon the severity of obstruction and may include bilateral flank masses, distended bladder, and poor urinary stream (with dribbling).

3. Diagnosis: many are diagnosed prenatally; voiding cystourethrogram (VCUG)

4. Interventions:

    a. Physical examination to assess the infant's general condition and evaluate the presence of enlarged kidneys and distended bladder. Note urine stream if voiding occurs.

    b. Emergent bladder drainage with 5 FR urinary catheter or infant feeding tube

    c. Urinalysis and urine culture; antibiotics empirically; serum electrolytes, blood urea nitrogen (BUN), and creatinine to assess hydration and renal function

    d. Ablation of valves is initial operative procedure; urinary diversion may be needed.

5. Outcome: approximately 50% of patients will progress to renal failure and transplantation despite treatment; approximately 46% have diurnal enuresis.

B. Ureteral pelvic junction (UPJ) obstruction (Coplen & Snyder, 2000; Kaplan & McAleer, 1999; Lantz, 2000):

1. Definition: blockage of the normal UPJ leading to hydronephrosis

2. Etiology: usually the result of narrowing of the ureter at the junction of the renal pelvis with the ureter. *Most common cause of antenatal hydronephrosis*

3. Clinical manifestations: flank mass (*most common cause of palpable abdominal mass in the newborn*)

4. Diagnosis: postnatal ultrasound at 10 to 14 days of life (when UPJ is observed on prenatal ultrasound); VCUG; and renal scan

5. Interventions: antibiotic prophylaxis (Amoxicillin); pyeloplasty for *significant obstruction* during the first 4 to 6 weeks of life

6. Outcome: due to the compliance of the pelvis, renal function is usually preserved even if the kidney is massively dilated behind the obstruction; surgery usually results in improvement in drainage and renal function.

C. Urinary tract infection (UTI) (Brion, Satlin, & Edelmann, 1999; Chiura, 1999; Lott, 1994):

1. Definition: presence of pathogenic bacteria or fungus in the urinary tract with or without symptoms of infection

2. Etiology: predominant organisms are gram-negative rods (*Kleb-*

siella, Pseudomonas, Proteus, and *Escherichia coli* [most common]); *Candida* species (nosocomially acquired UTI)

3. Risk factors: male gender (more common in uncircumcised males); indwelling urinary catheters; systemic sepsis; urinary tract obstructions; and neurogenic bladder

4. Clinical manifestations:
   a. May be asymptomatic.
   b. Subtle signs: lethargy, temperature instability, irritability, poor feeding, vomiting, jaundice, or failure to thrive
   c. Overt signs of sepsis: respiratory distress, apnea, bradycardia, poor perfusion, or abdominal distention

5. Diagnosis:
   a. Blood culture; urine culture and Gram stain (unnecessary during first 3 days of life because incidence of UTI during this time is low) (suprapubic aspiration or catheterization; microorganisms $> 10^3$/mL is indicative of infection; Gram stain will assist in identifying the microorganism)
   b. Complete blood count (CBC)
   c. Urinalysis: presence of leukocytes and bacteria suggestive of UTI, but absence does not rule it out. Yeast cells on microscopic examination suggestive of candiduria
   d. Renal ultrasound followed by VCUG to detect anomalies of the kidneys and urinary tract

6. Interventions: broad-spectrum antibiotics (ampicillin and gentamicin) until sensitivities are completed; repeat urine culture 36 to 48 hours after antibiotics are started.

7. Outcome: prognosis for isolated UTI is good; potential exists for injury to the kidneys and urinary tract; and recurrent UTIs may result from structural abnormalities of the urinary system.

D. Neurogenic bladder (Cartwright & Snow, 2000):
   1. Definition: bladder dysfunction resulting from congenital or acquired lesions that affect bladder innervation. The bladder's ability to store and/or empty urine may be affected.
   2. Etiologies:
      a. Congenital lesions: neural tube defect (*most common*), degenerative neuromuscular disorder, cerebral palsy, tethered cord, sacral agenesis, imperforate anus, VACTERAL association, and other causes
      b. Acquired lesions: trauma to the brain, spinal cord, or pelvic nerves *or* the result of tumor, infection, or vascular lesions affecting these same structures
   3. Diagnosis: renal and bladder ultrasound; VCUG; measurement of postvoid residuals; and urodynamic evaluation (measurement of bladder pressures)
   4. Interventions depend upon results of radiologic and urodynamic evaluations.
      a. For infants who spontaneously void: follow-up studies at 6 months
      b. For reflux or upper tract deterioration: intermittent catheterization, anticholinergic therapy, or temporary vesicostomy may be necessary.

    c. Clean intermittent catheterization (CIC); anticholinergic drug therapy is usually coupled with CIC.

    d. Diversion with cutaneous vesicostomy (reserved for infants with serious deterioration of the upper tract, or those who cannot be managed with CIC and anticholinergic drugs)

    e. Surgical treatment: bladder augmentation or enlargement; cutaneous urinary diversion by ileal or colon conduit or by cutaneous ureterostomy

  5. Outcomes: bacteriuria is common with CIC and may lead to upper tract deterioration.

Part B: Renal Defects and Disorders

I. Renal anatomic defects

  A. Bilateral renal agenesis (Gomella, 1994; Kaplan, 1994; Moore, 1988; Vogt and Avner, 2002):

    1. Definition: congenital absence of both kidneys

    2. Etiology: failure of ureteric bud to form the renal cortex and nephrons

    3. Clinical manifestations: oligohydramnios; severe oliguria or anuria; absence of distended bladder; Potter's facies (low-set ears, small chin, turned-down tip of nose, and skin creases from the inner canthus of the eye)

    4. Diagnosis: prenatal ultrasound shows absence of kidneys and absent bladder.

    5. Prognosis: incompatible with life; 40% are stillborn and those born alive die shortly after birth secondary to pulmonary hypoplasia or renal failure.

    6. Interventions: supportive care

  B. Unilateral renal agenesis (Kaplan, 1994; Kenner, Brueggemeyer, & Gunderson, 1993; Vogt & Avner, 2002):

    1. Definition: congenital absence of one kidney

    2. Clinical manifestations: asymptomatic unless contralateral kidney is injured, malformed, or diseased; suspect if infant is diagnosed with imperforate anus, congenital scoliosis, or vaginal/uterine agenesis

    3. Diagnosis: found in healthy infants during evaluation for other reasons; renal ultrasound; renal scan, and VCUG

    4. Outcome: excellent prognosis as long as the functional kidney remains disease free

  C. Polycystic kidney disease (Brion et al., 1999; Kaplan & McAleer, 1994; Vogt & Avner, 2002):

    1. Definition: bilateral asymmetrically enlarged spongy kidneys

    2. Etiology: autosomal-dominant polycystic disease (ADPKD) (*most common inherited renal disease*); autosomal-recessive polycystic kidney disease (ARPKD)

    3. Clinical manifestations: oligohydramnios; Potter's facies; fetal compression syndrome; enlarged abdomen; respiratory failure secondary to lung hypoplasia; hypertension (HTN); abnormal liver (liver failure); and stillborn

    4. Diagnosis: family history; prenatal or postnatal ultrasound; renal biopsy; and intravenous urography (IVU)

    5. Interventions: antihypertensives; check urine culture and treat UTIs; portacaval shunt secondary to development of portal hypertension; dialysis; renal transplantation

    6. Outcome: ADPKD (most survive early infancy; limited data regarding prognosis); ARPKD (supportive until end-stage renal disease; grim prognosis)

D. Multicystic kidney disease (Brion et al., 1997; Kaplan & McAleer, 1994; Pulito, 1994; Vogt & Avner, 2002):

    1. Definition: enlarged nonfunctional cystic kidneys

    2. Etiology: renal dysplasia secondary to intrauterine obstruction of the urinary tract; 90% are unilateral; may be associated with VACTERL syndrome.

    3. Clinical manifestations:

        a. Asymptomatic

        b. Flank mass; usually on left

        c. Potter's facies; anuria; pulmonary HTN

    4. Diagnosis: renal ultrasound (demonstrates multiseptated fluid-filled mass); intravenous pyelography (IVP)

    5. Treatment: controversial because disease is not progressive; nephrectomy indicated when there are complications such as HTN, infection, or renal cell carcinoma

E. Hydronephrosis (Chase, 2001; Spitzer, Bernstein, Borchus, & Edelman, 1992):

    1. Definition: dilation of the renal pelvis that includes any excess fluid within the collecting system

    2. Etiology:

        a. Fetal hydronephrosis: usually transient and secondary to hormonal effects, volume expansion, or inadequate bladder emptying

        b. Persistent hydronephrosis *secondary* to lower urinary tract obstruction, retrograde rise in hydrostatic pressure, or dilation of the urinary tract above the lesion

        c. Persistent hydronephrosis *limited* to the pelvis and calyces usually due to obstruction to urine outflow at the UPJ

    3. Diagnosis: renal ultrasound (prenatal or postnatal)

    4. Clinical manifestations: oligohydramnios; unilateral or bilateral flank mass in severe cases

    5. Interventions:

        a. Goal of treatment is to restore patency of the tract and allow adequate urine outflow; surgical correction of obstruction

        b. Monitor serum BUN and creatinine; urinary catheter may be necessary to monitor urine output.

        c. Amoxil prophylaxis (25 mg/kg/day) to prevent UTIs and scarring (Hirshfeld, Getachew, & Sessions, 2000)

    6. Outcome: high mortality; 20% die within the first 2 weeks of life; 50% die by 2 years of age.

F. Renal vein thrombosis (Brion et al., 1997; Heritage, 1994; Vogt & Avner, 2002):

1. Definition: venous obstruction secondary to dehydration and cell sludging causing renal enlargement, anuria or oliguria, and hematuria
2. Etiology:
   a. Antenatal thrombosis secondary to poorly treated diabetes; postnatal thrombosis secondary to nondiluted hypertonic radiocontrast agents; decreased thrombolytic pathway activity
   b. Hyperviscosity; decreased renal blood flow (RBF)
   c. Perinatal asphyxia; birth injury; adrenal hemorrhage
3. Clinical manifestations: congenital HTN; hematuria; flank mass; oliguria or anuria; thrombocytopenia; vomiting; lethargy; and erythrocyte fragmentation
4. Diagnosis: renal ultrasound (increased echogenicity and nephromegaly)
5. Treatment:
   a. Hydration; correction of fluid and electrolyte imbalances
   b. Treatment of renal failure; peritoneal dialysis in select cases
   c. Steroids (if associated with adrenal insufficiency)
   d. Aggressive treatment of polycythemia
6. Outcomes: renal insufficiency; tubular dysfunction; renal tubular acidosis (RTA); phosphaturia with rickets; systemic HTN; and symmetric involution of the thrombosed kidney
G. Renal tumors (Brion et al., 2002):
   1. Congenital mesoblastic nephroma (solitary unencapsulated tumor that is firm and rubbery): most common form; invades adjacent structures and recurs; may metastasize.
   2. Wilms tumor or nephroblastoma (mass of cysts, tubules, and glomeruli): invades adjacent kidney, renal veins, and contiguous organs; metastases are confined to lungs, liver, bones, and the opposite kidney; may coexist with other renal abnormalities; and associated with Beckwith-Wiedemann, Denys-Drash, and Perlmann syndromes
   3. Clinical manifestations: abdominal swelling or palpable mass; vomiting; hyperthermia; hematuria; elevated erythrocyte sedimentation rate; and HTN
   4. Diagnosis:
      a. Renal ultrasound shows distinctive ring sign (sharp demarcation between the tumor and the normal renal parenchyma).
      b. Scintigraphy and IVU: determine type and degree of invasiveness of the tumor.
      c. Computed tomography (CT) scan
      d. Renal angiography: defines extent of neoplasm and evaluates the condition of the contralateral kidney before surgery.
   5. Treatment:
      a. Surgical exploration; nephrectomy
      b. Malignancy treated with radiation and chemotherapy for 2 to 3 years
      c. Follow-up screening: high risk (ultrasound every 2 months for 1 year after diagnosis; CT scan every 6 months for 1 year after

diagnosis); low risk (Beckwith-Wiedemann and Denys-Drash syndrome) (ultrasound every 4 months for 1 year)
6. Outcome: good when found in the newborn period; 80% survival in infants < 1 year of age; substantial morbidity secondary to HTN and toxic effects of medication or radiation

II. Functional renal problems

A. Hypertension (Brion, et al., 1997; Ferris, Brennan, & Portman, 1993; Gomella, 1994):
  1. Definition:
     a. Term infants: a systolic blood pressure (BP) that is consistently > 90 torr and a diastolic > 60 torr
     b. Preterm infants: a systolic > 80 torr and a diastolic > 50 torr
     c. Also defined as a BP > 2 standard deviations above normal values for age and weight
  2. Etiology:
     a. Most common causes: renal artery thrombosis from umbilical artery catheter; aortic thrombosis; obstructive uropathy; infantile polycystic kidneys; renal failure; medications (steroids, theophylline); fluid overload; pain or agitation; BP decrease; and coarctation of the aorta
     b. Less common causes: renal artery stenosis; renal vein thrombosis; kidney hypoplasia or dysplasia; pyelonephritis; medications (Pavulon, dopamine, epinephrine, ocular phenylephrine); endocrine disorders (hyperaldosteronism, hyperthyroidism); renal tumors; adrenogenital syndrome; increased intracranial pressure (ICP) secondary to intravascular hemorrhage (IVH), subdural hemorrhage, meningitis, or hydrocephalus; closure of abdominal wall defects; and seizures
  3. Clinical manifestations: nonspecific, with the exception of an elevated systolic BP of > 90 torr in term infants and > 80 torr in preterm infants
  4. Diagnosis (Ferris et al., 1993):
     a. Renal ultrasound, renal scan, or angiography
     b. Serum creatinine (normal or slightly elevated)
     c. Urinalysis, hematuria, and proteinuria
  5. Treatment:
     a. Medications (IV dioxide, enalapril, oral captopril, calcium channel blockers [still under investigation])
     b. Surgical correction of the anatomic abnormality (eg, urinary tract obstruction, tumor, or a coarctation of the aorta)
  6. Outcome: excellent if BP is well controlled medically or cured surgically

B. Renal failure (Filmer, 1994):
  1. Definition: the absence of urinary output (anuria) or urinary output of < 0.5 mL/kg/hr (oliguria) with an elevated serum creatinine
  2. Etiology (Table 17.1)
  3. Clinical manifestations: oliguria or anuria; abdominal mass; Potter's facies; meningomyelocele with neurogenic bladder; pulmonary hypoplasia; urinary ascites; and prune-belly syndrome
  4. Diagnosis:

TABLE 17.1 Renal Failure Etiologies

	Causes	Conditions
Prerenal	Poor renal perfusion	Dehydration, poor feeding, and increased insensible water loss
		Perinatal asphyxia
		Hypotension, hemorrhage, and shock
		Sepsis
		Congestive heart failure
Intrinsic	Acute tubular necrosis	Aminoglycosides
	Nephrotoxins	Methoxyflurane anesthesia
	Congenital anomalies	Renal agenesis
	Disseminated intravascular coagulation	Polycystic kidney disease
	Renal vein thrombosis	
	Renal artery thrombosis	
Postrenal	Urinary outflow obstruction	Bilateral ureteropelvic obstruction
		Ureterovesical obstruction
		Posterior urethral valves

Adapted from Filmer, B. (1994). Renal diseases. In T. L. Gomella (Ed.), *Neonatology: management, procedures, on-call problems, diseases and drugs.* (3rd ed.). Stamford, CT: Appleton & Lange.

a. Family history of urinary tract or renal disease
b. Urinary catheterization to confirm inadequate urine output (large amounts suggest obstruction or a neurogenic bladder)
c. Laboratory studies:
(1) Serum creatinine (after 24 hours of age): term infant > 1 mg/dL; preterm infant > 1.6 mg/dL. (If the creatinine doubles, approximately half of the renal function is lost.)
(2) BUN (after 24 hours of age): term infant > 15–20 mg/dL; preterm infant > 15–20 mg/dL.
(3) Urinary studies to evaluate acute renal failure: urinalysis to check for hematuria and/or pyuria; obtain spot urine osmolality; check spot serum/urine sodium and creatinine; calculate the fractional excretion of sodium and the renal failure index. (Values are inaccurate if diuretics are used.)

$$\text{Fractional excretion of sodium (FeNa)} = \frac{\text{Urine Na} \times \text{Plasma Cr.}}{\text{Urine Cr.} \times \text{Plasma Na}} \times 100$$

$$\text{Renal failure index (RFI)} = \frac{\text{Urine Na}}{\text{Urine Cr.}} \times \text{Plasma Cr.}$$

(4) Indices of renal failure (Table 17.2)
(5) Monitor white blood count (WBC) and platelets for thrombocytopenia.
(6) Serum potassium levels to rule out hyperkalemia
d. Fluid challenge: administer 5–10 mL/kg NS IV bolus; if no response give a second bolus; follow saline bolus with Lasix 1

TABLE 17.2 Indices of Renal Failure in the Neonate

	Prerenal	Renal
Urine Na (mEq/mL)	31±19	63±3
Urine creatinine	29±16	10±4
Urine osmolality	> 400	< 400
Renal failure index	< 3	> 3
FeNa	< 2.5	> 2.5

Adapted from Filmer, B. (1994). Renal diseases. In T. L. Gomella (Ed.), *Neonatology: Management, procedures, on-call problems, diseases and drugs* (3rd ed.). Stamford, CT: Appleton & Lange.

mg/kg/dose; if urinary output does not increase, then obtain ultrasound to rule out bladder obstruction. If there is no obstruction, the cause is probably intrinsic renal failure.

   e. Radiologic studies:

   (1) Abdominal ultrasound: identifies hydronephrosis, dilated ureters, abdominal masses, distended bladder, or renal vein thrombosis.

   (2) Abdominal x-ray: identifies spina bifida or absent sacrum, which causes a neurogenic bladder.

   (3) Radionuclide scanning: delineates functioning renal parenchyma with DMSA (dimercaptosuccinic acid) and indicates renal flow and function (diethyltriamine pentaacetic acid [DTPA]).

5. Interventions:

   a. Replace insensible fluid losses (preterm infants 50–70 mL/kg/d; term 30 mL/kg/d) plus output.

   b. Daily weights and strict intake and output

   c. Follow serum sodium and potassium levels and replace cautiously as needed; remove potassium from parenteral fluids.

   d. Restrict protein intake to < 2 g/kg/day and provide adequate nonprotein caloric intake.

   e. Use breast milk or PM 60/40 for infants in renal failure.

   f. Treat hyperphosphatemia with oral aluminum hydroxide (50–150 mg/kg/day). When phosphorous is normalized, calcium with/without vitamin D supplements should be used as needed.

   g. Treat metabolic acidosis (pH < 7.25 *or* serum bicarbonate < 12 mEq) with oral bicarbonate supplements.

   HCO_3 deficit = (24 − <u>measured</u> serum bicarbonate) × 0.5 wt (in kg)

6. Definitive management:

   a. Prerenal failure: correct the specific condition as listed.

   b. Intrinsic renal disease: some renal function may recover over time if caused by toxins or acute tubular necrosis.

   c. Postrenal failure: depending upon the level of the obstruction, bypass the obstruction with a catheter or nephrostomy drainage tube. Surgical correction will be required.

   d. Dialysis or renal transplantation

C. Acute tubular necrosis (ATN) (Bilfield & Jordan, 1993; Seaman, 1995):
1. Definition: an intrinsic cause of renal failure due to renal parenchyma damage from primary ischemic injury
2. Etiology:
   a. Low glomerular filtration rate (GFR) secondary to damage to the tubular system resulting from asphyxia, hypoxia, or shock
   b. Tubular obstruction from cellular debris (eg, uric acid, myoglobin); nephrotoxins
   c. Any condition that decreases systemic BP, impairs cardiac output, or increases renal vascular resistance (Bissinger, 1995; Blifeld & Jordan, 1993)
3. Clinical manifestations (Chase, 1996; Kenner, et.al., 1998; Lewy, 1994): edema; lethargy; abdominal distention; cardiac arrhythmias; cardiac enlargement; oliguria; pulmonary edema; and hyponatremia with oliguria
4. Interventions (Blifeld & Jordan, 1993; Gomella, 1994):
   a. Follow labs (urine osmolality, urine Na, FeNa, serum electrolytes, BUN, and creatinine) to establish diagnosis and monitor/correct electrolyte imbalances.
   b. Prevent perinatal and delivery room situations that place the infant at risk; antenatal monitoring; timely delivery if fetus is compromised; skillful and effective delivery room resuscitation to prevent hypoxia and poor blood flow to the kidneys; minimal maternal and neonatal exposure to nephrotoxic drugs
   c. Correct hypovolemia; maintain proper fluid and electrolyte balance; insert catheter to obtain accurate urinary output.
   d. Administer Lasix or mannitol to clear tubular system.
5. Outcome (Blifeld & Jordan, 1993):
   a. Favorable prognosis with supportive care; recovery will take time.
   b. Long-term therapy may involve dialysis and subsequent kidney transplantation.

▼ References

Bissinger, R. (1995). Renal physiology: Part I—structure and function. *Neonatal Network*, *14*(4): 9–19.

Blifeld, L., & Jordan, S. (1993). Acute renal failure in the neonatal period. In J. J. Pomerance & C. J. Richardson, *Neonatology for the clinician*. Norwalk, CT: Appleton & Lange.

Brion, L. P., Satlin, L. M., & Edelmann, C. M., Jr. (1999). Renal disease. In G. B. Avery, M. A. Fletcher, & M. G. MacDonald (Eds.), *Neonatology: Pathophysiology and management of the newborn* (5th ed.). Philadelphia: Lippincott Williams & Wilkins.

Cartwright, P. C., & Snow, B. W. (2000). Bladder and urethra. In K.W. Ashcraft (Ed.), *Pediatric surgery* (3rd ed.). Philadelphia: WB Saunders.

Chase, M. (1996). The asphyxiated kidney. *Central Lines*, *12*(2), 19–20.

Chase, M. (2002). Physiology of the renal system. *Central Lines*, 17(1), 24–25.

Chirua, A. N. (1999). Renal diseases. In T. L. Gomella (Ed.), *Neonatology* (4th ed.). Stamford, CT: Appleton & Lange.

Coplen, D. E., & Snyder, H. M. (2000). Ureteral obstruction and malformations. In K.W. Ashcraft (Ed.), *Pediatric surgery* (3rd ed.). Philadelphia: WB Saunders.

Ferris, M. E, Brennan, P., & Portman, R. J. (1993). Neonatal nephrology. In G. B. Merenstein & S. L. Gardner (Eds.), *Handbook of neonatal intensive care*. (3rd ed.). St. Louis: Mosby.

Filmer, B. (1994). Renal diseases. In T. L. Gomella (Ed.), *Neonatology: Management, procedures, on-call problems, diseases and drugs* (3rd ed.). Stamford, CN: Appleton & Lange.

Gomella, T. L. (1993). *Neonatology: Management, procedures, on-call problems, diseases and drugs.* (3rd ed.). Stamford, CT: Appleton & Lange.

Heritage, C. K. (1994). Infant of diabetic mother. In T. L. Gomella (Ed.), *Neonatalogy: Management, procedures, on-call problems, diseases and drugs* (3rd ed.). Stamford, CT: Appleton & Lange.

Hirshfeld, A. B., Getachew, A., & Sessions, J. (2000). Drug doses. In G. K. Sidberry & R. Iannone (Eds.), *The Harriet Lane handbook* (15th ed.). St. Louis: Mosby.

Kaplan, G. W., & McAleer, I. M. (1999). Structural abnormalities of the genitourinary system. In G. B. Avery, M. A. Fletcher, & M.G. MacDonald (Eds.), *Neonatology: Pathophysiology and management of the newborn* (5th ed.). Philadelphia: Lippincott Williams & Wilkins.

Kenner, C., Amlanc, S., & Flandermeyer, A. (1998). *Protocols in neonatal nursing.* Philadelphia: W. B. Saunders.

Kenner, C., Brueggemeyer, A., & Gunderson, L. P. (1993). *Comprehensive neonatal nursing: A physiologic perspective.* Philadelphia: W. B. Saunders.

Lantz, K. E. (2000). Surgery. In G. K. Siberry & R. Iannone (Eds.), *The Harriet Lane Handbook* (15th ed.). St Louis: Mosby.

Lewy, J. (1994). Nephrology: Fluids and electrolytes. In R. Behrman & R. Kliegman (Eds.), *Nelson's essentials of pediatrics.* (2nd ed.). Philadelphia: W. B. Saunders.

Lott, J. W. (1994). *Neonatal infection: Assessment, diagnosis, and management.* Petaluma, CA: NICU Ink.

Moore, K. L. (1988). *Essentials of human embryology.* Illustrated by Herbst, M., & Thompson, M. Toronto: B. C. Decker, Inc.

Moore, K. L., Persaud, T. V. N., & Shiota, K. (1994). *Color atlas of clinical embryology.* Philadelphia: WB Saunders.

Murphy, J. P. (2000). Exstrophy of the bladder. In K.W. Ashcraft (Ed.), *Pediatric surgery* (3rd ed.). Philadelphia: WB Saunders.

Noseworthy, J. (2000). Neonatal torsion. In K.W. Ashcraft (Ed.), *Pediatric surgery* (3rd ed.). Philadelphia: WB Saunders.

Page, J. (1994). The newborn with ambiguous genitalia. *Neonatal Network 13*(5), 15–21.

Pulito, A. R. (1994). Surgical disease of the newborn. In T. L. Gomella (Ed.), *Neonatology: Management, procedures, on-call problems, diseases and drugs* (3rd ed.). Stamford, CT: Appleton & Lange.

Repetto, J. E. (1999). Ambiguous genitalia. In T. L. Gomella (Ed.), *Neonatology* (4th ed.). Stamford, CT: Appleton & Lange.

Seaman, S. (1995). Renal physiology: Part 2—Fluid and electrolyte regulation. *Neonatal Network, 14*(5), 5–11.

Spitzer, A., Bernstein, J., Borchus, H., & Edelman, C. (1992). Kidney and urinary tract. In A. Fanaroff & R. Martin (Eds.), *Neonatal-Perinatal medicine* (5th ed.). St Louis: Mosby.

Tappero, E., & Honeyfield, M. (1996). *Physical assessment of the newborn* (2nd ed.). Petaluma, CA: NICU Ink.

Vogt, B. A., & Avner, E. D. (2002). The kidney and urinary tract. In A. Fanaroff & R. Martin (Eds.), *Neonatal-Perinatal medicine* (7th ed., vol 2.). St. Louis: Mosby.

Wallen, E. M., & Shortliffe, L. (2000). Undescended testis and testicular tumors. In K. W. Ashcraft (Ed.), *Pediatric surgery* (3rd ed.). Philadelphia: WB Saunders.

Warner, B. W., & Ziegler, M. M. (2000). Exstrophy of the cloaca. In K. W. Ashcraft (Ed.), *Pediatric surgery* (3rd ed.). Philadelphia: WB Saunders.

Weber, T. R., & Tracy, T. F., Jr. (2000). Groin hernias and hydroceles. In K. W. Ashcraft (Ed.), *Pediatric surgery* (3rd ed.). Philadelphia: WB Saunders.

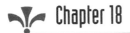 **Chapter 18**

Metabolic and Endocrine Disorders
Robin R. Maguire, MSN, RNC, NNP

I. Hereditary metabolic disorders
A. Introduction: there are more than 400 biochemical genetic disorders (Berry, 1998); most are X-linked or autosomal recessive.
B. Etiology (Stokowski, 1999):
    1. Can be related to the disruption of the synthesis or catabolism of complex molecules, which leads to permanent progressive symptoms.
    2. Can be related to the interference with the sequence of metabolism that leads to accumulation of toxic compounds.
    3. Can be related to deficiencies in energy production or use.
C. General clinical manifestations:
    1. May be present hours to months after birth.
    2. May mimic signs and symptoms of sepsis. Many people recommend a serum ammonia level for any infant < 3 months of age with suspected sepsis.
    3. Should be suspected in any infant who: appears healthy after birth but develops symptoms after the introduction of feeds; has unexplained severe metabolic acidosis; has recurrent vomiting; presents with an altered state of consciousness; has suspicion of sepsis; and has a family history of similar symptoms, mental retardation, sudden infant death syndrome (SIDS), or unexplained neonatal death.
    4. May present as an acute life-threatening event that is not responsive to the usual therapies.
    5. Clinical findings may include: gastrointestinal (**always suspect with vomiting**, poor feeding, poor weight gain, diarrhea, jaundice, or hepatomegaly); neurologic (lethargy, irritability, weak suck, tremors, seizures, hypertonicity, rigidity, or coma); cardiac (cardiomyopathy or arrhythmias); unusual odor or color of urine; respiratory (tachypnea, apnea, or respiratory distress); dysmorphic features; eyes (cataracts, ectopia lentis, cherry-red spot, corneal clouding, or pigmentary retinopathy); hair (alopecia, steely or kinky hair); skin (skin nodules, thick skin, ichthyosis, or skin lesions); and head (macrocephaly or microcephaly).
D. Diagnostic studies:
    1. State metabolic screening (refer to Section VII)
    2. Complete blood count (CBC) with differential
    3. Urinalysis: reducing substances, ketones, smell, and color
    4. Arterial blood gas (ABG): metabolic acidosis or respiratory alkalosis
    5. Serum electrolytes: increased anion gap usually > 16 (refer to

Chapter 7: Fluid and Electrolytes); anion gap is not present with all inborn errors of metabolism.

6. Blood glucose:

a. Hypoglycemia can be associated (Ozand, 2000): 3-Methylglutaconic aciduria; maple syrup urine disease; deficiency of 3-hydroxy-3-methylglutaryl CoA Lyase; propionic acidemia; methylmalonic acidemia; medium-chain Acyl-CoA dehydrogenase deficiency; glutaric aciduria Type 2; short-chain 3-hydroxyacyl-CoA dehydrogenase deficiency; carnitine/acylcarnitine translocase deficiency; and carnitine-palmityl transferase I and II deficiencies.

b. Hypoglycemia is not associated with glycogen storage disease type II.

7. Plasma ammonia level: frequently exceeds 1000 μmol/L (Burton, 1999).

8. Liver enzymes, including total and direct bilirubin levels

9. Plasma and urine amino acids; urine organic acids

10. Plasma lactate levels

11. May need more specialized testing (eg, skin biopsy and cerebrospinal fluid [CSF] testing).

E. Interventions:

1. Provide supportive care. Need to obtain results relatively quickly.

2. **Nothing by mouth (NPO) until diagnosis is obtained**

3. **Always make a metabolic/genetic referral and consider transfer to an institution that specializes in hereditary metabolic disorders.**

F. Outcomes: some inborn errors of metabolism are responsive to dietary changes; some inborn errors of metabolism are lethal and require palliative care.

II. Common inborn errors of carbohydrate metabolism

A. Galactosemia:

1. Etiology: GALK (galactokinase), GALT (galactose-1-phosphate uridyltransferase), and uridine 5-diphosphate galactose-4-epimerase are responsible for hepatic conversion of galactose to glucose following ingestion of dietary lactose (Berry, 1998). Deficiency in one or more of these enzymes results in the inability to digest lactose.

2. Clinical manifestations: presents with vomiting, poor feeding, jaundice, hepatomegaly, hypoglycemia, seizures, and lethargy. Cataracts usually develop by the second week of life. **Increased risk for *Escherichia coli* sepsis or gram-negative rod sepsis**

3. Diagnostic findings: may have positive urine reducing substances; high blood galactose levels, red blood cell (RBC) galactose-1-phosphate levels, and urine galactitol levels.

4. Interventions: treatment is a lifelong galactose-free diet.

B. Glycogen storage diseases:

1. Glycogen storage disease type I:

a. Etiology: decreased activity of glucose-6-phosphatase

b. Clinical manifestations: presents with poor growth, enlarged abdominal girth, hepatomegaly, and signs/symptoms of hypoglycemia

    c. Laboratory findings: fasting hypoglycemia, ketosis, lactic acidosis, hyperlipidemia, and hyperuricemia

    d. Diagnosis: based on hepatic enzyme analysis and/or molecular diagnostic testing

    e. Interventions: treatment consists of frequent feedings and restriction of lactose/sucrose.

  2. Glycogen storage disease type II (Pompe disease) (Tein,1999):

    a. Etiology: deficiency of the lysosomal enzyme α-glucosidase

    b. Clinical manifestations: presents with cardiomegaly with congestive heart failure (CHF), hepatomegaly, macroglossia, and hypotonia.

    c. Diagnosis is made on muscle biopsy.

    d. Interventions: high-protein diet; cardiac transplant is an option.

C. Hereditary fructose intolerance:

  1. Etiology: deficiency of the enzyme gructose-1,6-bisphosphate aldolase

  2. Clinical manifestations: usually does not present until infant ingests fruits or a formula that contains sucrose or fructose. Presents with poor feeding, vomiting, loose stools, poor growth, hepatomegaly, or signs/symptoms of hypoglycemia; may become pale and lethargic, with an altered state of consciousness soon after ingesting fruits or sucrose/fructose-containing formula.

  3. Laboratory findings: hypoglycemia, hypophosphatemia, elevation of serum alanine transferase and aspartate transaminase, reducing substances in the urine, and metabolic acidosis

  4. Diagnosis is made by an intravenous (IV) fructose test.

  5. Interventions: elimination of dietary fructose and sucrose

III. Common disorders of protein metabolism

A. Maple sugar urine disease (MSUD) (Berry, 1998):

  1. Etiology: deficiency of the enzyme BCKAD (branched-chain 2-keto dehydrogenase) complex

  2. Clinical manifestations: presents 2 to 3 days after birth with poor feeding, spitting, lethargy, high-pitched cry, hypotonia alternating with hypertonia, ophistotonic posturing, coma, and odor of maple syrup in urine, feces, breath, and cerumen.

  3. Diagnostic findings: metabolic acidosis, ketonuria, and elevated levels of amino acids, especially leucine

  4. Interventions: supportive care and formula without branched-chained amino acids. May need supplemental isoleucine and valine solutions to maintain normal plasma levels.

  5. Outcome: depends upon on how early the diagnosis is made.

B. Phenylketonuria (Berry, 1998; Burlina, Bonafe, & Zacchello, 1999):

  1. Etiology: deficiency in the activity of phenylamine hydrolase that converts phenylalanine into tyrosine

  2. Clinical manifestations: presents as vomiting, poor feeding, irritability or overactivity, seizures, hypopigmented skin/hair, eczema, and musty-smelling urine.

  3. Diagnostic findings: positive ferric chloride test of urine and elevated serum phenylalanine levels

  4. Intervention: low-protein diet and phenylalanine-absent formula

  5. Outcome: dependent upon how early the diagnosis is made

C. Nonketotic hyperglycinemia (Berry, 1998; Burlina, Bonafe, & Zacchello, 1999):

1. Clinical manifestations: presents as well newborn that manifests hiccups, seizures, and hypotonia within 12 to 36 hours and becomes comatose with an absence of tendon reflexes.
2. Laboratory findings: excessive serum and urine glycine levels; CSF glycine is elevated and out of proportion to serum glycine level (Berry, 1998).
3. Interventions: there is no effective treatment.

IV. Urea cycle defects

A. Most common defects: ornithine transcarbamylase (OTC) deficiency (most common); argininosuccinate lyase deficiency; argininosuccinate synthetase deficiency; carbamoylphosphate synthetase I deficiency

B. Etiology (Berry, 1998): defect within the five steps of the urea cycle; results in accumulation of ammonia; OTC is X-linked; all other urea cycle defects are autosomal recessive.

C. Clinical manifestations (Berry 1998; Burlina, Bonafe, & Zacchello, 1999): poor feeding and/or vomiting; hyperventilation; lethargy followed by coma within 12 to 24 hours of life

D. Clinical findings (Berry 1998; Burlina, Bonafe, & Zacchello, 1999): respiratory alkalosis; hyperammonemia; absence of metabolic acidosis; abnormal levels of plasma citrulline levels; abnormal levels of urinary orotate and argininosuccinic acid

E. Interventions:

1. Supportive care
2. Decrease dietary protein; hemodialysis to decrease serum ammonia levels
3. Alternative waste nitrogen therapy with sodium benzoate and sodium phenylacetate combined with arginine (Berry, 1998). Food and Drug Administration (FDA) approval for emergency use is required.

F. Outcome: death can occur despite dialysis; alternative waste nitrogen therapy with high-calorie intake can decrease mortality (Barry, 1998).

1. Liver transplant is recommended (Scaglia et al., 2002).

V. Common defects in organic acid metabolism

A. Isovaleric acidemia (Berry, 1998; Burlina, Bonafe, & Zacchello, 1999):

1. Etiology: selective deficiency of isovaleryl-CoA dehydrogenase
2. Clinical manifestations: poor feeding, vomiting, lethargy, seizures, coma, and an odor of sweaty feet
3. Laboratory findings: markedly elevated level of isovalerylglycine in the urine
4. Interventions: dialysis, protein restriction, intravenous (IV) fluids with glucose and sodium bicarbonate, and glaucine
5. Outcome: most do not survive.

B. Propionic acidemia (Berry 1998; Burlina, Bonafe, & Zacchello, 1999):

1. Etiology: selective deficiency of propionyl-CoA carboxylase. Precursors for propionyl-CoA carboxylase are isoleucine, valine, methionine, threonine, pyrimidine compound, thymine, and odd-chain fatty acids.

2. Clinical manifestations: poor feeding, vomiting, lethargy, hypotonia, seizures, hepatomegaly, ketosis, leukopenia, thrombocytopenia, and metabolic acidosis with/without increased anion gap

3. Laboratory findings: excessive concentrations of methylcitrate, propionylglycine, 2-methyl-3-hydroxybutyrate, 2-methylacetoacetate in the urine. Plasma glycine levels may be elevated. Propionyl-CoA carboxylase may be assayed in the WBC or skin fibroblasts (Berry, 1998).

4. Interventions: eliminate protein, correct the acidosis and thrombocytopenia, and provide dialysis if necessary.

5. Outcome: despite low-protein diet, most neonates do not survive the first decade of life (Berry, 1998).

VI. Common disorders of fatty acids

A. Most common defects: medium-chain Acyl-CoA dehydrogenase deficiency (one of the most common disorders) (Burton, 1999); very-long-chain Acyl-CoA dehydrogenase deficiency; short-chain Acyl-CoA dehydrogenase deficiency; glutaric acidemia type 2; carnitine palmitoyltransferase type I deficiency; acylcarnitine translocase deficiency; carnitine palmitoyltransferase type II deficiency; and long-chain 3-Hydroxyzcyl-CoA dehydrogenase deficiency

B. Etiology (Barry, 1998; Burton, 1999): deficiency of the enzymes responsible for oxidizing fatty acids during periods of fasting

C. Clinical manifestations: hypoglycemia; metabolic acidosis; cardiomyopathy; hypotonia (except for the carnitine deficiencies)

D. Clinical findings (Tein, 1999): hypoglycemia; metabolic acidosis; moderate hyperammonemia; organic acidemia; abnormal liver functions; elevated CPK; and diagnosis may be assayed on WBC, muscle or liver biopsy, or skin fibroblasts.

E. Treatment (Tein, 1999): prognosis is dependent upon the defect; goal is prevention of hypoglycemia using high carbohydrate, low fat diets; may need carnitine supplementation.

VII. Hereditary metabolic screening

A. Testing: performed in all 50 states and Washington, DC; great individuality between states. Only PKU and hypothyroidism are tested in each state. It is important to know which screening tests are done in your state or country; tandem mass spectrometry is the newest development in neonatal screening. This method measures many different molecules in a single test and allows for more accurate testing as well as more accurately identifying specific disorders. At present, 50 inherited disorders are being screened. For more information, go to *http://www.neogenscreening.com*.

B. Procedure: it is recommended that the sample be obtained after 24 hours of age or within seven days if not feeding; repeat specimens are required if the neonate is discharged before 24 hours of age or had not established feedings before the initial screening.

VIII. Metabolic bone disease

A. Risk factors:

1. Fetal or congenital rickets is rare but may occur with the following conditions: maternal causes (severe maternal nutritional osteomalacia, hypoparathyroidism or hyperparathyroidism, and prolonged treatment with magnesium or phosphate); inherited

defects (renal tubular disorders, vitamin D or parathyroid disorders, and lysosomal storage disease [eg, I-cell]).

2. Premature infants are at risk secondary to the following reasons: did not receive active transport of calcium and phosphorus during the last trimester; prolonged exposure of total parental nutrition (TPN) with low calcium and phosphorus supplementation; long-term loop diuretic therapy; and feedings with soy formula or human milk without supplementation.

3. Rare for term infants and is usually associated with limited calcium and vitamin D intake.

B. Clinical manifestations: usually asymptomatic and found serendipitously; may have pain with handling.

C. Diagnosis:

1. Classic radiographic features are generalized bone demineralization (washed-out appearance), and widening, cupping, and fraying of the distal metaphyses.

2. Testing includes serum calcium (normal), serum phosphorus (low), serum alkaline phosphatase (high), and 1,25-dihydroxyvitamin D level (high).

D. Interventions:

1. Responds to nutritional therapy; maintain Ca/P ratio of 1.3:1 to 1.7:1 in total parental nutrition; calcium and phosphorus supplementation. **Phosphorus must always be added to calcium supplementation to diminish the risk of nephrocalcinosis**.

2. Use premature formulas or supplement maternal breast milk with human milk fortifier.

3. Rickets of prematurity needs a daily maintenance dose of vitamin D (Umpaichitra, Bastian, & Castells, 2001).

IX. Disorders of the parathyroid gland

A. Function: parathyroid gland is located by the thyroid gland; secretes parathyroid hormone (PTH), which is the primary regulator of serum calcium; PTH increases serum calcium by mobilizing calcium from the bone, increasing calcium reabsorption in the kidneys, and indirectly acting on the formation of vitamin D.

B. Hypoparathyroidism (Steffensrud, 2000):

1. Risk factors: congenital (eg, familial isolated hypoparathyroidism, DiGeorge syndrome, or Kerry-Caffy syndrome); transient or secondary (eg, maternal hypoparathyroidism, premature infants, infants of a diabetic [IDM] mother, and birth asphyxia)

2. Diagnosis: low serum calcium and high serum phosphorus with normal renal function; PTH levels will be low or high if the underlying problem is end-organ responsiveness.

3. Clinical manifestations: may be subtle; muscle jerking, twitching, and seizures; lethargy; poor feeding; apnea; prolonged bleeding; decreased cardiac contractility, poor perfusion, tachycardia, and/or hypotension; decreased bone mineralization; and suspect if not able to maintain normal serum calcium levels

4. Treatment:

   a. Transient hypoparathyroidism requires short-term calcium supplementation.

    b. Congenital disorder requires lifelong calcium and vitamin D supplementation with reduction in phosphorus intake. (Umpaichitra et al., 2001).

    c. PTH administration is experimental (Steffensrud, 2000).

C. Hyperparathyroidism (Steffensrud, 2000):

  1. Etiology: rare but life-threatening; primary hyperparathyroidism is characterized by hyperplasia of all four glands and may be inherited (Steffensrud, 2000); secondary hyperparathyroidism is usually the result of maternal hypoparathyroidism.

  2. Diagnosis: family history; high serum calcium, low serum phosphorus, and high PTH; increased renal excretion of sodium, potassium, and bicarbonate

  3. Clinical manifestations: constipation, poor feeding, dehydration, and failure to thrive; lethargy, hypotonia, and exaggerated tendon reflexes; respiratory distress; metabolic acidosis; hematuria; and radiographic subperiosteal bone reabsorption with generalized bone demineralization, and unexplained bone fractures

  4. Treatment:

    a. Immediate therapy: maintain respiratory status and blood pressure; correct acidosis; lower serum calcium levels with furosemide administration

    b. Long-term therapy secondary to primary hyperparathyroidism: restriction of calcium and vitamin D (including restricting sunlight exposure) and phosphorus supplementation

    c. Total parathyroidectomy with autotransplantation is possible (Steffensrud, 2000).

X. Disorders of the thyroid gland

  A. Function (Stokowski, 1999): thyroid gland has two lobes joined by the isthmus and located below the cricoid cartilage; assists with thermogenesis, cardiac output, erythropoiesis, respiratory drive, gut motility, and carbohydrate, protein, and lipid metabolism; growth of organs, tissues, and the central nervous system (CNS), especially the brain; and potentiates the actions of catecholamines by means of increased β-adrenergic receptor binding.

  B. Hormonal regulation:

    1. Thyroid stimulating hormone (TSH) is released from the pituitary in response to thyrotropin-releasing hormone (TRH).

    2. TSH stimulates the thyroid to release thyroxine (T4) and tri-iodothyronine (T3).

    3. T4 and T3 bind with thyroid-binding globulin (TBG), which carries 70% of circulating hormone (Stokowski, 1999).

    4. T4 is converted to T3 (metabolically active form).

    5. Requirements for hormonal regulation are an intact Hypothalamic-Pituitary Axis, adequate iodine supply within the thyroid gland, deiodinase enzymes to convert T4 to T3, and sufficient TBG.

  C. Hypothyroidism:

    1. Congenital hypothyroidism:

      a. Etiology (Moshang & Thorton, 1999; Stokowski, 1999): thyroid dysgenesis (absent, hypoplastic, or ectopic [most common]); thyroid or end-organ unresponsiveness to hormones; familial dyshormonogenesis; maternal exposure to radioiodine, pro-pylthiouracil (PTU), or methimazole during pregnancy; defects in the pituitary gland; and TBG deficiency (X-linked)

b. Clinical manifestations:
  (1) Symptoms usually not seen until later unless infant is severely affected
  (2) Large open fontanel; large birth weight (> 4 kg) or gestation longer than 42 weeks
  (3) Hypothermia; hypotonia; lethargy
  (4) Poor feeding, abdominal distention, and jaundice lasting longer than 3 days
  (5) Goiter
  (6) Late signs: dry skin, macroglossia, coarse hair, puffy eyelids, hoarse cry, myxedema, and constipation (Stokowski, 1999)

c. Diagnostic studies:
  (1) Usually diagnosed by newborn screening: low T4 and high TSH; rarely, low T4 and low TSH; low T4 and normal TSH can be seen with ectopic or hypoplastic thyroids (Stokowski, 1999)
  (2) Thyroid functions are elevated in the newborn period (Moshang & Thorton, 1999): obtain T4, free T4, TSH, T3, and TGB; thyroid scan

d. Treatment:
  (1) Consult an endocrinologist.
  (2) Levothyroxine (Synthyroid) (Zenk, Sills, & Koepel, 2000): should be instituted as soon as possible and continued throughout life; dosage is adjusted according to T4 and TSH levels and should be monitored frequently.
  (3) TBG deficiency has no treatment (Stokowski, 1999).

e. Outcome: prognosis of mental development is dependent upon the onset of therapy; children whose treatment started within 1 month of age have a good prognosis for mental development (Moshang & Thorton, 1999).

2. Transient conditions:
  a. Euthyroid sick syndrome occurs in acute and chronic illnesses. Presents with low T4, very low T3, elevated reversed T3, and normal TSH levels (Fisher, 1998; Moshang & Thorton, 1999). Usually, no treatment is necessary.
  b. Transient primary hypothyroidism is rare; occurs more frequently in Europe than the United States. Presents with low T4 and high TSH. Temporary administration of iodine is recommended (Polk & Fisher, 1998).
  c. Transient hypothyroxinemia (Fisher, 1998; Kok, Briet, & van Wassenar, 2001; Paul Leef, Stefano, & Bartoshesky, 1998; Ruess, Paneth, Pinto-Martin, Lorenz & Susser, 1996): common among preterm infants

(1) Etiology: presumed to be due to immature H-P-T axis, low/high iodine, and other factors related to immaturity. Usually, by 4 to 6 weeks of age the T4 will be trending toward normal.

(2) Laboratory findings: **low** T4 and **normal** TSH

(3) Interventions: it is believed that no treatment is recommended at this time but studies are ongoing. If etiology is unclear (ie, transient versus congenital), follow thyroid levels and weigh the risk/benefits of starting Levothyroxine.

(4) Outcome: premature infants with low T4 may be at risk for intravascular hemorrhage (IVH), increased mortality, lower scores on neurodevelopmental outcomes, and cerebral palsy.

D. Hyperthyroidism:

1. Etiology: rare in neonates; usually born to mothers with Grave's disease (Moshang & Thorton, 1999) or born to mothers with Hashimoto thyroiditis

2. Clinical manifestations (onset of symptoms is usually within the first 2 weeks of age): irritability, tremors, and hyperactivity; hyperthermia, sweating, and flushing; vomiting and diarrhea; CHF, tachycardia, and hypertension (HTN); hepatosplenomegaly and jaundice; and exophthalmos, staring, and lid retraction

3. Diagnostic studies: total and free T4 are elevated; TSH low; antibody levels can be measured.

4. Interventions: maintain airway (thyroid may be pressing against the trachea); use β-adrenergic blockers or Digoxin; maintain cardiac output; sedatives; agents to suppress thyroid function (10% potassium iodide or Lugol's iodine solution); and monitor thyroid functions.

5. Outcomes: most cases resolve within 9 months (Moshang & Thorton, 1999); may have rapid bone growth and premature craniosynostosis.

XI. Disorders of the pituitary gland

A. Function: hypothalamus regulates the anterior pituitary by secreting stimulating hormones and inhibiting hormones (Moshang & Thorton, 1999); anterior pituitary secretes growth hormone, TSH, ACTH, prolactin (PR), luteinizing hormone (LH), and follicle-stimulating hormone (FSH); posterior pituitary secretes vasopressin and oxytocin.

B. Disorders of the anterior pituitary:

1. Etiology (Moshang & Thorton, 1999): malformations (may be associated with cleft lip and palate, optic nerve atrophy, septooptic dysplasia, transphenoidal encephalocele, holoprosencephaly, and anencephaly); trauma; congenital infection; tumor; isolated or combined familial or idiopathic pituitary hormone deficiency; and autosomal-recessive or X-linked recessive familial panhypopituitarism

2. Clinical manifestations: suspect with midline defects; may not be evident in neonatal period; most common symptoms are hypo-

glycemia, micropenis, and cholestatic jaundice (Moshang & Thorton, 1999).

3. Diagnostic studies: imaging of brain; ophthalmologic examination; hormone levels (ACTH, thyroid, and growth hormone); and ACTH stimulation and growth hormone testing

4. Treatment:
   a. Consult endocrinologist.
   b. Treatment based on severity of symptoms
   c. May require growth hormone, glucocorticoid replacement, human chorionic gonadotropin (HCG), testosterone, and thyroxine.

5. Outcome: outcome dependent on etiology; administering HCG and/or testosterone may increase penile growth (Moshang & Thorton, 1999).

C. Disorders of posterior pituitary gland:
   1. Diabetes insipidus (DI) (Moshang & Thorton, 1999):
      a. Etiology: primary causes (autosomal dominant, X-linked, and idiopathic); secondary causes (malformation sequences, birth trauma, periventricular hemorrhage, and infection)
      b. Clinical manifestations: may have history of polyhydramnios; may present with failure to thrive, irritability, fever, vomiting, weight loss, and hypernatremia; always suspect in symptomatic, cachectic-appearing, and hypernatremic infant; continued output greater than 60% of fluid intake and/or single void greater than 6 mL/kg/hr.
      c. Diagnostic studies:
         (1) Urine electrolytes, specific gravity, and osmolarity
         (2) Serum electrolytes and osmolarity
         (3) Diagnosis: inappropriately diluted urine in the presence of hyperosmolar serum *and* appropriate urine output after vasopressin administration
      d. Interventions:
         (1) Treat shock with fluid resuscitation; administer several times the maintenance of free water.
         (2) Severe dehydration: administer aqueous vasopressin because it is short acting.
         (3) Long-term treatment: administer long-acting analog of vasopressin.
         (4) Avoid rapid shifts in serum sodium secondary to excessive intake or output.
         (5) Consider one-third diluted formula to provide free water while maintaining caloric content for growth.
         (6) Follow serum electrolytes and urine output closely.
   2. Syndrome of inappropriate antidiuretic hormone secretion (SIADH) (Moshang & Thorton, 1999):
      a. Etiology: ADH levels are increased in premature infants; sick neonates (birth asphyxia, pneumothorax, pulmonary interstitial emphysema, artificial ventilation, hemorrhage, surgery, pain, and periventricular hemorrhage)
      b. Clinical manifestations: history of being ill or premature; low urine output with high specific gravity; may have edema,

weight gain, tachycardia, increased pulse pressures, and increased work of breathing.

   c. Diagnostic studies:

     (1) Urinary sodium, specific gravity, and osmolarity: urine sodium may be > 20–30 mEq/L; urine osmolarity > serum osmolarity

     (2) Serum electrolytes and osmolarity: serum sodium (low); serum osmolarity < urine osmolarity

     (3) Low urine output, high urinary sodium and osmolarity in the presence of low serum sodium and lower serum osmolarity

   d. Treatment: fluid restriction (40–60 mL/kg/day); follow serum sodium and osmolarity, urine sodium and osmolarity; urine output; determine cause for SIADH.

XII. Disorders of the adrenal glands

   A. Function: adrenal glands are located above, behind, and medial to the kidneys. Two separate glands: adrenal medulla secretes epinephrine and norepinephrine in response to sympathetic stimulation. It is rare to have disorders in the neonatal period; adrenal cortex secretes glucocorticoids (cortisol or hydrocortisone), mineralocorticoids (aldosterone and desoxycorticosterone), and androgenic hormones via negative feedback from the hypothalamus-pituitary axis.

   B. Congenital adrenal hyperplasia (CAH):

     1. Etiology (Polk, 1998):

       a. Inherited defects in the enzymes of cortisol synthesis: 21-Hydroxylase deficiency (most common); 11-β-hydroxylase deficiency; 17-hydroxylase deficiency; 3-β-hydroxysteroid dehydrogenase deficiency; and 20,22-desmolase deficiency

       b. Impaired cortisol secretion results in hypersecretion of ACTH and consequent hyperplasia of the adrenal cortex, thereby causing excessive production of adrenal androgens.

     2. Clinical manifestations (Collett-Solberg, 2001; Moshang & Thorton, 1999):

       a. Depends upon the site and severity of enzyme block: simple virilizing form (salt-loss is mild; adrenal insufficiency occurs only under stress); salt-losing form (usually leads to adrenal crisis during the neonatal period)

       b. Suspect CAH in any child with ambiguous genitalia (including isolated bilateral cryptorchidism), newborns presenting with shock and dehydration, or males/females with signs of inappropriate virilization

       c. Symptoms for adrenal crisis usually present within 5 to 30 days of life and may include vomiting, poor feeding, dehydration, dehydration, failure to thrive, hyponatremia, hyperkalemia, hypoglycemia, and acidosis.

       d. Hypertension is possible with 11-hydroxylase deficiency and 17 α-hydroxylase defect.

     3. Diagnostic studies:

       a. Newborn screening (some states and countries measure 17-OH progesterone)

       b. Physical examination (Collett-Solberg, 2001):

(1) Females may have urogenital sinus, scrotalization of the labia majora, labial fusion, clitoromegaly, or formation of penile urethra. They may appear normal in some forms of CAH.

(2) Males may appear undervirilized, hypospadias, or normal in appearance.

(3) Hyperpigmentation, especially the extensor creases and genitalia (Moshang & Thornton, 1999)

  c. Testing:

    (1) Chromosomes

    (2) Serum electrolytes (hyponatremia and increased potassium are suggestive of mineralocorticoid deficiency); serum glucose

    (3) Specific enzymes: 17-hydroxyprogesterone; 17-OH pregnenolone; 11-hydroxylase; 3 β-hydroxysteroid dehydrogenase; dehydroepiandrosterone (DHEA); and androstenedione

    (4) ACTH and renin levels

    (5) Adrenal and pelvic ultrasounds

4. Interventions:

  a. Fluid resuscitation with 20 mL/kg of normal saline; begin IV administration at twice the maintenance volume and use D5W/0.9NSS.

  b. Draw specific enzymes (see above) before administering ACTH; administer ACTH stimulation test; repeat ACTH and other specific enzymes and cortisol levels; if ACTH is elevated after test, give hydrocortisone.

  c. Will require long-term cortisol (hydrocortisone) and mineralocorticoid (9 α-fludrocortisone) replacement.

  d. Always consult a pediatric endocrinologist and consider transport to an institution that specializes in endocrinology and has the medical, surgical, and psychologic support services needed.

5. Outcomes: will need extra cortisol during times of stress; follow bone growth; for virilized females, a team approach will be necessary to determine each individual's need for and timing of reconstructive surgery (Collett-Solberg, 2001).

C. Adrenal insufficiency:

  1. Etiology (Polk, 1998): adrenal hemorrhage; transient or iatrogenic adrenal insufficiency; congenital adrenal hypoplasia; isolated aldosterone deficiency; pseudohypoaldosteronism; congenital adrenal ACTH resistance; neonatal adrenoleukodystrophy; infantile glycerol kinase deficiency

  2. Clinical manifestations:

    a. Congenital hypoplasia will present as a neonate with profound hypoglycemia, poor feeding, and failure to thrive.

    b. Transient insufficiency may present as hyponatremia, hyperkalemia, polyuria, dehydration, and failure to thrive.

  3. Diagnostic studies:

    a. Serum electrolytes; serum glucose; serum and urinary cortisol levels

    b. ACTH and renin levels; ACTH stimulation testing

    c. Adrenal ultrasounds

4. Interventions: supportive care; may consider short course of glu-cocorticoid treatment if transient. Congenital hypoplasia will require lifelong cortisol replacement.
   5. Outcomes: transient insufficiency does not require lifelong replacement therapy; outcome for other causes is dependent upon the etiology.
D. Adrenal hemorrhage:
   1. Etiology: usually from mechanical trauma during the birth process
   2. Clinical manifestations:
      a. May be asymptomatic.
      b. Usually presents with pallor, apnea, hypothermia with falling hematocrit (Hct), and jaundice (Polk, 1998). May present in hypovolemic shock if severe enough.
      c. Flank mass (usually the right side)
      d. Signs of adrenal insufficiency do not usually present unless there is bilateral bleeding with 90% of the adrenocortical tis-sue destroyed (Black & Williams as cited by Polk, 1998).
   3. Diagnostic testing: adrenal ultrasound
   4. Interventions:
      a. No intervention if asymptomatic; treat shock with volume replacement.
      b. Steroid replacement is recommended if there is bilateral hem-orrhage and symptoms of adrenal insufficiency.
      c. ACTH stimulation testing should be done after the acute phase.
   5. Outcomes (Polk, 1998): calcification formation; adrenal function generally improves.

▼ References

Berry, G. T. (1998). Inborn errors of carbohydrate, ammonia, amino acids and organic acid metabolism. In H. W. Taeusch & R. A. Ballard (Eds.), *Avery's diseases of the newborn* (7th ed., pp. 245–274). Philadelphia: WB Saunders.

Burlina, A. B., Bonate, L., & Zacchello, F. (1999). Clinical and biochemical approach neonate with a suspected inborn error of amino acid and organic acid metabo-lism. *Seminars in Perinatology, 23*(2), 162–173.

Burton, B. K. (1999). Inherited metabolic disorders. In G. B. Avery, M. A. Fletcher, & M. G. MacDonald (Eds.) *Neonatology: Pathophysiology and management of the newborn* (5th ed., pp. 839–858). Philadelphia: Lippincott Williams & Wilkins.

Chen, Y. T. (2000). Defects in metabolism of carbohydrates: Defects in galactose metabolism. In R. E. Behrman, R. M. Kliegman, & H. B. Jenson (Eds.), *Nelson textbook of pediatrics* (16th ed., pp. 413). Philadelphia: WB Saunders.

Collett-Solberg, P. F. (2001). Congenital adrenal hyperplasia from genetics and bio-chemistry to clinical practice: Part 2. *Clinical Pediatrics, 40,* 125–132.

Fisher, D. A. (1998). Thyroid function in premature infants: The hypothyroxinemia of prematurity. *Clinics in Perinatology: Emerging Concepts in Perinatal Endocrinology, 25*(4), 999–1014.

Kok, J. H., Briet, J. M., & vanWassenar, A. G. (2001). Postnatal thyroid hormone replacement in very preterm infants. *Seminars in Perinatology, 25*(6), 417–425.

Moshang, T., & Thorton, P. S. (1999). Endocrine disorders of the newborn. In G. B. Avery, M. A. Fletcher, & M. G. MacDonald (Eds.), *Neonatology: Pathophysiology and management of the newborn* (5th ed., pp. 859–886). Philadelphia: Lippincott Williams & Wilkins.

Ozand, P. T. (2000). Hypoglycemia in association with various organic and amino acid disorders. *Seminars in Perinatology, 24*(2), 172–193.

Paul, D. A., Leef, K. H., Stefano, J. L., & Bartoshesky, L. (1998). Low serum thyroxine on initial newborn screening is associated with intraventricular hemorrhage and death in very low birth weight infants. *Pediatrics, 101*(5), 903–907.

Polk, D. H. (1998). Disorders of the adrenal gland. In H. W. Tauesch & R. A. Ballard (Eds.), *Avery's diseases of the newborn* (7th ed., pp. 1027–1214). Philadelphia: WB Saunders.

Polk, D. H., & Fisher, D. A. (1998). Disorders of the thyroid gland. In H. W. Tauesch & R. A. Ballard (Eds.), *Avery's diseases of the newborn* (7th ed., pp. 1224–1234). Philadelphia: WB Saunders.

Rezvani, J. (2000). Defects in metabolism of amino acids. In R. E. Behrman, R. M. Kliegman, & H. B. Jenson (Eds.), *Nelson textbook of pediatrics* (16th ed., pp. 344–376). Philadelphia: WB Saunders.

Reuss, M. L., Paneth, N., Pinto-Martin, J. A., Lorenz, J. J. M., & Susser, M. (1996). The relation of transient hypothyroxinemia in preterm infants to neurologic development at two years of age. *New England Journal of Medicine, 334*, 821–827.

Scaglia, F., Zheng, Q., O'Brien, W. E., Henry, J., Rosenberger, J., Reeds, P., & Lee, B. (2002). An integrated approach to the diagnosis and prospective management of partial orthithine transcarbamylase deficiency. *Pediatrics, 109*(1), 150–152.

Steffensrud, S. (2000). Parathyroids: The forgotten glands. *Neonatal Network, 19*(1), 9–16.

Stokowski, L. C. (1999). Endocrine disorders. In J. Deacon & P. O'Neill (Eds.), *Core curriculum for neonatal intensive care nursing* (2nd ed., pp. 357–382). Philadelphia: WB Saunders.

Stokowski, L. C. (1999). Metabolic disorders. In J. Deacon & P. O'Neil (Eds.), *Core curriculum for neonatal intensive care nursing,* (2nd ed., pp. 326–356). Philadelphia: WB Saunders.

Tein, I. (1999). Neonatal metabolic myopathies. *Seminars in Perinatology, 23*(2), 125–151.

Umpaichitra, V., Bastian, W., & Castells, S. (2001). Hypocalcemia in children: Pathogenesis and management. *Clinical Pediatrics, 40*, 305–312.

Zenk, K. E., Sills, J. H., & Koeppel, R. M. (2000). Neonatal medications and nutrition: A comprehensive guide (2nd ed.). Santa Rosa, CA: NICU Ink.

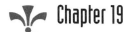 **Chapter 19**

Dysmorphism

Paulette S. Haws, MSN, RNC, NNP

Because approximately 3% of live-born infants have a major anomaly and there are at least 500 known developmental anomalies (Halle, 1993), it is not possible to discuss each one. This chapter contains definitions that clarify types of problems in morphogenesis, patterns of malformation and the etiology of dysmorphism, and information regarding some of the more commonly recognized patterns of dysmorphism. Key physical features observable during the neonatal period appear in italics.

I. Dysmorphism: abnormality of shape

A. General terms:
   1. Phenotype: the observable physical features present in an individual that are the manifestation of his or her genotype
   2. Genotype: the specific genetic makeup of an individual
   3. Congenital anomaly: an abnormal structural defect present at birth; an anomaly does not denote the etiology of a defect.

B. Types of problems in morphogenesis (Hudgins & Cassidy, 1997; Kirby, 1993):
   1. Malformation: primary structural defect in tissue formation secondary to abnormal development of the tissue caused by genetic or teratogenic reasons (eg, neural tube defects, congenital heart defects)
   2. Deformation: structural defect caused by abnormal mechanical forces, often due to the intrauterine environment, exerting pressure on normally developed tissues (eg, clubfoot, abnormal head shape)
   3. Disruption: refers to an interruption of development of intrinsically normal tissue and affects a body part rather than a specific organ (eg, amniotic bands).
   4. Dysplasia: a primary defect resulting in the lack of normal organization of cells into tissues (eg, bronchopulmonary dysplasia—iatrogenic lung disease secondary to positive pressure ventilation)

C. Patterns of malformation:
   1. Syndrome: a recognizable pattern of multisystem anomalies stemming from a single specific cause (eg, trisomy 21) (Kirby, 1993)
   2. Sequence: a single defect during development (variable etiology) that can be identified as the causal factor for other anomalies (eg, Potter's [oligohydramnios sequence], Pierre Robin Sequence)
   3. Association: a combination of defects occurring together but in a less fixed group than a syndrome; no specific or known etiology is identified (eg, VACTERL Association).

D. Etiology of dysmorphism (Hudgins & Cassidy, 1997):

1. Genetic: single gene; chromosomal; and multifactorial (interaction of multiple genetic and environmental factors)
2. Teratogens: anything external to the fetus that leads to postnatal structural or functional disability: chemicals, drugs, and radiation; infectious agents; and uterine factors (eg, decreased amniotic fluid, uterine anatomic abnormalities)
3. Unknown etiology

II. Commonly observed patterns of dysmorphism

A. Achondroplasia (Cooperman & Thompson, 1997; Jones, 1997): most common of the skeletal dysplasias, ie, a group of disorders that produces short stature, many recognizable at birth and others only recognizable during growth and development
1. Etiology: a defect in a gene that encodes fibroblast growth factor receptor 3 (FGFR3) located at chromosome 4p16.3; autosomal-dominant inheritance; approximately 90% are new mutations.
2. Physical manifestations:
  a. Extremities: *short limbs and normal trunk*; bowed bilateral lower extremities; *short trident hand, fingers similar in length* (Cooperman & Thompson, 1997)
  b. Facial: *megalocephaly*; *low nasal bridge with prominent forehead*; *mild midfacial hypoplasia*; and narrow nasal passages
  c. Vertebral: small cuboid-shaped vertebra; lumbar lordosis; thoracolumbar kyphosis
  d. Central nervous system (CNS): mild hypotonia and normal intelligence
3. Outcome:
  a. Increased risk for osteoarthritis as an adult
  b. Respiratory complications secondary to small thorax and possible upper airway obstruction; "sleep-disordered breathing"
  c. There are lethal forms of skeletal dysplasias (eg, thanatophoric dysplasia, achondrogenesis, and type II osteogenesis imperfecta).

B. Apert syndrome (acrocephalosyndactyly) (Jones, 1997):
1. Etiology: autosomal dominant; the majority of cases are sporadic and associated with older paternal age. The gene that is responsible is a mutation in the fibroblast growth factor receptor 2 (FGFR2) gene located on chromosome 10q25-q26 (same loci as Crouzon syndrome).
2. Physical manifestations:
  a. CNS: *absent corpus callosum*; nonprogressive ventriculomegaly; progressive hydrocephalus; and gyral, hippocampal, and septum pellucidum abnormalities
  b. Craniofacial: *craniosynostosis*; *large fontanels* may be present; and *midface hypoplasia; hypertelorism; down-slanting palpebral fissures*
  c. Skeletal: *syndactyly of fingers and toes* (often with complete fusion of second, third, and fourth fingers); *broad distal thumb and great toe*; and *cervical vertebrae fusion* (usually C5-C6)
3. Outcome:
  a. Airway compromise secondary to small nasopharynx, decreased patency of nares, and tracheal cartilage abnormalities

    b. Surgical repair of craniosynostosis
    c. Mental deficiency in most patients
    d. Dental abnormalities; malocclusion
C. Beckwith-Wiedemann syndrome (Jones, 1997; Kalhan & Saker, 1997; Shephard & Kupke, 1998):
    1. Etiology: many have normal chromosomes; abnormal karyotypes have been noted (eg, duplication of chromosome 11p15.5, balanced translocation of chromosomes 11p and 22q, duplication of distal two third of chromosome 8q, and deletion of upper half of chromosome 12p)
    2. Physical manifestations:
        a. *Macrosomia*; visceromegaly (liver, kidney, and spleen)
        b. Facial: *macroglossia*; *midface hypoplasia*; prominent occiput; *large fontanels*; *nevus flammeus*; and ear creases/pits
        c. Abdominal wall defects: *omphalocele*; hernia; diastasis recti; and prune belly
        d. *Hypoglycemia* probably secondary to hyperinsulinemia (most resolve spontaneously)
        e. Occasional cardiac defects
        f. Neonatal polycythemia
    3. Outcome: may have normal intelligence; infants are predisposed to adrenal carcinomas and nephroblastomas.
D. CHARGE Association (Jones, 1997; Shephard & Kupke, 1998):
    1. Etiology: unknown; many of the anomalies stem from a problem in morphogenesis during the second month of gestation. Many anomalies overlap with those found in VACTERL(S) Association.
    2. Associated physical manifestations:
        a. *C*oloboma
        b. *H*eart defects: tetralogy of Fallot; atrial septal defect (ASD), ventricular septal defect (VSD), patent ductus arteriosus (PDA); and double outlet right ventricle with atrioventricular (AV) canal
        c. Choanal *a*tresia
        d. *R*etarded growth and development; CNS abnormalities
        e. *G*enital hypoplasia (in males)
        f. *E*ar anomalies; deafness
    3. Outcome:
        a. Death during the perinatal period with severe defects
        b. Decreased linear growth during first 6 months of life possibly due to growth hormone deficiency
        c. Most infants have some degree of mental deficiency; visual and/or auditory handicaps
E. Cri-du-chat syndrome (5p deletion syndrome) (Jones, 1997):
    1. Etiology: partial deletion of the short arm of chromosome 5; approximately 85% of the cases are sporadic new mutations whereas the remaining 15% are secondary to an unequal segregation of a parental translocation.
    2. Physical manifestations:
        a. *Cat-like cry during infancy*

        b. *Low birth weight* and slow postnatal growth

        c. Hypotonia

        d. Craniofacial: *microcephaly*; *hypertelorism*; *epicanthal folds; downward slant of palpebral fissures*; and low-set and/or malformed ears

        e. Occasional congenital heart defect

        f. *Simian crease*

    3. Outcome: mental deficiency in all affected patients; scoliosis frequently occurs.

F. Crouzon syndrome (Jones, 1997):

    1. Etiology: autosomal dominant; approximately 25% represent fresh mutation; variable expression; caused by a mutation in the FGFR2 gene located at chromosome 10q25-q26 (same loci as Apert syndrome)

    2. Physical manifestations: *craniosynostosis*; *hypertelorism; exophthalmos secondary to shallow orbits; frontal bossing*; and *curved parrot-like nose* (possible)

    3. Outcome:

        a. Poor visual acuity

        b. Surgical repair of craniosynostosis to relieve increased intracranial pressure (ICP) and allow proper brain growth; elective repair for cosmetic reasons

        c. Mental deficiency (occasional)

G. Ellis van Creveld syndrome (chondroectodermal dysplasia) (Jones, 1997):

    1. Etiology: autosomal recessive; found mainly in the Amish population

    2. Physical manifestations:

        a. *Small stature; small thorax*

        b. Teeth and mouth: *neonatal teeth*; partial anodontia (congenital absence of the teeth); and *short upper lip* bound by frenula to alveolar ridge

        c. Extremities: *polydactyly of fingers and/or toes*; *hypoplastic nails; irregularly short extremities; hypoplasia of upper lateral tibia; extra and malformed carpal bones*; and talipes equinovarus

        d. Cardiovascular: *ASD*, often with single atrium

        e. Other: mental retardation (occasionally); Dandy-Walker malformation; scant or fine hair; cryptorchidism; epispadius; renal agenesis

    3. Outcome:

        a. Approximately 50% die in infancy secondary to cardiorespiratory compromise.

        b. Most of those who survive have normal intelligence; some limitation in hand function; dental problems

H. Fanconi's pancytopenia syndrome (Kisker, 1998; Jones, 1997):

    1. This syndrome should be considered with any anemic infant/child with chromosome breaks in the absence of dysmorphism *or* with characteristically dysmorphic children in the absence of hematologic abnormalities. Onset of hematologic abnormalities ranges from birth to 31 years (mean age = 7 years).

2. Etiology: autosomal recessive with four complementation groups (A, B, C, and D); disorder is genetically heterogeneous; gene for group A linked to distal region of chromosome 20q and gene for group C mapped to chromosome 9q22.3

3. Physical manifestations:
   a. Intrauterine growth restriction (IUGR); *microcephaly; short stature*
   b. *Hypoplastic or aplastic thumbs and radii*; congenital hip dislocation
   c. Abnormal *brown skin pigmentation*
   d. *Eye abnormalities*: ptosis of eyelid; strabismus; nystagmus; and microphthalmos
   e. *Renal defects*: hypoplastic or malformed kidneys; double uterus; small penis; small testes; cryptorchidism
   f. *Pancytopenia*: reticulocytopenia; thrombocytopenia; leukopenia; poikilocytosis (irregular red blood cell [RBC] shape); and anisocytosis (RBCs are unequal in size)
   g. Chromosomal breaks and fragmentation

4. Outcome: frequent respiratory infections; bleeding diathesis; and bone marrow transplantation is the only actual cure.

I. Fetal alcohol syndrome (FAS) (Evans, 2000):
   1. Etiology: the exact amount of alcohol required to produce FAS or FAE (fetal alcohol effect, which is an incomplete expression of FAS) has not been defined. "The level of consumption at which the risk becomes negligible is unknown . . .binge drinking or single episodes of ingestion of large quantities of alcohol may also place the fetus at risk for FAS" (Evans, 2000, p. 30).
   2. Physical manifestations (Evans, 2000; Jones, 1997; Rosen, 1997):
      a. CNS: *prenatal and postnatal growth deficiency*; *microcephaly*; neonatal abstinence syndrome; tremor and irritability lasting from months to years; mild to moderate mental retardation; developmental delays; and apnea and seizures
      b. Abnormal midline facial features: *flattened nasal bridge and philtrum*; *thin upper lip*; *short palpebral fissures*; and *microphthalmia*
      c. Cardiovascular: VSD; ASD
      d. Orthopedic: *joint defects*; decreased elbow and phalangeal joint movement; hip dysplasia
      e. Genitourinary: anomalous external genitalia; labial hypoplasia; hypospadias
      f. Other: generalized hirsutism; skin hemangiomas
   3. Outcome (Jones, 1997):
      a. Variable outcome depending upon systemic involvement
      b. Decreased number of brain cells, faulty neural migration and malformation of the early brain, and decreased intelligence
      c. Irritable infants; hyperactive children
      d. Poor judgment, distractibility, and difficulty recognizing social cues

J. Goldenhar syndrome (ocular-auricular-vertebral) (Hamming & Miller, 1997; Jones, 1997):
   1. Etiology: unknown; a nonrandom association of anomalies rep-

resenting problems in morphogenesis of the first and second branchial arches. It is a variant of hemifacial microsomia (a group of patients with microtia, macrostomia, and mandibular anomalies). Occurrence is usually sporadic, with approximately 2% recurrence in first-degree relatives.

2. Physical manifestations:
    a. Anomalous findings are usually asymmetric and approximately 70% are unilateral.
    b. Facial: *hypoplastic malar, mandibular, and/or maxillary regions*; macrostomia; and hypoplastic facial muscles
    c. Eye: *epibulbar dermoid*; lipodermoid; upper eyelid *coloboma* (usually on the more affected side); strabismus; and microphthalmia
    d. Ear: *microtia*; preauricular tags and/or pits; and middle ear anomalies with variable *deafness*
    e. Oral: *decreased or absent parotid secretions*; abnormal tongue structure and function; and *cleft lip/palate*
    f. Vertebral: *hemivertebra* or vertebral hypoplasia
    g. Cardiovascular: VSD, PDA, Tetrology of Fallot (TOF), and coarctation of the aorta

3. Outcome: usually normal intelligence; decreased mental capacity when microphthalmia is present; and deafness

K. Marfan syndrome (Shephard & Kupke, 1998):
1. Etiology (Zahka, 1997; Jones, 1997): Autosomal dominant; single gene defect. Marfan syndrome is a connective tissue disorder caused by mutations in the fibrillin gene located on chromosome 15q21.1.
2. Physical manifestations:
    a. Extremities: *arachnodactyly*; *dolichostenomelia* (long, slender extremities); and *joint laxity*
    b. Anterior chest wall deformities
    c. Cardiac anomalies: *aneurysms or dissecting ascending aorta*; aortic valve incompetence; and mitral and tricuspid regurgitation leading to congestive heart failure (CHF)
    d. Eye: *anteriorly dislocated ocular lens*; detached retina; and large, deep-set eyes
    e. *Spontaneous pneumothoraces* in neonatal period
    f. Other: scoliosis and kyphosis; inguinal and/or femoral hernias
3. Outcome:
    a. Normal intelligence
    b. Increased risk for aortic dilation. β-Adrenergic blockers are recommended when the diagnosis is made.
    c. Ocular lens dislocation and retinal detachment

L. Neurofibromatosis (von Recklinghausen disease) (Cooperman & Thompson, 1997; Jones, 1997):
1. Etiology (Cole, 1998): autosomal dominant; 50% are fresh gene mutations. The neurofibromatosis type 1 gene is located on the long arm of chromosome 17.
2. Physical manifestations:
    a. *Six or more café au lait spots or spots measuring > 1.5 cm* (most common on trunk)
    b. Anterolateral bow of the tibia

    c. *Dysplastic benign tumors* made up of connective tissue, neurilemma cells, and/or mast cells; occurs along nerves, in subcutaneous tissue, and in eyes and/or meninges.

    d. Cardiovascular: pulmonary stenosis or coarctation of the aorta (occasionally)

    e. Diagnosis criteria include the presence of two or more of the following (Cooperman & Thompson, 1997): multiple café au lait spots; positive family history; definitive biopsy; pseudoarthrosis of tibia; hemihypertrophy (abnormal enlargement of one side of the body); and short angulated spinal curvature.

  3. Outcomes (Jones, 1997):

    a. Majority of patients have a benign course.

    b. Tumors rarely occur before 6 years of age. Tumors increase during puberty, pregnancy, and between 50 and 70 years of age.

    c. Complications from neurofibromas depend upon whether the tumors interfere with tissue structure (eg, macrocephaly, cardiac defects), tissue function (eg, seizures, speech, hypertension [HTN]), or neoplasias. Frequent comprehensive physical examination is recommended to evaluate structural and functional complications.

M. Noonan syndrome (Shephard & Kupke, 1998):

  1. Etiology: autosomal dominant; up to 50% of the cases may be sporadic.

  2. Physical manifestations:

    a. Prenatal diagnosis of cystic hygroma, polyhydramnios, or hydrops fetalis is common.

    b. *Excessive neck skin and/or webbing*

    c. *Chest deformity* (eg, pectus excavatum or carinatum)

    d. *Congenital heart defect* (approximately 50% of the cases): pulmonary valve stenosis, hypertrophic cardiomyopathy

    e. *Facial abnormalities*: hypertelorism; broad, sloping forehead; antimongoloid slant of the palpebral fissures; deeply grooved philtrum; and low-set posteriorly rotated ears

  3. Outcome:

    a. Early feeding difficulties that usually resolve with time

    b. Short stature

    c. Males have cryptorchidism with increased infertility problems

    d. May have neurologic problems, including seizures, hearing deficits, peripheral neuropathy, and schwannomas.

    e. If cognitive and motor problems are mild, then normal development may occur.

N. Osteogenesis imperfecta (Cooperman & Thompson, 1997; Jones, 1988):

  1. Etiology and physical manifestations: osteogenesis imperfecta is a group of genetic bone diseases divided into four types (Types III and IV are rare), all of which result in *brittle and frail bones*.

  2. Associated features include: *multiple fractures*; *deafness*; *blue sclera*; *kyphosis and kyphoscoliosis*; *tooth abnormalities*; *chest deformities*; and *short stature*.

   3. Type I: autosomal dominant with sporadic familial occurrence
   a. Physical characteristics:
      (1) Increased bone fragility and increased risk for fractures
      (2) Hyperextensible joints and ligaments; kyphoscoliosis
      (3) Thin translucent skin and blue sclera
      (4) Presenile hearing loss secondary to otosclerosis
      (5) Defective dentinogenesis: dentin and pulp hypoplasia
         with translucent, bluish-gray teeth
   4. Type II (three groups): the majority of cases are Type II A and
   due to sporadic mutations of an autosomal dominant gene. Type
   II B and Type II C are rare and due to autosomal-recessive inheritance.
   a. Physical manifestations:
      (1) Most die prenatally or in early infancy secondary to respi-
         ratory failure.
      (2) Bones crumble in utero; short broad long bones; multiple
         fractures and callus formation
      (3) Blue sclera
   5. Type III: autosomal dominant
   a. Physical manifestations:
      (1) Infants are born with multiple fractures; macrocephaly
         with triangular facial appearance; progressive bone defor-
         mity; kyphoscoliosis; abnormal dentinogenesis; presenile
         hearing loss; and early in life infant has blue sclera that
         improves with increasing maturity.
   6. Type IV: autosomal dominant
   a. Physical manifestations:
      (1) Modest bone fragility secondary to osteoporosis; moder-
         ately short to normal stature; modest bowing of bones
      (2) White sclera
      (3) Possible defective dentinogenesis
O. Pentalogy of Cantrell (Flake & Ryckman, 1997):
   1. Etiology: failure of growth and fusion of the lateral and cephalic
   folds before the fifth week of gestation
   2. Physical manifestations: epigastric omphalocele; lower cleft ster-
   num; anterior diaphragmatic defect; pericardial defects; congenital cardiac abnormalities, including ectopia cordi
P. Pierre Robin sequence:
   1. Etiology (Jones, 1997; Prows & Bender, 1999): 80% of patients
   have an underlying genetic abnormality, whereas 20% of cases
   are isolated findings. Early mandibular hypoplasia, the primary
   defect, causes the tongue to be located posteriorly, thereby preventing closure of the posterior palatal shelves.
   2. Physical manifestations: *micrognathia; glossoptosis* (tongue falls
   downward from its normal position); *U-shaped palate or cleft
   palate*; and *airway obstruction*
   3. Outcome:
   a. Normal individuals who survive the early period of airway
   obstruction have a favorable prognosis.
   b. Pierre Robin sequence, when associated with other malformation syndromes, such as trisomy 18, has a graver prognosis.

Q. Potter sequence (oligohydramnios sequence) (Aase, 1992; Kaplan, 1998; Kaplan & McAleer, 1999; Jones, 1988):
   1. Etiology: the primary defect (either renal dysplasia/agenesis or chronic leakage of amniotic fluid) leads to oligohydramnios.
   2. Physical manifestations are secondary to oligohydramnios.
      a. Fetal compression leading to: IUGR; limb contractures; *Potter's facies* (Bernhardt, 1999) (hypertelorism; depressed nasal bridge and blunted nose; low-set malformed ears; and recessed chin) and breech presentation
      b. Pulmonary hypoplasia: small bell-shaped chest
   3. Outcome: death secondary to respiratory insufficiency
R. Shprintzen syndrome (velo-cardio-facial syndrome) (Jones, 1997; Prows & Bender, 1999; Shephard & Kupke, 1998):
   1. Etiology: autosomal dominant (microdeletion of chromosome region 22q11.21-q11.23; same region of deletion as DiGeorge syndrome; both syndromes have phenotypic overlap); approximately 90% of cases are new deletions. Deletion may be detected by fluorescent in situ hybridization (FISH).
   2. Physical manifestations:
      a. Dysmorphic facies: hypertelorism, short palpebral fissures; *malformed low-set ears*; *micrognathia, cleft palate*; and *prominent nose with square nasal root*
      b. Cardiac defects: *tetralogy of Fallot*; transposition of the great vessels; truncus arteriosus; and VSD
      c. IUGR
      d. *Hypotonia*; hyperextensible hands and fingers
   3. Outcome:
      a. *Transient neonatal hypocalcemia*
      b. Mild mental deficiency; learning disabilities; speech delays; conductive hearing loss
S. Smith-Lemli-Opitz syndrome (Berry, 1998; Jones, 1997):
   1. Etiology: autosomal recessive; there is a severe defect with cholesterol biosynthesis (primary metabolic defect) with resultant low plasma cholesterol levels and high levels of the cholesterol precursor, 7-dehydrocholesterol.
   2. Physical manifestations:
      a. *Microcephaly* with narrow frontal area
      b. Craniofacial dysmorphic features: *ptosis of eyelids*; *inner epicanthal folds*; *slanted low-set ears*; and *anteverted nostrils*
      c. Limb malformations; *syndactyly of second and third toes.*
      d. Genitourinary abnormalities: *hypospadias; cryptorchidism*; ureteropelvic junction obstruction; hydronephrosis; and renal dysplasia/agenesis
   3. Outcome:
      a. Most are born in breech presentation; stillbirth and neonatal demise is common; 20% die during the first year.
      b. Progressive liver disease secondary to 7-dehydrocholesterol reductase deficiency; failure to thrive; and moderate to severe mental deficiency
T. Sturge-Weber sequence (encephalooculofacial angiomatosis) (Hamming & Miller, 1997; Jones, 1997)

1. Etiology: unknown; there is aberrant vasculature in the facial skin, eyes, and meninges.
2. Physical manifestations:
   a. *Port wine stains* (pink to purplish-red nonelevated cutaneous hemangiomas) of face, usually unilateral, that may or may not be confined to the second or third division of the trigeminal nerve
   b. Meningeal hemangioma with seizures
   c. Congenital glaucoma
3. Outcome:
   a. Onset of seizures (grand mal, often asymmetric) is usually between 2 and 7 months of age.
   b. Approximately 30% have paresis; 56% have seizures; 39% have normal intelligence.
   c. Onset of glaucoma frequently after 5 years of age
U. Thrombocytopenia and absent radius syndrome (TAR) (Jones, 1997; Kisker, 1998):
   1. Etiology: autosomal recessive
   2. Physical manifestations:
      a. Hematologic abnormalities: *thrombocytopenia* with absent/hypoplastic megakaryocytes (worst in the first few months and then improves); transient "leukemoid" granulocytosis > 100,000; eosinophilia; and anemia
      b. Bilateral upper extremity deformities: *absent or hypoplastic radii*; short, absent, or malformed ulna bones; and *thumbs are always present*.
      c. Cardiac lesions
      d. Failure to thrive
   3. Outcome: many die during early infancy secondary to hemorrhage. With advancing age the hematologic disorder improves; delayed motor development secondary to skeletal anomalies
V. Treacher-Collins syndrome (mandibulofacial dystocia) (Hamming & Miller, 1997; Jones, 1997):
   1. Etiology: autosomal dominant; 60% of cases are presumed new mutations.
   2. Physical manifestations:
      a. Bilateral *coloboma* of lower eyelid
      b. *Malar and mandibular hypoplasia*
      c. *Downward slant of palpebral fissures*; partial/total absence of lower eyelids
      d. *Macrostomia*
      e. *Ear anomalies*: malformed auricles; external ear canal defects; and conductive deafness
      f. Cleft palate
      g. Scalp hair projecting onto lateral cheek
   3. Outcome:
      a. Respiratory compromise secondary to narrow airway requiring, at times, tracheostomy
      b. Deafness and visual loss
      c. Most patients have normal intelligence.
W. Trisomy 13 (Dickerman, Park, & Clark, 1997; Jones, 1997):
   1. Etiology: trisomy of all or a large part of chromosome 13

2. Physical manifestations:

    a. CNS: *midline defects* (eg, holoprosencephaly); *microcephaly*; seizures

    b. *Head and face*: cutis aplasia; microphthalmia; coloboma; low-set ears; abnormal auricles; and cleft lip and/or palate

    c. Cardiac defects: VSD; PDA; ASD; dextrocardia

    d. Skeletal: simian crease; hyperconvex narrow fingernails; *polydactyly* of hands and/or feet; *camptodactyly* (permanent flexion of fingers and/or toes); and pelvic hypoplasia

    e. Genitalia: cryptorchidism; abnormal scrotum; bicornate uterus

3. Outcome: most patients (80%) die within the first month; only 5% live more than 6 months; severe mental deficiency for survivors

X. Trisomy 18 (Dickerman, et al., 1997; Jones, 1997):

  1. Etiology: trisomy of all or a large part of chromosome 18

  2. Physical manifestations:

    a. *IUGR*; poor tone during neonatal period

    b. *Craniofacial*: prominent occiput; short palpebral fissures; cataracts; partial fusion of eyelids; micrognathia; and low-set ears, malformed auricles

    c. Cardiovascular: VSD; ASD; PDA

    d. Skeletal: *rocker-bottom feet; overlapping fingers; hypoplastic nails*

    e. Thrombocytopenia

  3. Outcome: half of those affected die during the first week of life; only 5% to 10% survive past the first year; survivors have severe mental deficiency.

Y. Trisomy 21 (Jones, 1997; Dickerman, et al., 1997; Shephard & Kupke, 1998):

  1. Etiology: trisomy for all or large part of chromosome 21; 21 trisomy and normal mosaicism and translocations. The risk for trisomy 21 increases with advancing maternal age.

  2. Physical manifestations:

    a. *Hypotonia*; poor Moro reflex

    b. Down's facies: *Brushfield spots; epicanthal folds; up-slanted palpebral fissures; flattened nasal bridge; midfacial hypoplasia; protuberant tongue; small round low-set ears*; and *webbed neck*

    c. *Short fingers and toes; fifth finger clinodactyly; simian crease; wide space between great and second toes*

    d. *Gastrointestinal (GI) anomalies*: duodenal atresia; esophageal atresia; imperforate anus; and Hirschsprung disease

    e. *Cardiac anomalies*: endocardial cushion defect; ASD; VSD; PDA

    f. Other: *dysplastic pelvis; joint hyperflexibility*; eleven paired ribs (occasionally); and leukocytosis

  3. Outcome:

    a. Early mortality secondary to congenital heart defects

    b. Mental deficiency

    c. Muscle tone improves with advancing age.

    d. Pleasant personalities

    e. Cataracts in adulthood; hearing loss

Z. Turner's syndrome (45, XO) (Jones, 1988; Shephard & Kupke, 1998):
   1. Etiology: abnormal chromosome distribution leading to a 45 chromosome, XO individual (paternal sex chromosome is more likely to be missing)
   2. Physical manifestations: *webbed neck*; *lymphedema of hands and feet*; *epicanthal folds*; *strabismus*; *high arched palate*; *prominent ears*; *cardiac defects* (coarctation of the aorta, aortic stenosis, mitral valve prolapse); *broad chest with wide spaced nipples*; and *renal anomalies* (horseshoe kidney; double or cleft renal pelvis)
   3. Outcome:
      a. Infertility secondary to ovarian dysgenesis
      b. Short stature; tendency for obesity
      c. Mental deficiency (occasional); hearing impairment
AA. VACTERL(S) association (Kirby, 1993; Shephard & Kupke, 1998):
   1. Etiology: unknown, with a nonrandom association of multiple defects
   2. Physical manifestations:
      a. *V*ertebral defects
      b. *A*nal anomalies/atresia
      c. *C*ardiac defects (ASD is most common, VSD)
      d. *T*racheoesophageal fistula
      e. *E*sophageal atresia
      f. *R*enal defects (agenesis—unilateral or bilateral)
      g. *L*imb (radius) dysplasia
      h. *S*ingle umbilical artery
   3. Outcome: early developmental delays secondary to physical defects; most have favorable brain function.
BB. Zellweger syndrome (cerebro-hepato-renal) (Jones, 1997; Kaplan, 1998; Vosatka, 1998):
   1. Etiology: autosomal recessive; two identified loci, chromosome 7q11.23 and chromosome 1p21-p22. Zellweger syndrome is a peroxisomal disorder (inborn error of metabolism) that affects lipid metabolism.
   2. Physical manifestations:
      a. CNS: *profound hypotonia; seizures*; and *gross brain developmental abnormalities*
      b. Craniofacial: large *fontanel; high forehead; flat occiput; flat facies; hypertelorism; up-slanting palpebral fissures; hypoplastic supraorbital ridges; congenital cataracts; Brushfield spots;* anteverted nares; redundant skin on neck; micrognathia; and abnormal ears
      c. *Hepatosplenomegaly; multicystic kidneys*
      d. *PDA; VSD*
   3. Outcome:
      a. Most infants are born in breech position; most infants die within the first year of life.
      b. Survivors have severe mental deficiency; seizures; deafness.

▼ References

Aase, J. M. (1992). Dysmorphologic diagnosis for the pediatric practitioner. *Pediatric Clinics of North America, 39*(1), 135.

Bernhardt, J. (1999). Renal and genitourinary disorders. In J. Deacon & P. O'Neill (Eds.), *Core curriculum for neonatal intensive care nursing* (2nd ed., pp. 442–473). Philadelphia: WB Saunders.

Berry, G. T. (1998). Introduction to the metabolic or biochemical genetic diseases. In H. W. Taeusch & R. A. Ballard (Eds.), *Avery's diseases of the newborn* (7th ed., pp. 239–244). Philadelphia: WB Saunders.

Cole, F. S. (1998). Immunology. In H. W. Taeusch & R. A. Ballard (Eds.), *Avery's diseases of the newborn* (7th ed., pp 435–452). Philadelphia: WB Saunders.

Cooperman, D. R., & Thompson, G. H. (1997). Neonatal orthopedics, part 3: Congenital abnormalities of the upper and lower extremities and spine. In A. A. Fanaroff & R. J. Martin (Eds.), *Neonatal-Perinatal medicine: Diseases of the fetus and infant* (6th ed., pp. 1721–1742). St. Louis: Mosby.

Dickerman, L. H., Park, V. M., & Clark, B. A. (1997). Genetic aspects of perinatal disease and prenatal diagnosis. In A. A. Fanaroff & R. J. Martin (Eds.), *Neonatal-Perinatal medicine: Diseases of the fetus and infant* (6th ed., pp. 57–83). St. Louis: Mosby.

Evans, A. T. (2000). Perinatal drug use. In A. T. Evans & K. R. Niswander (Eds.), *Manual of obstetrics* (6th ed., pp. 27–39). Philadelphia: Lippincott Williams & Wilkins.

Flake, A. W., & Ryckman, F. C. (1997). Selected anomalies and intestinal obstruction. In A. A. Fanaroff & R. J. Martin, (Eds.), *Neonatal-Perinatal medicine: Diseases of the fetus and infant* (6th ed., pp. 1307–1330). St. Louis: Mosby.

Halle, J. N. (1993). Diagnostic evaluation of high-risk pregnancies. In S. Mattson & J. E. Smith (Eds.), *Core curriculum for maternal-newborn nursing* (pp. 157–184). Philadelphia: WB Saunders.

Hamming, N. A., & Miller, M. T. (1997). Neonatal eye disease, part 2: The eye. In A. A. Fanaroff & R. J. Martin (Eds.), *Neonatal-Perinatal medicine: Disease of the fetus and infant* (6th ed., pp. 1677–1701). St. Louis: Mosby.

Hudgins, L., & Cassidy, S. B. (1997). Congenital anomalies. In A. A. Fanaroff & R. J. Martin (Eds.), *Neonatal-Perinatal medicine: Disease of the fetus and infant* (6th ed., pp. 455–477). St. Louis: Mosby.

Jones, K. L. (1997). *Smith's recognizable patterns of human malformation* (5th ed.). Philadelphia: WB Saunders.

Kalhan, S. C., & Saker, F. (1997). Metabolic and endocrine disorders, part 1: Disorders of carbohydrate metabolism. In A. A. Fanaroff & R. J. Martin (Eds.), *Neonatal-Perinatal medicine: Disease of the fetus and infant* (6th ed., pp. 1439–1463). St. Louis: Mosby.

Kaplan, B. S. (1998). Developmental abnormalities of the kidneys. In H. W. Taeusch & R. A. Ballard (Eds.), *Avery's diseases of the newborn* (7th ed., pp. 1136–1143) Philadelphia: WB Saunders.

Kaplan, G. W., & McAleer, I. M. (1999). Structural abnormalities of the genitourinary system. In G. B. Avery, M. A. Fletcher, & M. G. MacDonald (Eds.), *Neonatology: Pathophysiology and management of the newborn* (5th ed., pp. 975–1003). Philadelphia: Lippincott Williams & Wilkins.

Kisker, C. T. (1998). Pathophysiology of bleeding disorders in newborns. In R. A. Polin & W. W. Fox (Eds.), *Fetal and neonatal physiology* (2nd ed., pp. 1848–1868). Philadelphia: WB Saunders.

Kirby, E. (1993). Assessment of the dysmorphic infant. In E. P. Tappero & M. E. Honeyfield (Eds.), *Physical assessment of the newborn* (pp. 147–162). Petaluma, CA: NICU Ink.

Prows, C. A., & Bender, P. L. (1999). Beyond Pierre Robin sequence. *Neonatal Network 18*(5), 13–19.

Rosen, T. S. (1997). Infants of addicted mothers. In A. A. Fanaroff & R. J. Martin (Eds.), *Neonatal-Perinatal medicine: Disease of the fetus and infant* (6th ed., pp. 672–682). St. Louis: Mosby.

Shephard, B., & Kupke, K. G. (1998). Special genetic disorders presenting in the newborn. In H. W. Taeusch & R. A. Ballard (Eds.), *Avery's diseases of the newborn* (7th ed., pp 209–228). Philadelphia: WB Saunders.

Vosatka, R. J. (1998). Modes of inheritance. In H. W. Taeusch & R. A. Ballard (Eds.), *Avery's diseases of the newborn* (7th ed., pp 175–183). Philadelphia: WB Saunders.

Zahka, K. G. (1997). The cardiovascular system, part 2: Causes and associations. In R. A. Polin & W. W. Fox (Eds.), *Fetal and neonatal physiology* (2nd ed., pp. 1119–1121). Philadelphia: WB Saunders.

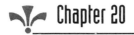 **Chapter 20**

Skin and Mucous Membrane Lesions

Karen M. O'Leary, MSN, RNC, NNP

I. Introduction

Careful assessment of the skin is an important part of the newborn physical examination and can give the practitioner valuable information about gestational age and nutritional status and the presence of cutaneous or systemic disease (Lund, Kuller, Lane, Lott, & Raines, 1999; Witt, 1996).

A. Functions of the skin include: physical protection against mechanical, chemical, and bacterial invasion; thermoregulation, fat storage, and insulation; maintenance of water and electrolyte balance; and sense perception.

B. Anatomy of the skin (three main layers):

    1. Epidermis: outermost layer (stratum corneum) functions as a barrier; retains water, heat, and other substances; prevents penetration and absorption of toxins and microorganisms. Lower layers of the epidermis contain keratinocytes and melanocytes.

    2. Dermis: directly under epidermis; composed of fibrous and elastic tissue that imparts great mechanical strength and elasticity to withstand frictional stress while still able to extend freely over joints. The dermis contains blood and lymph vessels, mast cells, inflammatory cells, and cutaneous nerves.

    3. Subcutaneous layer: fatty tissue layer functions as insulation, protection of internal organs, and calorie storage. Fat deposition occurs primarily in the last trimester.

C. Differences in the skin of premature infants:

    1. Premature skin is thinner and appears gelatinous in extremely immature infants.

    2. There are fewer layers of stratum corneum; therefore, less protection against toxins and infectious agents; skin is more permeable and may absorb topical chemicals and drugs.

    3. There are fewer connections between epidermis and dermis, thereby placing the infant at a higher risk for epidermal stripping when adhesive is removed.

    4. Premature infants have edema and decreased blood flow due to less collagen and fewer elastic fibers in the dermis, thereby increasing the risk of tissue injury.

    5. Premature babies have decreased brown fat deposits and are at increased risk for temperature instability.

D. Definitions of terms used to describe skin lesions:

    1. Bulla: a fluid-filled lesion larger than 1 cm

    2. Ecchymosis: a large area of subepidermal hemorrhage that does not blanch with pressure

    3. Lesion: area of altered tissue

    4. Macule: a pigmented, flat spot < 1 cm in diameter. It is visible but not palpable.

5. Nodule: a papule > 1 cm in diameter
6. Papule: a solid, elevated, palpable lesion < 1 cm in diameter
7. Patch: a flat pigmented spot > 1 cm in diameter
8. Petechiae: subepidermal hemorrhages, pinpoint in size, that do not blanch with pressure
9. Plaque: elevated palpable lesion with circumscribed borders > 1 cm *or* a fusion of several papules
10. Purpura: small hemorrhagic spot larger than a petechia; 1 to 3 mm in size
11. Pustule: a vesicle filled with cloudy or purulent fluid
12. Scale: exfoliation of dead or dying bits of skin; can also result from excess keratin.
13. Vesicle: elevated lesion or blister filled with serous fluid < 1 cm in diameter

II. Skin and mucous membranes

A. Blueberry muffin rash (Hagay, Biran, Ornoy, & Reece, 1996; Mellinger, et al., 1995; Witt, 1996):
  1. Description: petechiae and purpuric macules (resembling a "blueberry muffin") observed on the head, trunk, and extremities of infants who are affected. Lesions are caused by extramedullary hematopoietic tissue within the skin.
  2. Significance: lesions are associated with congenital TORCH infections (toxoplasmosis, syphilis, rubella, cytomegalovirus [CMV], and herpes), as well as gram-negative bacillary infections. Infants with congenital CMV or rubella may shed virus for many months after birth, thereby posing a risk to other susceptible individuals.
      a. May be associated with other signs of congenital infections, including hepatosplenomegaly, thrombocytopenia, anemia, heart defects, deafness, glaucoma, cataracts, optic atrophy, chorioretinitis, jaundice, pneumonia, bone changes, somatic growth restriction, immunologic abnormalities, hydrocephalus, seizures, periventricular calcifications, and developmental delays.
B. Cutis aplasia (Weston, Lane, and Morelli, 2002; Witt, 1996):
  1. Description: refers to a congenital absence of skin, making cutis aplasia a developmental defect rather than a birthmark. These lesions occur mainly on the scalp, although they may be found on the face, trunk, or extremities. They heal slowly over several months, leaving hypertrophic or atrophic scars.
  2. Significance: may be associated with trisomy 13; may occur as an autosomal-dominant trait; may be associated with dystrophic forms of epidermolysis bullosa.
C. Café au lait spots (Sahn & Esterly, 2002; Witt, 1996):
  1. Areas of hyperpigmentation (tan or brown) with well-defined borders; more common on trunk
  2. Significance: no significance unless there are more than six lesions; lesions more than or equal to six in number and larger than 0.5 to 3 cm in length, especially when accompanied with freckling of the axilla, are strongly associated with neurofibromatosis. These lesions may be the only finding of neurofibro-

matosis in the newborn period. (Refer to Neurofibromatosis in Chapter 19: Dysmorphism.) Café au lait spots, usually found along with white macules, may be found in patients with tuberous sclerosis. Café au lait spots, multiple endocrine disorders, and polycystic bone dysplasia are found in patients with McCune Albright syndrome.

D. Epstein's pearls (Gomella, 1999; Witt, 1996):

   1. Description: small grayish-white or white firm nodules, usually multiple in number, found at the juncture of the soft and hard palates or on the alveolar ridge. They are keratin-containing cysts. Epstein's pearls are the oral counterpoint of facial milia.

   2. Significance: normal finding. They resolve spontaneously within a few weeks and are found in approximately 85% of newborns.

E. Erythema toxicum neonatorum (Cohen, Mallory, Davis, & Zitelli, 1997; Weston, Lane, & Morelli, 2002; Witt, 1996):

   1. Description: the rash is described as *"flea-bite"* dermatitis because of the characteristic intense erythema with a central papule or pustule that resembles a flea bite. Lesions occur on the face, chest, back, and extremities; not found on the palms or soles. Lesions are 2 to 3 cm in diameter and vary greatly in number from a few to a few hundred. Lesions typically appear at 24 to 48 hours of age and occur in 70% of term infants. Individual lesions clear in 4 to 7 days, but new lesions may appear up to 10 days of life or later. Handling or rubbing may exacerbate the rash.

   2. Significance: benign; cause unknown; no treatment necessary. Smear of a central pustule will reveal many eosinophils on Wright-stained preparations. A peripheral blood eosinophilia of up to 20% may also be seen in addition to the tissue eosinophil accumulation, especially in those infants with many lesions.

F. Hemangiomas (Gomella, 1999; Orlow, Isakoff, & Blei, 1997; Powell, 1999; Sahn & Esterly, 2002; Weston, Lane, & Morelli, 2002):

   1. Description (by type):

   a. Strawberry hemangioma: characterized by dilated newly formed capillaries occupying the entire subdermal and dermal layers. It is a sharply demarcated, raised, bright or dark-red swelling with a rough surface resembling the outside of a ripe strawberry. They usually occur alone; may be multiple; commonly found on the head. They may be present at birth, but more likely start appearing during the first few months of life; more common in premature infants < 1,500 g. After a period of growth, sometimes extremely rapid, the majority of these lesions spontaneously involute and then regress. Most stop growing by 8 months of age and disappear by 7 years of age; many disappear sooner.

   b. Cavernous hemangioma: characterized by a poorly circumscribed soft deep-seated, compressible swelling described by some as feeling like a *"bag of worms."* The swelling may elevate and give a bluish color to the overlying skin. Composed of a communicating meshwork of interconnected venules, with or without a few large sinuses, and may be found anywhere on the body. It is present at birth, or soon afterward. It usually enlarges before beginning to involute and regress.

2. Significance:

   a. Most infants with hemangiomas require no treatment other than monitoring for complications and providing reassurance for anxious parents. Hemangiomas that interfere with important functions (eg, airway or vision) need intervention, such as corticosteroid therapy or surgical resection.

   b. Kasabach-Merritt syndrome: giant cavernous hemangiomas associated with sequestration of platelets and thrombocytopenia. Clinical manifestations (spontaneous ecchymosis, petechiae, prolonged bleeding from intravenous [IV] sites or orifices, or oozing from the umbilicus or circumcision) or extremely rapid growth of the hemangioma require intervention. Interventions include: hematologic workup (clotting studies; fibrinogen; fibrin split products; factors II, V, and VIII levels; hemoglobin [Hb]; hematocrit [Hct]; platelet count; and smear) and red blood cell (RBC), platelet, and fresh frozen plasma administration

   c. PHACE syndrome associated with extensive facial hemangiomas: *p*osterior fossa malformation, large *h*emangioma of the face, *a*rterial abnormalities, *c*ardiac defects, *e*ye abnormalities.

   d. Blue-rubber bleb syndrome: consists of multiple small raised blue to blue-black cutaneous hemangiomas; may or may not be associated with other hemangiomas in the lungs, gastrointestinal (GI) system, liver, and central nervous system (CNS).

G. Herpetic lesions (Brown et al., 1997; Riley, 1998; Sahn & Esterly, 2002; Weston, Lane, & Morelli, 2002):

   1. Description: grouped or clustered viral vesicles on an erythematous base. Involvement of any area of the skin is possible; most commonly found on the scalp or buttocks. Vesicles may be noted at birth, but more likely, the onset occurs days after birth (6 days is the mean age of onset). Some babies with neonatal herpes (HSV) will not have skin lesions; 70% of infants will display lesions.

   2. Diagnosis: nasopharyngeal, eye, rectal, and urine cultures. If lesions are present, culture or direct fluorescent antibody (DFA) is indicated. A smear prepared by carefully scraping the base of a fresh vesicle and staining with Giemsa or Wright stain (Tzank test) will reveal characteristic multinucleated giant and balloon cells. In all infants with suspected herpes, send cerebrospinal fluid PCR for herpes.

   3. Significance:

      a. Localized involvement: 30% of babies have sequelae.

      b. CNS involvement: decreased activity and lethargy, irritability, tremors, vomiting, fever, and/or seizures; infants may also exhibit localized lesions; 40% mortality rate and 70% of survivors have sequelae.

      c. Disseminated involvement: jaundice, respiratory distress, purpura, apnea, shock, and/or disseminated intravascular coagulation; infants may have localized and CNS involvement; 80% mortality rate and 50% of survivors have sequelae.

d. Infants born to mothers with a primary herpes genital infection at the time of delivery are more likely to develop neonatal herpes simplex than babies born to mothers with recurrent herpes genital lesions. A high degree of suspicion should be maintained with the following: cesarean section delivery after more than 4 to 6 hours of ruptured membranes or vaginal delivery through maternal herpes lesions → send cultures, start acyclovir, and maintain contact isolation; onset of neonatal sepsis during the first 5 to 10 days of life, or infant does not respond to the antibiotic regimen already in place → add acyclovir to the regimen; baby is positive for HSV → continue acyclovir for 21 days.

e. Outcomes: survivors have a poor prognosis even with antiviral treatment. More than half develop spasticity, paralysis, microcephaly, seizures, blindness, or deafness; those with skin involvement often exhibit recurrent crops of skin vesicles for several years.

H. Milia (Gomella,1999; Weston, Lane, & Morelli, 2002; Witt, 1996):

1. Description: multiple white papules (epidermal inclusion cysts), 1 to 2 mm in diameter, occurring on the cheeks, nose, forehead, and oral cavity (Epstein's pearls). Sebaceous gland hyperplasia is characterized by tiny (1 mm) yellow macules or yellow papules noted on the nose and cheeks of newborn.

2. Significance: benign; no treatment necessary. Milia exfoliate their contents within a few weeks of birth; sebaceous gland hyperplasia disappears completely by 4 to 6 months of age.

I. Mongolian spots (Witt, 1996):

1. Description: gray, blue-green, dark-blue, or purple macules noted most commonly on buttocks, flanks, or shoulders; occurs in 90% of Black, Asian, and Hispanic infants, and < 5% of Caucasian infants; caused by the presence of melanocytes in the dermis

2. Significance: benign; no treatment necessary; usually fade by 2 to 4 years after birth.

J. Nevus (Cohen et al., 1997; Moss, 2000; Powell, 1999; Sahn & Esterly, 2002; Weston, Lane, & Morelli, 2002; Witt, 1996):

1. Nevus simplex (or "stork bites," "salmon patches," or "Unna's naevus"): salmon or pink macular areas of distended capillaries found on the upper eyelids, the glabella, forehead, upper lip, or the nape of the neck. They have diffuse borders, become pinker with crying, and blanch with pressure. They are considered a normal variant, and lesions fade by 1 to 2 years; those on the nape of the neck may persist.

2. Nevus flammeus (or port-wine stain): macular vascular pale pink to purple nevus noted at birth; usually sharply demarcated and flat in infancy, but, in time, may develop a slightly thickened pebbly appearance. Consists of mature capillaries that are congested and dilated directly below the epidermis; range in size from a few millimeters to large lesions, occasionally involving up to half the body surface. It does not grow in area or size; it is permanent and will not fade. Pulsed dye laser surgery has been somewhat successful cosmetic treatment.

   a. Significance:

      (1) Sturge-Weber syndrome: facial port-wine stains found in a pattern similar to that of the branches of the trigeminal nerve. Outcomes include developmental delays, seizures, glaucoma, and hemiplegia. 8% of infants with port-wine stains will develop Sturge-Weber syndrome, but the incidence is higher if the lesion is bilateral or the lesion covers the upper and lower eyelids.

      (2) Kleppel-Trenaunay-Weber syndrome: port-wine stains noted on an extremity and associated with soft tissue or bony hypertrophy of that extremity. Hypertrophy of an extremity can cause orthopedic deformity. Arteriovenous fistulas are found in 25% of these patients.

      (3) A midforehead port-wine stain is an occasional and fairly nonspecific finding in many different genetic syndromes, including trisomy 13 and Beckwith-Wiedemann.

3. Nevus sebaceous of Jadassohn (Jang, Choi, Park, & Kim, 1999): noted at birth as a slightly raised oval or linear plaque; yellow or orange; found most commonly on face, neck, or scalp. They are without hair, producing a congenital circumscribed hair loss. Interventions include regular long-term observation or prophylactic surgical removal.

4. Nevus spilus: macular hairless nevus that varies in color from pale yellow to brown or black. It rarely requires removal, except when rapid change in color or size is noted or when its position makes constant irritation inevitable.

5. Nevus pilosis: hairy nevus covered with short fine or coarse hair. When found at the base of the spine, may be associated with spina bifida.

6. Congenital giant melanocytic nevi (or giant hairy or "garment" nevus): the skin affected (most commonly the trunk) may be smooth, nodular, or leathery; color is often variegated from light brown to black. Numerous satellite nevi may be found elsewhere on the body. Giant hairy nevus may be associated with leptomeningeal melanocytosis and manifested by seizures.

K. Pustular melanosis (Cohen et al., 1997; Gomella, 1999; Sahn & Esterly, 2002):

   1. Description: transient neonatal pustular melanosis is a rash that may appear on any body surface, including the palms, soles, and scalp, characterized by three stages: superficial vesiculopustules; ruptured vesiculopustules with collarettes of scale; and hyperpigmented macules. All three types of lesions may be present at birth, but the macules are noted more frequently.

   2. Significance: benign, transient condition requiring no therapy; the hyperpigmentation fades in approximately 3 weeks to 3 months.

L. Scalded skin syndrome (Ladhani, 2001; Weston, Lane, & Morelli, 2002; Witt, 1993):

   1. Description: presents as an abrupt onset of widespread, tender erythema, followed by blisters varying from small vesicles to large bullae, with subsequent exfoliation of large sheets of skin within 48 hours. The blisters frequently begin in the diaper area and spread to the rest of the body. Blister, nasopharyngeal, and rectal cultures are likely to show staphylococci or streptococci.

2. Significance: *highly contagious*. Isolation of the newborn who is affected is essential in order to prevent nursery epidemics. With early diagnosis and intervention, mortality remains low; long-term complications are rare because the lesions are superficial and heal rapidly without scarring.

3. Interventions include systemic antibiotics (eg, penicillin G; unless the organism is resistant); locally applied antibiotic ointment; fluid and electrolyte replacement; and strict isolation.

M. Other common lesions:

1. Mottling and Cutis marmorata (Cohen et al., 1997; Gomella, 1999; Weston, Lane, & Morelli, 2002):

   a. Mottling: a lace-like pattern of dusky erythema that appears on the extremities and trunk when exposed to a decreased environmental temperature. This phenomenon may be sensitive to small increments of temperature change. If normal color returns with rewarming, mottling is considered a normal response in a healthy infant. Also occurs with cold stress, hypovolemia, or sepsis.

   b. Cutis marmorata: this lesion may mimic mottling but the color change will not disappear with rewarming. Cutis marmorata, or mottling that persists beyond 6 months of life, may be associated with hypothyroidism, Down syndrome, trisomy 13, and trisomy 18.

2. Hypopigmentation lesions (Cohen et al., 1997; Moss, 2000):

   a. Vitiligo: macular lesions that show a complete loss of pigmentation, with a characteristic distribution around the mouth, eyes, elbows, hands, feet, and genitals. Spontaneous repigmentation may be noted in areas around hair follicles, imparting a speckled appearance. May represent an autoimmune response.

   b. Ash leaf spots: white oval macules noted either at birth or shortly thereafter as 1 to 3 cm macular lesions; not as ivory white or as sharply demarcated as those of vitiligo. They are an early marker for tuberous sclerosis ([autosomal-dominant neurocutaneous disorder], hypopigmented ash leaf spots, shagreen patches, and fibromas)

   c. Albinism and generalized reduction of pigment: Type I oculocutaneous albinism ([autosomal dominant] pink eyes and nystagmus. Nystagmus does not usually appear until 2 to 3 months of age. Severe strabismus and poor visual acuity are common); Type II oculocutaneous albinism ([heterogeneous disorder] melanin production is decreased but not absent; eyes are light blue rather than pink; associated with Prader-Willi syndrome)

   d. Relative hypopigmentation may be associated with other congenital syndromes: Chediak-Hegashi syndrome (patients exhibit diluted pigment and susceptibility to infection); Hermansky-Pudlak syndrome (decreased pigment, bleeding diathesis, pulmonary fibrosis, and granulomatous colitis); phenylketonuria (characteristic fair skin and hair); Waardenburg syndrome ([autosomal dominant] characterized by a triangular white patch with white overlying hair on the central forehead, facial dysmorphism, and deafness); Piebaldism (patchy hypopigmentation usually associated with a white forelock); and Naevus depigmentosus (congenital depigmentation in a linear or segmental distribution that is usually an isolated cutaneous anomaly)

3. Ichthyosis (Moss, 2000; Sahn & Esterly, 2002):
   a. Description: disease characterized by excessive scaling of skin; usually an isolated skin disorder but may be associated with other congenital syndromes. There are four types:
      (1) X-linked ichthyosis: characterized by skin, eye (corneal opacities), placental, and testicular abnormalities; may be present at birth or later in the first year and occurs only in males.
      (2) Lamellar ichthyosis (autosomal recessive): presents at birth with bright red erythema and generalized desquamation. Scales are large and plate-like; eversion of the lips and eyelids may occur; palms and soles may be thickened.
      (3) Bullous ichthyosis (autosomal dominant): characterized by recurrent formation of bullous lesions, erythema, dryness and peeling; infection is the main concern in the neonatal period.
      (4) Ichthyosis vulgaris: most common and benign of this group; characterized by excessively dry skin and fine white scales
   b. Ichthyotic neonatal conditions:
      (1) Collodion infant: presents at birth with a tight shiny epidermis that cracks across the flexures as the baby moves. Mucous membranes are unaffected and thus are stretched outward by the adjacent skin. The collodion membranes start to crack and peel within the first few days; complete shedding may take weeks. Major complications include dehydration, electrolyte imbalance secondary to increased water loss, and pneumonia. Liberal use of emollients is used for lubrication during the neonatal period.
      (2) Harlequin ichthyosis: characterized by diamond-shaped thick plates of scale separated by deep fissures, resembling the pattern on a harlequin's costume; severe and usually fatal neonatal condition
4. Subcutaneous fat necrosis:
   a. Description: firm sharply demarcated purple or reddish nodules found on cheeks, arms, thighs, or buttocks within the first 2 weeks of life; spontaneously resolve in several weeks.

Cold injury is believed to be responsible. It is occasionally associated with hypercalcemia, with or without irritability, vomiting, and failure to thrive. Serum calcium levels should be checked frequently in infants who have large amounts of involved skin or who have renal disease.

5. Sucking blisters: single oval blister on a nonerythematous base may be noted at birth. Vigorous sucking in utero is believed to be the etiology.

6. Caput succedaneum: subcutaneous edema of the presenting part of the infant's head. The caput tends to be soft and crosses suture lines. Occurs mainly in vertex deliveries and resolves spontaneously.

7. Cephalohematoma: subperiosteal collection of blood, bounded by the suture lines of the skull and may be fluctuant. If the bleeding is extensive, it can serve as a source of hyperbilirubinemia. May take weeks to resolve.

8. Congenital epulis: benign smooth-surfaced nonhemorrhagic tumor attached to the alveolar mucous membrane by a pedicle. Occurs most frequently in the area of the maxilla; easily treated by local excision

9. Abnormal hair (Jones, 1997; Moss, 2000): hair is so variable at birth that it is difficult to say if it abnormal; fair tightly curled hair in a male may suggest Menke's kinky hair syndrome; multiple or abnormal hair whorls or a pronounced anterior upsweep may be associated with a congenital syndrome (eg, trisomy 13 or Prader-Willi).

III. Skin care (Lund et al., 1999; Nopper, Horii, Sookdeo-Drost, Wang, Mancini, & Lane, et al., 1996)

A. Bathing and skin disinfection:

1. Avoid soaps containing hexachlorophene.

2. Choose cleansing agents that have a neutral pH and minimal dyes and perfumes to reduce the risk of future allergic sensitization to topical agents; frequency need be only two to three times per week.

3. For extremely premature infants (< 26 weeks' gestation) sterile water alone is the safest choice when bathing the infant.

4. Rubbing skin surfaces should be avoided to prevent chafing and irritation. Excessive vernix may be removed; however, removal of all vernix is not necessary.

5. Immersion bathing may be helpful, when clinically feasible, from a developmental standpoint and may be beneficial in facilitating the removal of sloughed cells and excess creams and rehydrating skin surfaces.

6. The first bath should wait until the baby's temperature has normalized for 1 to 2 hours to reduce the possibility of hypothermia.

7. For babies born to mothers with hepatitis or HIV disease, administer vitamin K after the first bath.

8. Routine use of an emollient such as Aquaphor (a preservative-free petrolatum-based water-miscible product) can prevent excessive drying, skin cracking, and fissures in premature infants and can also be used to treat areas of extreme dryness in full-term

infants. Avoid perfumed lotions or creams because they can irritate newborn.

9. Increased permeability of newborn or premature skin may allow absorption of medications or products such as alcohol or povidone-iodine (Betadine). After procedures using any of these products for skin disinfection, the product should be completely removed, using sterile saline solution or sterile water, to prevent further absorption.

10. Involve the parents in the bathing of their infant for effective developmental care and positive family bonding.

B. Adhesive application and removal:

1. Avoid use of adhesive removal solvents. The safest way of removing adhesive is to use warm water and cotton balls and slowly and carefully remove the adhesive.

2. Skin-bonding products such as Mastisol used on the premature infant's skin may create a stronger bond between adhesive and epidermis than between epidermis to dermis and could result in epidermal stripping when the adhesive is removed.

3. Pectin barriers placed under adhesives may be beneficial because they mold to body contours and help the adhesive to work better in a moist environment.

C. Cord care: cord care options include triple dye, isopropyl alcohol, povidone-iodine solutions, antimicrobial ointment, or no intervention at all. The use of antimicrobial interventions were instituted to control nosocomial streptococcal and staphylococcal infections in hospital nurseries. Today, these practices continue based on nursery tradition. Teach parents to maintain diaper below the baby's cord to keep the cord dry. Tub bathing is delayed until the cord has fallen off, usually by 2 weeks of age.

D. Circumcision care:

1. At circumcision, the penis is prepared with antimicrobial solutions, which may be absorbed. The solution should be completely removed after the procedure is completed.

2. After circumcision, emollients such as petrolatum-impregnated gauze, petrolatum alone, or Aquaphor ointment can facilitate healing, prevent pain during urination, and prevent the penis from sticking to the diaper. Antimicrobial ointments are not recommended because of lack of benefit and increased risk of sensitization.

3. Emollients or other topical agents are not recommended with the use of the Plastibell, according to the manufacturer. Simple cleansing of the penis with clean water for 3 to 4 days after the circumcision is all that is necessary.

▼ References

Brown, Z. A., Selke, S., Zeh, J., Kopelman, J., Maslow, A., Ashley, R. L., Watts, H., Berry, S., Herd, M., & Corey, L. (1997). The acquisition of herpes simplex virus during pregnancy. *The New England Journal of Medicine, 337*(8), 509–515.

Cohen, B., Mallory, S., Davis, H., & Zitelli, J. (1997). Dermatology. In B. J. Zitelli & H. W. Davis (Eds.), *Atlas of pediatric physical diagnosis* (3rd ed., pp. 246–257). St. Louis: Mosby-Year Book.

Gomella, T. L. (1999). Newborn physical exam. In T. L. Gomella, M. D. Cunningham, F. G. Eyal, & K. E. Zenk (Eds.), *Neonatology: Management, procedures, on-call problems, diseases, drugs* (4th ed., pp. 29–37). Stamford, CT.: Appleton & Lange.

Hagay, Z. J., Biran, G., Ornoy, A., & Reece, A. E. (1996). Congenital cytomegalovirus infection: A long-standing problem still seeking a solution. *American Journal of Obstetrics and Gynecology, 174*(1), 241–245.

Jang, I., Choi, J., Park, K., & Kim, S. (1999). Nevus sebaceous syndrome. *International Journal of Dermatology, 38*(7), 531–533.

Jones, K. L. (1997). *Smith's recognizable patterns of human malformations* (5th ed.). Philadelphia: WB Saunders.

Ladhani, S. (2001). Recent developments in staphylococcal scalded skin syndrome [review] [[63 references]]. *Clinical Microbiology and Infection, 7*(6), 301–307.

Lund, C., Kuller, J., Lane, A., Lott, J., & Raines, D. (1999). Neonatal skin care: The scientific basis for practice. *Journal of Obstetric, Gynecologic, & Neonatal Nursing, 28*(3), 241–254.

Mellinger, A. K., Cragan, J. D., Atkinson, W. L., Williams, W. W., Kieger, B., Kimber, R. G., & Travis, D. (1995). High incidence of congenital rubella syndrome after a rubella outbreak. *Pediatric Infectious Disease Journal, 14*(7), 573–578.

Moss, C. (2000). Genetic skin disorders. *Seminars in Neonatology, 5*(4), 311–320.

Nopper, A., Horii, K., Sookdeo-Drost, S., Wang, T., Mancini, A., & Lane, A. (1996). Topical ointment therapy benefits premature babies. *Journal of Pediatrics, 128*(5), 660–669.

Orlow, S. J., Isakoff, S. M., Blei, F. (1997). Increased risk of symptomatic hemangiomas in a "beard" distribution. *Journal of Pediatrics, 131*, 643–646.

Powell, J. (1999). Update on hemangiomas and vascular malformations. *Current Opinion in Pediatrics, 11*, 457–463.

Riley, L. E. (1998). Herpes simplex virus. *Seminars in Perinatology, 22*(4), 284–292.

Sahn, E., & Esterly, N. (2002). The skin. In A. A. Fanaroff & R. J. Martin (Eds.), *Neonatal-Perinatal medicine: Diseases of the fetus and infant* (Vol. 2, 7th ed., pp. 1637–1670). St. Louis: Mosby-Year Book.

Weston, W. L., & Lane, A. T, & Morelli, J. G. (2002). *Color textbook of pediatric dermatology,* (3rd ed.). St. Louis: Mosby-Year Book.

Witt, C. (1996) Skin assessment. In E. Tappero & M. E. Honeyfield (Eds.), *Physical assessment of the newborn: A comprehensive approach to the art of physical examination* (pp. 39–52). Petaluma, CA: NICU Ink.

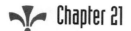 **Chapter 21**

Eyes and Ears

Ann Marie Bodi, MSN, RNC, NNP

I. Eyes
  A. Appearance of various components of the eye:
   1. Sclera (Gomella, Cunningham, Eyal, & Zenk, et al., 1999; Kenner, Lott, & Flandermeyer, 1998):
      a. Normal: white
      b. Deep blue: consider osteogenesis imperfecta.
      c. Bluish tint: seen in premature infants, whose sclera is thin
      d. Jaundiced: hyperbilirubinemia
      e. Hemorrhage: trauma
   2. Conjunctiva (Gomella et al., 1999):
      a. Normal: clear
      b. Red: seen in 5% of deliveries; common after traumatic delivery but can occur in normal delivery; resolves in 24 to 48 hours.
      c. Pink: conjunctivitis (see Conjunctivitis)
   3. Iris (Fanaroff & Martin, 1997; Gomella et al., 1999; Tappero & Honeyfield, 1996):
      a. Normal: even color (eg, gray, blue, or brown) at birth with final pigment at approximately 6 months of age
      b. Brushfield spots: salt and speckling of iris; may be normal variant or associated with Down syndrome
      c. Coloboma: defect in the normal continuity resulting in a key-hole-shaped structure of the iris; may be associated with anomalies such as CHARGE Association.
   4. Pupils (Kenner et al., 1998):
      a. Normal: equal size bilaterally and reactive to light. Unequal or nonreactivity to light indicates increased intracranial pressure (ICP) or brain damage.
      b. Best viewed by cross-illumination
   5. Cornea (Kenner et al., 1998):
      a. Normal: clear, bright, and shiny
      b. Haziness may be due to prematurity or edema; usually resolves without treatment; if haziness persists, suspect rupture of Descemet's membrane (see Trauma).
      c. Cloudy cornea may be due to the following: congenital cataracts (may be hereditary *or* secondary to maternal diabetes, x-ray exposure, malnutrition, retinopathy of prematurity [ROP], inborn errors of metabolism, or congenital rubella; early surgery is necessary); congenital glaucoma (symptoms include tearing, light sensitivity, eyelid spasm, and large cloudy cornea; surgical treatment necessary).
   6. Retina (Kenner et al., 1998):
      a. Usually transparent
      b. Red: indicates retinal hemorrhage (see Trauma).

    c. Red reflex: should be present bilaterally; may look pale in infants who are dark skinned; absent red reflex (suspect cataracts); white ([or leukokoria] most common presenting symptom of retinoblastoma)

  7. Lacrimal duct (Gomella et al., 1999; Taeusch & Ballard, 1998; Tappero & Honeyfield, 1996):

    a. Tear formation begins at approximately 2 to 3 months of age.

    b. Nasolacrimal duct not fully patent until 5 to 7 months of age; purulent or mucoid eye drainage is common.

    c. Treatment: most eye drainage clears without treatment; use lacrimal massage and gentle cleansing with water and cotton ball if not accompanied by redness or swelling. If a problem persists, consult an ophthalmologist.

  8. Eyelids (Fanaroff & Martin, 1997; Tappero & Honeyfield, 1996):

    a. Ptosis: paralytic drooping of the eyelids when fully open

    b. Coloboma of eyelid margin (present with Treacher-Collins syndrome)

  9. Eyebrows: normally the length of the palpebral fissure

    a. If eyebrows meet at glabella or are abnormally long or tangled, consider a syndrome, such as Cornelia de Lange.

    b. Synophrys: fusion of eyebrows in the midline; common in hirsute infants; may also be familial.

B. Size, position, and abnormal findings (Fanaroff & Martin, 1997; Kenner et al., 1998; Tappero & Honeyfield, 1996):

  1. Normal size can be calculated by dividing the distance between the outer canthi into thirds. The inner canthal distance equals one palpebral fissure length.

  2. Exophthalmus (abnormal protrusion of eyeball): associated with hyperthyroidism and congenital glaucoma.

  3. Epicanthal fold (a vertical fold of skin extending from the root of the nose to the median end of the eyebrow and hides the inner canthus and caruncle): it is a normal finding in certain Asiatic races and may occur as a congenital anomaly in others (Venes, 2001).

  4. Mongolian slant ([outer canthus is higher than inner canthus] common in trisomy 21); antimongolian slant ([inner canthus is higher that outer canthus] present with Treacher-Collins Syndrome)

  5. Sunset slant (lid retraction and a downward gaze): commonly seen with hydrocephalus

  6. Palpebral fissure (the opening for the eyes between the eyelids): abnormal eye placement or small palpebral fissures may occur with syndromes or chromosomal anomalies (eg, fetal alcohol syndrome [FAS] and trisomy 18).

  7. Hypertelorism (wide spaced eyes) occurs with several syndromes; even when severe it is less likely to be related to underlying brain malformation; hypotelorism (closely spaced eyes) is often associated with holoprosencephaly.

C. Movement (Taeusch & Ballard, 1998):

  1. Usually coordinated

  2. Nystagmus: rapid searching movement of eyeballs; usually disappears by 3 to 4 months of age.

3. Strabismus (muscular incoordination that gives the appearance of crossed eyes); pseudostrabismus (firm flat nasal bridge or epicanthal folds, usually resolves by 1 year of age)

4. Doll's eye response: while rotating the infant's head from side to side the eyes should deviate away from the direction of the rotation. An abnormal response, ie, the eyes move in the direction of head rotation, may indicate damage to trochlear, abducens, and oculomotor nerves.

D. Neonatal conjunctivitis (Gomella et al., 1999; Kenner et al., 1998; Pickering, 2000): etiologies include:

1. Chemical conjunctivitis secondary to silver nitrate administration; reactions start within a few hours and lasts up to 48 hours; no treatment necessary

2. Chlamydia: the most common cause and is transmitted from infected mother; clinical manifestations include swollen eyelids and mucopurulent discharge appearing in 4 to 14 days and bilateral involvement; diagnosis confirmed by conjunctival scraping for Giemsa staining; treatment is oral erythromycin 50 mg/kg/day in divided doses for 14 days; topical treatment is ineffective.

3. Gonorrhea: clinical manifestations include acute purulent bilateral conjunctivitis with eyelid edema presenting 1 to 4 days after birth; diagnosis confirmed with gram stain and culture; treatment includes lavaging eye with sterile saline and Ceftriaxone 50 mg/kg (maximum dose = 1 g) intramuscular (IM) × 1 dose.

4. Herpes simplex may be part of localized or systemic infection. Clinical manifestations include eyelid swelling, conjunctival inflammation, corneal opacities, and epithelial dendrites presenting 2 to 14 days after birth; diagnosis made by epithelial scrapings for Giemsa staining and tissue cultures; treatment includes Acyclovir intravenous (IV) 60 mg/kg/day in 3 divided doses for 14 days for skin, eye, and mouth disease; 21-day course for disseminated disease or central nervous system (CNS) involvement

5. Staphylococcal: transmission occurs during a vaginal delivery or contact with infected caregiver. Clinical manifestations include mild conjunctivitis with purulent discharge; may progress to corneal ulcer, endophthalmitis, or generalized skin infection; usually unilateral. Diagnosis made on culture and gram stain; treatment includes topical bacitracin or erythromycin ointment.

E. Trauma:

1. Eyelids (Fanaroff & Martin, 1997; Gomella et al., 1999): edema/bruising may occur secondary to forcing swollen eyelids open to examine eye; resolves within 1 week; laceration may require microsurgery.

2. Orbital fracture (Fanaroff & Martin, 1997; Gomella et al., 1999): may occur with high forceps delivery; usually results in immediate death; surviving infants will demonstrate traumatic eyelid changes and disturbances of extraocular muscle movement and exophthalmos requiring immediate ophthalmologic evaluation.

3. Horner's syndrome (Fanaroff & Martin, 1997; Gomella et al., 1999): cervical sympathetic nerve trauma frequently accompanied by lower brachial plexus injury. Clinical manifestations

include miosis (pupil constriction), partial ptosis (drooping eyelid), enophthalmos (sunken eyeball), anhidrosis (sweating) of ipsilateral side of the face, and delayed pigment of ipsilateral iris.

4. Cornea (Fanaroff & Martin, 1997; Gomella et al., 1999): abrasion is suggested by unilateral tearing. Persistent haziness may be secondary to rupture of Descemet's membrane; results in permanent damage that leads to scarring and eventually astigmatism and amblyopia.

5. Intraocular hemorrhage (Gomella et al., 1999):
   a. Retinal hemorrhage: flame-shaped or streaked hemorrhage found near the optic disc; no treatment is required and usually disappears within 1 week.
   b. Hyphema: gross blood in anterior chamber of the eye; no treatment is required and resolves within 1 week.
   c. Vitreous hemorrhage: floaters, absent red reflex, and blood pigment seen with slit lamp. If resolution does not occur by 1 year of age, consult surgery.

6. Eyelid trauma results in edema, suffusion, or ecchymosis (Fanaroff & Martin, 1997).

7. Lagophthalmos: inability to close the eye; usually unilateral; results from facial nerve injury by forceps pressure (Fanaroff & Martin, 1997).

F. ROP:
1. Definition: ROP is a disorder of the developing retinal vasculature in premature infants. An injurious event (hypoxia, hyperoxia, prolonged mechanical ventilation and oxygen exposure, acidosis, sepsis, and shock) causes the proliferation of abnormal blood vessels in the retina, resulting in scar tissue. This process can lead to retinal detachment and blindness (Lee, 1999).

2. Classification: stages, zones, and clock hours are used to describe the location and extent of the disease (Cloherty & Stark, 1998):
   a. Stage 1: demarcation line between vascular and avascular retina
   b. Stage 2: ridge of scar tissue replaces the demarcation line in Stage 1.
   c. Stage 3: extraretinal fibrovascular proliferative tissue develops at the ridge.
   d. Stage 4: partial retinal detachment occurs by traction. Stage 4A occurs outside the macula and chance of vision is good with retinal reattachment. Stage 4B: involves the macula and limits likelihood of useable vision.
   e. Stage 5: complete retinal detachment
   f. Plus disease: presence of vascular dilation and tortuosity
   g. Threshold: 5 or more contiguous or 8 cumulative clock hours of Stage 3 with plus disease in either Zones 1 or 2

3. Zones and clock hours (Figure 21.1)

4. Screening (American Academy of Pediatrics, 2001):
   a. Birth weight < 1,500 g or < 28 weeks' gestation *or* 1,500 to 2,000 g with unstable clinical course should have at least two funduscopic examinations. First examination should be performed 4 to 6 weeks postnatally or 31 to 33 weeks postcon-

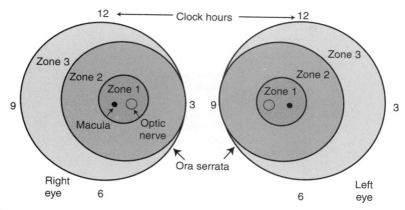

Figure 21.1. Zones of the retina and clock hours. Used with permission from Siberry, G. K., & Iannone, R. (2000). *The Harriet Lane handbook* (15th ed.). St. Louis: Mosby.

ception, whichever is later. Follow-up examinations should occur every 2 to 3 weeks until normal vascularization proceeds to Zone III and the risk for ROP has passed.

   b. If ROP is found, follow-up examinations should be performed at least every 1 to 2 weeks until retinal vascularization has reached Zone III or until threshold conditions are reached.

   c. Once threshold disease/Zone I has occurred, the infant should have ablative surgery for at least one eye within 72 hours of diagnosis.

   d. Follow-up examinations should occur weekly.

5. Treatment (Lee, 1999):

   a. Prevent prematurity!

   b. Mild ROP (Stages 1, 2, and most of 3): spontaneous regression occurs.

   c. Severe ROP (threshold ROP and Stages 4 and 5): surgical ablation of the peripheral avascular retina using laser photocoagulation or cryotherapy to retain macular vision

   d. Retinal detachment: scleral buckling and vitrectomy

II. Ears

A. Appearance (Kenner et al., 1998; Taeusch & Ballard, 1998):

   1. Development of the ears, ie, cartilage formation and recoil, is an indication of maturity.

   2. Length of ears at greatest vertical point is < 3 cm for a term infant.

B. Placement and position (Gomella et al., 1999; Kenner et al., 1998; Taeusch & Ballard, 1998).

   1. Normal position: helix of the ear is above an imaginary line drawn circumferentially around the head through the inner and outer canthus of eye.

   2. Low-set: helix of the ear falls below the imaginary line mentioned previously. Often occurs with congenital anomalies (eg, Treacher-Collins syndrome, triploidy, trisomies 9 and 18, and fetal aminopterin effects) and abnormalities of urinary system.

3. Posterior rotation: may also occur with major anomalies.

C. Malformations:

1. May be an isolated trait, part of a syndrome, or indicative of renal anomalies.

2. Hairy ears: occurs in infants of diabetic mothers (IDM) (Gomella et al., 1999).

3. Hypoplastic or square-shaped lobes (may be inherited innocently rather that part of genetic syndrome) (Pomerance & Richardson, 1993).

4. Auricular tags and sinuses (Taeusch & Ballard, 1998): common mild malformation; usually isolated and unilateral. It occurs more often in Asians and African American infants.

   a. Auricular tags: skin-covered nodules, often contain cartilage, and are usually benign; typically located anterior to pinna. Tags may occur anywhere from temple to tragus *or* anterior to tragus to angle of the mouth. Mild to moderate hearing loss is seen in 13% of infants with isolated ear tags. They may be associated with syndromes such as: oculo-auriculo-vertebral spectrum (Goldenhar syndrome); Towne-Brocks syndrome; cat-eye syndrome; Wolf-Hirschorn syndrome; and cri-du-chat syndrome.

   b. Auricular sinuses (Taeusch & Ballard, 1998): shallow dimples, pits, or depressions ranging in size from 1 to 3 mm; typically located on anterior margin of ascending helix or, less often, in preauricular area; may be associated with conductive and sensorineural hearing loss; usually an isolated anomaly but can be associated with the following: oculo-auriculo-vertebral spectrum; Beckwith-Wiedemann syndrome; branchio-oto-renal syndrome (Melnick-Fraiser syndrome); Pickering-plus syndrome; and other chromosomal aberrations.

5. Injuries:

   a. May occur secondary to forceps placement near the ears (Gomella et al., 1999).

   b. Abrasions and bruising: usually mild and require no treatment other than keeping the area clean; spontaneous resolution

   c. Hematomas: liquefy slowly and may develop into a cauliflower ear; therefore, they may need to by incised and evacuated (Kenner et al., 1998).

   d. Avulsion (tearing away) of the auricle: consult surgery if auricle is involved.

   e. Laceration of the ear: most lacerations can be sutured with 7-0 nylon sutures.

D. Hearing loss (AAP, 1999; Kenner et al., 1998; Taeusch & Ballard, 1998):

1. Significant hearing loss is one of most common major abnormalities present at birth. Early diagnosis is important. If diagnosis is undetected, then speech, language, cognitive, social, and emotional development will be impeded. The American Academy of

Pediatrics supports the statement of the Joint Committee on Infant Hearing (1994), ie, it endorses the goal of universal detection of hearing loss by screening all infants before 3 months of age with appropriate intervention no later than 6 months of age.

2. May have either inappropriate or excessive startle patterns.
3. Risk factors (Gomella et al., 1999): family history of childhood hearing impairment; congenital perinatal infection (eg, TORCH [toxoplasmosis, syphilis, rubella, cytomegalovirus [CMV], and herpes]); congenital malformation of head or neck; birth weight < 1,500 g; hyperbilirubinemia requiring exchange transfusion; bacterial meningitis; severe perinatal asphyxia; and ototoxic drugs (eg, furosemide, gentamicin, and vancomycin)
4. Diagnostic testing:
   a. High false-positive results make it difficult to diagnose hearing loss in neonatal period (Gomella et al., 1999).
   b. Brain stem auditory evoked potentials (ABR or BAER) (Kenner et al., 1998): disk electrodes are attached to vertex mastoid areas and repetitive sounds are presented to the ear in the form of clicks caused by a direct current pulse. The response recorded is a sequence of waves representing the action potential of the auditory nerve. The ABR is sensitive; no false negatives reported; requires specialized personnel and 1 to 2 hours to perform the test.
   c. Otoacoustic emissions (OAE) (AAP, 1999; Kenner et al., 1998): by using a sensitive microphone placed in an infant's ear canal, the OAE measures sound waves generated in response to emitted low-intensity sounds; quick and relatively inexpensive; debris or fluid in middle or external ear may affect results.

▼ References

American Academy of Pediatrics. (1999). Newborn and infant hearing loss: Detection and intervention. *Pediatrics, 103*(2), 527–530.

American Academy of Pediatrics. (2001). Screening examination of premature infants for retinopathy of prematurity. *Pediatrics, 108*(3), 809–811.

Cloherty, J. P., & Stark, A. R. (Eds.) (1998). *Manual of neonatal care* (4th ed.). Philadelphia: Lippincott-Raven.

Fanaroff, A., & Martin, R. (1997). *Neonatal-Perinatal medicine: Diseases of the fetus and infant* (6th ed.). St. Louis: Mosby.

Gomella, T. L., Cunningham, M. D., Eyal, F. G., & Zenk, K. E. (Eds.). (1999). *Neonatology: Management, procedures, on-call problems, diseases, and drugs* (4th ed.). Norwalk, CT: Appleton & Lange.

Kenner, C., Lott, J. W., & Flandermeyer, A. A. (Eds.). (1998). *Comprehensive neonatal nursing: A physiologic perspective* (2nd ed.). Philadelphia: WB Saunders.

Lee, S. (1999). Retinopathy of prematurity in the 1990s. *Neonatal Network* (18)2, 31–38.

Pickering, L. K. (Ed.). (2000). *Red book: Report of the committee on infectious diseases* (25th ed.). Elk Grove Village, IL: American Academy of Pediatrics.

Pomerance, J. J., & Richardson, C. J. (Eds.). (1993). *Neonatology for the clinician*. Norwalk, CT: Appleton & Lange.

Taeusch, H. W., & Ballard, R. A. (Eds.). (1998). *Avery's diseases of the newborn* (7th ed.). Philadelphia: WB Saunders.

Tappero, E. P., & Honeyfield, M. E. (1996). *Physical examination of the newborn: A comprehensive approach to the art of physical exam* (2nd ed.). Petaluma, CA: NICU Ink.

Venes, D. (Ed.). (2001). *Taber's cyclopedic medical dictionary*. Philadelphia: F. A. Davis Company.

Pounds/Ounces to Grams Conversion Table

| | | | | | | | Pounds | | | | | | |
Ounces	0	1	2	3	4	5	6	7	8	9	10	11	12
0	0	454	907	1361	1814	2268	2722	3175	3629	4082	4536	4990	5443
1	28	482	936	1389	1843	2296	2750	3203	3657	4111	4564	5018	5471
2	57	510	964	1417	1871	2325	2778	3232	3685	4139	4593	5046	5500
3	85	539	992	1446	1899	2353	2807	3260	3714	4167	4621	5075	5528
4	113	567	1021	1474	1928	2381	2835	3289	3742	4196	4649	5103	5557
5	142	595	1049	1503	1956	2410	2863	3317	3770	4224	4678	5131	5585
6	170	624	1077	1531	1984	2438	2892	3345	3799	4252	4706	5160	5613
7	198	652	1106	1559	2013	2466	2920	3374	3827	4281	4734	5188	5642
8	227	680	1134	1588	2041	2495	2948	3402	3856	4309	4763	5216	5670
9	255	709	1162	1616	2070	2523	2977	3430	3884	4337	4791	5245	5698
10	283	737	1191	1644	2098	2551	3005	3459	3912	4366	4819	5273	5727
11	312	765	1219	1673	2126	2580	3033	3487	3941	4394	4848	5301	5755
12	340	794	1247	1701	2155	2608	3062	3515	3969	4423	4876	5330	5783
13	369	822	1276	1729	2183	2637	3090	3544	3997	4451	4904	5358	5812
14	397	850	1304	1751	2211	2665	3118	3572	4026	4479	4933	5386	5840
15	425	879	1332	1786	2240	2693	3147	3600	4054	4508	4961	5415	5868

1 pound = 16 ounces
1 pound = 453.59 grams
1 ounce = 28.2395 grams
1 kilogram = 1000 grams
1 kilogram = 2.2 pounds

273

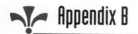

Fahrenheit to Centigrade Conversion Table

°F	°C	°F	°C	°F	°C	°F	°C
95	35	98	36.7	101	38.3	104	40
95.2	35.1	98.2	36.8	101.2	38.4	104.2	40.1
95.4	35.2	98.4	36.9	101.4	38.6	104.4	40.2
95.6	35.3	98.6	37	101.6	38.7	104.6	40.3
95.8	35.4	98.8	37.1	101.8	38.8	104.8	40.4
96	35.6	99	37.2	102	38.9	105	40.6
96.2	35.7	99.2	37.3	102.2	39	105.2	40.7
96.4	35.8	99.4	37.4	102.4	39.1	105.4	40.8
96.6	35.9	99.6	37.6	102.6	39.2	105.6	40.9
96.8	36	99.8	37.7	102.8	39.3	105.8	41
97	36.1	100	37.8	103	39.4	106	41.1
97.2	36.2	100.2	37.9	103.2	39.6	106.2	41.2
97.4	36.3	100.4	38	103.4	39.7	106.4	41.3
97.6	36.4	100.6	38.1	103.6	39.8	106.6	41.4
97.8	36.6	100.8	38.2	103.8	39.9	106.8	41.6

Centigrade to Fahrenheit: $(°C \times 1.8) + 32$

Fahrenheit to Centigrade: $\dfrac{(°F - 32)}{1.8}$

$1°C = 1.8°F$

$1°F = 0.555°C$

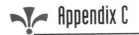

Recommended Childhood Immunization Schedule, United States, 2002

Vaccine ▼	Age ► Birth	1 mos	2 mos	4 mos	6 mos	12 mos	15 mos	18 mos	24 mos	4-6 yrs	11-12 yrs	13-18 yrs
Hepatitis B[1]	Hep B #1 *only if mother HBsAg (-)*	Hep B #2			Hep B #3				Hep B series			
Diphtheria, Tetanus, Pertussis[2]			DTaP	DTaP	DTaP		DTaP			DTaP	Td	
Haemophilus influenzae Type b[3]			Hib	Hib	Hib	Hib						
Inactivated Polio (IPV)			IPV	IPV	IPV					IPV		
Measles, Mumps, Rubella[5]						MMR #1				MMR #2	MMR #2	
Varicella[6]						Varicella				Varicella		
Pneumococcal[7]			PCV	PCV	PCV	PCV	PCV		PCV	PPV		
Hepatitis A[8]									Hepatitis A series			
Influenza[9]						Influenza (yearly)						

Vaccines below this line are for selected populations

range of recommended ages · catch-up vaccination · preadolescent assessment

This schedule indicates the recommended ages for routine administration of currently licensed childhood vaccines, as of December 1, 2001, for children through age 18 years. Any dose not given at the recommended age should be given at any subsequent visit when indicated and feasible. ▢ Indicates age groups that warrant effort to administer those vaccines not previously given. Additional vaccines may be licensed and recommended during the year. Licensed combination vaccines may be used whenever any components of the combination are indicated and the vaccine's other components are not contraindicated. Providers should consult the manufacturers' package inserts for detailed recommendations.

275

1. Hepatitis B vaccine (Hep B). All infants should receive the first dose of hepatitis B vaccine soon after birth and before hospital discharge; the first dose may also be given by age 2 months if the infant's mother is HBsAg-negative.Only monovalent hepatitis B vaccine can be used for the birth dose. Monovalent or combination vaccine containing Hep B may be used to complete the series; four doses of vaccine may be administered if combination vaccine is used. The second dose should be given at least 4 weeks after the first dose, except for Hib-containing vaccine which cannot be administered before age 6 weeks. The third dose should be given at least 16 weeks after the first dose and at least 8 weeks after the second dose. The last dose in the vaccination series (third or fourth dose) should not be administered before age 6 months.

Infants born to ABsAG-positive mothers should receive hepatitis B vaccine and 0.5 mL hepatitis B immune globulin (HBIG) within 12 hours of birth at separate sites. The second dose is recommended at age 1–2 months and the vaccination series should be completed (third or fourth dose) at age 6 months.

Infants born to mothers whose HBsAg is unknown should receive hepatitis B vaccine within 12 hours of birth. Maternal blood should be drawn at the time of delivery to determine the mother's HBsAg status; if the HBsAg test is positive, the infant should receive HBIG as soon as possible (no later than age 1 week).

2. Diptheria and tetanus toxoids and acellular pertussis vaccine (DTaP). The fourth dose of DtaP may be administered as early as age 12 months, provided 6 months have elapsed since the third dose and the child is unlikely to return at age 15–18 months. **Tetanus and diptheria toxoids (Td)** is recommended at age 11–12 years if at least 5 years have elapsed since the last dose of tetanus and diptheria toxoid-conataining vaccine. Susequent routine Td boosters are recommended every 10 years.

3. *Haemophilus influenzae* Type b (Hib) conjugate vaccine. Three Hib conjugate vaccines are licensed for infant use. If PRP-OMP (PedvaxHIB® or ComVax® [Merck]) is administered at ages 2 and 4 months, a dose at age 6 months is not required. DTaP/Hib combination products should not be used for primary immunization in infants at age 2, 4, or 6 months, but can be used as boosters following any Hib vaccine.

4. Inactivated poliovirus vaccine (IPV). An all-IPV schedule is recommended for routine childhood poliovirus vaccination in the United States. All children should receive four doses of IPV at age 2 months, 4 months, 6–18 months, and 4–6 years.

5. Measles, mumps, and rubella vaccine (MMR). The second dose of MMR is recoommended routinely at age 4–6 years but may be adminstered during any visit, provided at least 4 weeks have elapsed since the first dose and that both doses are administered beginning at or after age 12 months. Those who have not previously received the second dose should complete the schedule by the visit at 11–12 years.

6. Varicella vaccine. Varicella vaccine is recommended at any visit at or after age 12 months for susceptible children (i.e., those who lack a reliable history of chicken pox). Susceptible persons aged ≥ 13 years should receive two doses, given at least 4 weeks apart.

7. Pneumococcal Vaccine. The heptavalent pneumococcal conjugate vaccine (PCV) is recommended for all children aged 2–23 months and for certain children aged 24–59 months. Pneumococcal polysaccaride vaccine (PPV) is recommended in addition to PCV for certain high-risk groups. See *MMWR* 2000;49(RR-9);1–37.

8. Hepatitis A vaccine. Hepatitis A vaccine is recommended for use in selected states and regions, and for certain high-risk groups; consult your local public health authority. See *MMWR* 1999;48(RR-12);1–37.

9. Influenza vaccine. Influenza vaccine is recommended annually for children age ≥ 6 months with certain risk factors (including but not limited to asthma, cardiac disease, sickle cell disease, HIV, and diabetes; see *MMRW* 2001;50(RR-4);1–44), and can be administered to all others wishing to obtain immunity. Children age ≤ 12 years should receive vaccine in a dosage appropriate for their age (0.25 mL if age 6-36 months or 0.5 mL if aged ≥ 3 years). Children aged ≤ 8 years who are receiving influenza vaccine for the first time should receive two doses separated by at least 4 weeks.

For additional information about vaccines, vaccine supply, and contraindications for immunization, please visit the National Immunization Program Website at www. cdc.gov/nip or call the National immunization Hotline at 800-2332-2522 (English) or 800-232-0233 (Spanish).

Approved by the Advisory Committee on Immunization Practices (www.cdc.gov/nip/acip),
the American Academy of Pediatrics (www.aap.org), **and**
the American Academy of Family Physicians (www.aafp.org)

INDEX

Page references followed by the letters *b*, *f*, or *t* indicate material that is located in a box, figure, or table.

A

a/A (arterial/alveolar) ratio, 150–151
A-aDO₂ (alveolar-arterial gradient), 150, 151*t*
Abdominal wall defects
    bladder exstrophy, 212
    cloacal exstrophy, 212–213
    gastroschisis, 197–198
    omphalocele, 197
    prune belly syndrome, 198–199
ABO and Rh typing, 2, 25, 129
ABO hemolytic disease of the newborn, 2, 25, 109
Absolute neutrophil count (ANC) calculations, 99, 100*t*
Accelerations, in heart rate, 19
Achondroplasia, 242
Acid-base deficit/excess, 152*b*, 153*b*
Acidemia, 230–231
Acidosis, 53, 157
Acrocephalosyndactyly, 242–243
Activated partial thromboplastin time (aPTT), 121*t*
Activated protein C resistance, 122–123
Acute tubular necrosis (ATN), 225
Acyanotic heart lesions
    endocardial cushion defect, 165
    patent ductus arteriosus, 163–164
    ventricular septal defect, 164–165
Adenomatoid malformation, congenital, 148
Adhesive application and removal, 264
Admission procedures, 50–51
Adrenal glands
    congenital adrenal hyperplasia, 237–238
    disorders of, 237–239
    function of, 237
    hemorrhage in, 107, 239
    insufficiency, 238–239
Advanced maternal age (AMA)
    chromosomal abnormalities in relation to, 26*t*
AFP (α-fetoprotein), 8, 9*t*, 30
AG (Anion gap), 53
Agyria, 182
Air leak syndromes
    defined, 137
    etiology of, 137
    pneumomediastinum, 138
    pneumopericardium, 138–139
    pneumoperitoneum, 139–140
    pneumothorax, 137–138
    pulmonary interstitial emphysema, 139
Airways
    equipment for resuscitation, 40
    obstructions of, 140–142
Alanine aminotransferase (ALT), 128
Albinism, 261
Albumin, 129

Alcohol use and abuse, 35, 245
Alkaline phosphatase, 128
Alkalosis, 157
Alport's syndrome, 118
Alprostadil (PGE₁), 72*t*, 73*t*
ALT (alanine aminotransferase), 128
Alveolar-arterial gradient (A-aDO₂), 150, 151*t*
AMA. *See* Advanced maternal age
Ambiguous genitalia, 213–216
Amino acid metabolism, defects in, 134
Ammonia (NH₃), 128
Amniocentesis
    indications for procedure, 30
    in screening for fetal hemolytic disease, 2
    in screening for genetic defects, 8–9
Amniotic band syndrome, 193–194
Amniotic fluid
    creatinine level of, 9
    ΔOD 450 of, 2, 9, 25
    volume of, 12*t*
Amphetamines, 3
Analgesia, during labor and delivery, 20
ANC (absolute neutrophil count) calculations, 99, 100*t*
Androgen receptor, defect in, 214
Anemia
    due to acute and chronic blood loss, 112–114
    due to hemorrhage, 107, 108*t*, 109
Anemia *(continued)*
    etiology of, 3
    hemolytic, 109, 110*b*, 111–112
    hypoplastic, 112
    pathologic, 107
    physiologic, 106
    of prematurity, 106–107
    screening for, 3
Anencephaly, 185
Anesthesia, during labor and delivery, 20–22
Aneurysm, arterial, 181
Anion gap (AG), 53
Antenatal bleeding
    fetofetal transfusion in, 27
    fetomaternal transfusion in, 27
    placenta accreta in, 27
    placenta previa in, 26–27
    placental abruption in, 26
    umbilical cord conditions in, 28
    uterine rupture in, 27–28
Antenatal testing
    bacterial, protozoan and viral screenings, 4–8
    for fetal well-being, 10–12
    genetic testing, 8–10
    serology, 2–4
    urine testing, 4

H